PENGUIN BOOKS

THE CHALLENGE OF PAIN

Ronald Melzack is Professor of Psychology at McGill University and Research Director of the Pain Center at the Montreal General Hospital. After receiving his Ph.D. from McGill, he carried out research at the University of Oregon Medical School, the University of Pisa and University College London. When he was Associate Professor at the Massachusetts Institute of Technology, he and Professor Wall began an exchange of ideas which led to the publication of the gate-control theory of pain in 1965. The theory has subsequently had a profound impact on research and treatment related to pain. Professor Melzack is the author and editor of several books and many scientific articles on pain. He is a former President of the International Association for the Study of Pain and has won many awards for his contributions to understanding pain.

Patrick D. Wall is Professor Emeritus at the University of London and does research on the physiology of pain at United Medical and Dental Schools, St Thomas's Campus, London. After receiving his medical degree from Oxford, he worked at the Universities of Yale, Chicago and Harvard, and at the Massachusetts Institute of Technology. It was his research which established the physiological basis of the gate-control theory of pain and he continues his physiological studies particularly in relation to the chronic as well as to the acute effects of injury. Professor Wall is editor, with Professor Melzack, of the *Textbook of Pain*, and has published numerous articles on pain. He has received many honours for his work from a number of countries and is the founding editor of the journal *Pain*. He is a Fellow of the Royal Society.

The Challenge of Pain

RONALD MELZACK and
PATRICK D. WALL

UPDATED SECOND EDITION

PENGUIN BOOKS

PENGUIN BOOKS

Published by the Penguin Group
Penguin Books Ltd, 80 Strand, London WC2R 0RL, England
Penguin Putnam Inc., 375 Hudson Street, New York, New York 10014, USA
Penguin Books Australia Ltd, 250 Camberwell Road, Camberwell, Victoria 3124, Australia
Penguin Books Canada Ltd, 10 Alcorn Avenue, Toronto, Ontario, Canada M4V 3B2
Penguin Books India (P) Ltd, 11 Community Centre, Panchsheel Park, New Delhi – 110 017, India
Penguin Books (NZ) Ltd, Cnr Rosedale and Airborne Roads, Albany, Auckland, New Zealand
Penguin Books (South Africa) (Pty) Ltd, 24 Sturdee Avenue, Rosebank 2196, South Africa

Penguin Books Ltd, Registered Offices: 80 Strand, London WC2R 0RL, England

www.penguin.com

First published in Penguin Books 1982
Second edition published in Pelican Books 1988
Reprinted in Penguin Books 1991
Reprinted with updated references 1996

8

Set in Times Monophoto
Printed in England by Clays Ltd, St Ives plc

To the millions of people in every country who live and die in needless pain.

'We must all die. But if I can save [a person] from days of torture, that is what I feel is my great and ever new privilege. Pain is a more terrible lord of mankind than even death itself.'

Albert Schweitzer, 1953

Contents

Preface

Pain is one of the most challenging problems in medicine and biology. It is a challenge to the sufferer who must often learn to live with pain for which no therapy has been found. It is a challenge to the physician or other health professional who seeks every possible means to help the suffering patient. It is a challenge to the scientist who tries to understand the biological mechanisms that can cause such terrible suffering. It is also a challenge to society, which must find the medical, scientific and financial resources to relieve or prevent pain and suffering as much as possible.

We consider ourselves extremely privileged to have taken part in a genuine scientific revolution in the past two decades. Until the middle of this century, pain was considered primarily to be a symptom of disease or injury. We now know that chronic, severe pain is a problem in its own right that is often more debilitating and intolerable than the disease process which initiated it. The problem of pain was therefore transformed from a mere symptom to be dealt with by the various medical specialities to a speciality in its own right which is now one of the most exciting, rapidly advancing fields of science and medicine.

When we proposed the gate-control theory in 1965, we hardly dreamed of the explosion in research studies and new therapeutic approaches that followed. It was our unexpected good fortune that the theory came at a time when the field was ripe for change. In the 1960s, a wave of new facts and ideas (that had evolved gradually) was beginning to crest, and the gate-control theory rode in on the wave of the times. No one was more astounded at its success than we were. Naturally, acceptance was not immediate or total, but in spite of continuing controversy about details, the *concept* that injury signals can be radically modified and even blocked at the earliest stages of transmission in the nervous system is virtually universally accepted.

In recent years, our understanding of pain mechanisms has

increased enormously and new, effective treatments for pain have evolved. There is now an urgent need for education. Despite the obvious progress in our knowledge, many people who suffer cancer pain, post-surgical pain, labour pain and various chronic pains are inadequately treated. We are appalled by the needless pain that plagues so many people. Part of the problem lies with the health professionals who have failed to keep up with the advances in our field. Part lies with the patient who is often too meek to demand the basic human right to pain relief. Every human being has a right to freedom from pain to the extent that our knowledge permits health professionals to achieve this goal.

Our purpose in this book is to describe the current status of pain research and treatment as well as to point to future goals and ways to achieve them. The book contains four major sections. The first section describes the psychological and clinical aspects of pain and outlines the scope of the challenges of pain. The second section presents the physiological evidence regarding pain, which continues to grow at a breathtaking pace. The third section examines the major theories of pain in terms of their ability to explain pain phenomena and their implications for the control of pain. The final, fourth section describes the exciting new approaches to pain control and the rapidly evolving conception that the terrible suffering of patients with chronic pain, such as pain due to nerve injury or cancer, need an entirely new approach characterized by the pain clinic and the hospice.

We are grateful to many colleagues and friends who have worked with us and helped us in our attempt to understand pain. Their names appear in the pages of this book and in the bibliography. We are also grateful to Elizabeth Loggie and Julia Millard, who provided outstanding secretarial assistance in preparing this book.

Preface to the Updated Second Edition

The Challenge of Pain was written to provide a broad overview of a feature of life – pain and suffering – that touches all of us. Its purpose is to examine the major theories of pain as well as the exciting research advances that have occurred in recent years. It also describes forms of therapy for the varieties of pain that plague us.

Recent research has focused primarily on the complex mechanisms of the transmission of pain signals from the skin to the brain. We have learned a great deal about the multitude of transmitter substances and the mechanisms of transmission of pain signals at synaptic sites, especially in the spinal cord. Despite this impressive accumulation of detailed information, however, the basic concepts and facts in the field of pain have remained unchanged. In general, the earlier evidence is supported by more detailed, meticulous investigation. Most of this information is highly technical and is beyond the aims of this book.

This book was written for the reader who desires to know more about pain. The book's exposition of the important facts and concepts remains up to date. An attempt to provide all relevant recent references in this new printing would confuse rather than illuminate. The references have therefore been updated by citing reviews that cover recent advances in all the major fields of research and therapy. Readers who wish to follow specialized topics in greater detail will be able to find references to recent articles by outstanding scientists searching for a better understanding of pain and ways to control it.

Part One
The Puzzle of Pain

'... physicians too readily claim that *pain is a reaction of defence, a fortunate warning, which puts us on our guard against the risks of disease* ... Reaction of defence? Against whom? Against what? Against the cancer which not infrequently gives little trouble until quite late? Against heart afflictions, which always develop quietly? ... One must reject, then, this false conception of beneficient pain.'

René Leriche, 1939

1   Pain and Injury: the Variable Link

The link between pain and injury seems so obvious that it is widely believed that pain is always the result of physical damage and that the intensity of pain we feel is proportional to the severity of the injury. In general, this relationship between injury and pain holds true: a pinch of a finger usually produces mild pain, while a door slammed on it is excruciating; a small cut hurts a little, while a laceration can be agonizing. However, there are many instances in which the relationship fails to hold up. For example, some people are born without the ability to feel pain even when they are seriously injured (congenital analgesia), and many of us have injuries such as cuts and bruises without feeling any pain until many minutes or hours later (episodic analgesia). In contrast, there are severe pains that are not associated with any known tissue damage or that persist for years after an injury has apparently healed. Clearly, the link between injury and pain is highly variable: injury may occur without pain, and pain without injury.

This is the essence of the puzzle of pain. Why are pain and injury not always related? What activities of the nervous system intervene between injury and pain perception that make the relationship so variable? We shall begin to answer these questions by describing some extreme examples of the variability of the link between injury and pain. These examples challenge our intuitive feelings about pain and reveal the subtlety of the mechanisms which we will need to explain. Each example also contains clues for the control of pain.

Injury without pain

Congenital analgesia

People who are born without the ability to feel pain provide convincing testimony on the value of pain (Sternbach, 1968). Many of these people sustain extensive burns, bruises and lacerations during childhood, frequently bite deep into the tongue while chewing food, and learn only with difficulty to avoid inflicting severe wounds on themselves. The failure to feel pain after a ruptured appendix, which is normally accompanied by severe abdominal pain, led to near-death in one such man. Another man walked on a leg with a cracked bone until it broke completely.

The best-documented of all cases of congenital insensitivity to pain is Miss C., a young Canadian girl who was a student at McGill University in Montreal. Her father, a physician in western Canada, was fully aware of her problem and alerted his colleagues in Montreal to examine her. The young lady was highly intelligent and seemed normal in every way except that she had never felt pain. As a child, she had bitten off the tip of her tongue while chewing food, and had suffered third-degree burns after kneeling on a hot radiator to look out of the window. When examined by a psychologist (McMurray, 1950) in the laboratory, she reported that she did not feel pain when noxious stimuli were presented. She felt no pain when parts of her body were subjected to strong electric shock, to hot water at temperatures that usually produce reports of burning pain, or to a prolonged ice-bath. Equally astonishing was the fact that she showed no changes in blood pressure, heart rate, or respiration when these stimuli were presented. Furthermore, she could not remember ever sneezing or coughing, the gag reflex could be elicited only with great difficulty, and corneal reflexes (to protect the eyes) were absent. A variety of other stimuli, such as inserting a stick up through the nostrils, pinching tendons, or injections of histamine under the skin – which are normally considered as forms of torture – also failed to produce pain.

Miss C. had severe medical problems. She exhibited pathological changes in her knees, hip and spine, and underwent several orthopaedic operations. Her surgeon attributed these changes to the lack of protection to joints usually given by pain sensation. She apparently failed to shift her weight when standing, to turn over in her sleep, or to avoid certain postures, which normally prevent inflammation of joints.

The condition of the joints that Miss C. suffered from, because of her failure to feel pain, is called the 'Charcot joint'. It has long been known that if the nerves which normally innervate a joint are missing or defective, a condition develops in which the joint surface is damaged and the ligaments and other tissues are stretched. This happens particularly to those joints which are frequently subject to minor injuries in everyday life – ankles, knees, wrists and elbows.

All of us quite frequently stumble, fall or wrench a muscle during ordinary activity. After these trivial injuries, we limp a little or we protect the joint so that it remains unstressed during the recovery process. This resting of the damaged area is an essential part of its recovery. But those who feel no pain go on using the joint, adding insult to injury. Apparently, this is eventually sufficient to produce the Charcot joint with its severely eroded tissues. Dead or dying tissue is the perfect culture medium for bacteria and is the most likely place for infection to develop. Because blood flow is impaired by the injuries, the tissue is isolated from the body's own defence mechanisms. The infection is then free to extend into nearby bone and eventually into marrow, producing osteomyelitis where even the most powerful antibiotics cannot penetrate from the bloodstream. These are the conditions that led to Miss C.'s death.

Miss C. died at the age of twenty-nine of massive infections that could not be brought under control. During her last month, she complained of discomfort, tenderness and pain in the left hip. The pain was relieved by analgesic tablets. There is little doubt that her inability to feel pain until the final month of her life led to the 'extensive skin and bone trauma that contributed in a direct fashion to her death' (Baxter and Olszewski, 1960).

Astonishingly, examination of Miss C.'s nervous system by the best means available at the time failed to reveal any abnormality. The nerve endings and specialized receptors in her skin and joints appeared completely normal, as did her nerves, spinal cord and brain. Clearly, however, her nervous system was abnormal in some unknown way. Somewhere, the injury signals that normally ascend to the brain through the spinal cord were blocked at one or more of the many junctions (synapses) through which they pass. We shall examine the possibilities in later chapters.

While Miss C.'s case is the most thoroughly documented one, there are reports of several families with the same problem. In fact, there is strong evidence that some forms of this condition are inherited. However, it is now clear that congenital insensitivity to pain may be due to many causes (Comings and Amromin, 1974). In some cases, there is evidence of neurological damage. Even this is puzzling, though. In one form of insensitivity, examination of small pieces of excised nerve (nerve 'biopsies') showed that the large fibres in nerves are highly abnormal. In other cases, the small fibres in nerves are damaged or missing. This form occurs almost solely in Jewish families and is known as dysautonomia (or the Riley-Day syndrome). It is a tragic disease because all physical development is abnormal and these people rarely live to adulthood. One form of pain insensitivity is accompanied by the inability to sweat. In still another form, the nerve roots that fan out from a peripheral nerve and enter the spinal cord are damaged (sensory radicular neuropathy). Other kinds of insensitivity to pain are associated with severe mental retardation. However, many cases remain a mystery. Recently, a meticulous study of a sixteen-year-old boy with insensitivity to pain concluded that the boy's failure to feel pain could not be attributed to abnormal nerve activity or cerebrospinal endorphins ('the body's own opiates') (Manfredi *et al.*, 1981).

The importance of pain for survival becomes clear when we consider what happens to people who are insensitive to pain (Comings and Amromin, 1974). One woman, for example, reported only a 'tight feeling' during an appendicitis attack and was saved when her family doctor, who knew of her condition, suspected the worst and admitted her to hospital. After the operation, she had no pain but reported 'a pulling sensation' in the region of the fresh scar. Throughout her life, this woman had sustained numerous cuts and burns without feeling pain. Her mouth was scarred from blisters as a result of drinking beverages that were too hot, and her hands were calloused from frequent burns. During two pregnancies, she reported 'a funny, feathery feeling' rather than pain.

Her seven-year-old daughter had the same condition. At the age of three she broke her arm and at five she broke her nose, and felt no pain at any time. At seven, after taking a bath, 'she leaned over and her buttocks pressed up against a grated bathroom heater; she was branded with five large crosshatches over the buttocks but felt no pain'. Interestingly, during a careful neurological examination, it was found that the girl felt no pain when pinpricked on all parts of her body except a small circular area over the lower (lumbar) spine. Yet all the tests indicated no other neurological abnormality in any of the areas insensitive to pain. This girl had one brother who had a mild form of insensitivity and two sisters who perceived pain normally.

Consider another family, some of whose members were normal in every respect except that they felt no pain. The mother was once near death during a pregnancy because of a dangerous complication (eclampsia) which is normally accompanied by severe headache and discomfort. Her doctor, knowing that she did not feel pain, diagnosed the problem from her other symptoms and saved her life. Because of her condition, the woman was especially alert to signs of disease in her children. Indeed, one child developed appendicitis and peritonitis without any pain, and was saved by his mother's prompt reaction to his casual remark about a 'stiff stomach' (Sternbach, 1963).

Most people who are insensitive to pain learn, with difficulty, to avoid damaging themselves severely. However, they survive because they have language to symbolize potential danger and to communicate. Animals, who have no such verbal communication, would have died. It is amply clear, then, that pain plays an important role in survival.

Episodic analgesia

Cases of congenital analgesia are rare. However, there is a much more common condition which most of us have experienced at one time or another: being injured but not feeling pain until many minutes or hours afterwards. The injuries may range from minor cuts and bruises to broken bones and even the loss of a limb.

During the Second World War, Beecher (1959) observed the behaviour of soldiers severely wounded in battle. He was astonished to find that when the injured men were carried into combat hospitals, only one out of three complained of enough pain to require morphine. Most of the soldiers either denied having pain from their extensive wounds or had so little that they did not want any medication to relieve it. These men, Beecher points out, were not in a state of shock, nor were they totally unable to feel pain, for they complained as vigorously as normal men at an inept vein puncture. Beecher attributed their failure to feel pain to a sense of relief or euphoria at having escaped alive from the battlefield in spite of the injury.

A similar study (Carlen *et al.*, 1978) of Israeli soldiers with traumatic amputations after the Yom Kippur War provided comparable observations. Most of the wounded men spoke of their initial injury as painless and used neutral terms such as 'bang', 'thump' or 'blow' to describe their first sensation. They often volunteered their surprise that the injury did not hurt. These men were fully aware of the sad consequences of losing a limb, and some spoke during their pain-free state of feeling guilt at letting down their comrades, annoyance at allowing the injury to occur, and misery about the future. These soldiers were depressed (rather than euphoric), an emotional state which is normally associated with increased pain, yet they felt no pain whatever until many hours later.

This episodic analgesia involving major injury is not confined to soldiers. A recent study (Melzack *et al.*, 1982) found that thirty-seven per cent of the people who arrived at the emergency clinic of a large urban hospital with a variety of injuries, including amputated fingers, major lacerations of the skin and fractured bones, reported that they did not feel any pain until many minutes – even hours – after the injury.

There are six important characteristics of episodic analgesia. First, the condition has no relation to the severity or location of the injury. It may occur with small skin cuts or with an arm or a leg blown off by explosives. Second, it has no simple relation to the circumstances. It may occur in the heat of battle or when a craftsman cuts off the tip of his finger while trying to make an accurate cut. Diversion of attention to some other event sometimes appears to be involved, but it is not essential: the person's attention can be focused on the injury but no pain is felt. Third, the victim can be fully aware of the nature of the injury and of its consequences and yet feel no pain. A young woman with her leg blown off at the knee said, 'Who is going to marry me now?' A machine-shop foreman who had his foot amputated in an accident in his shop said, 'What a fool they will say I am to let this happen,' and later, 'Well, there goes my holiday.' Fourth, the analgesia is instantaneous. The victim does not first feel pain and then bring it under control. The injury may not be noticed or is described in neutral terms such as 'a bang' or 'a blow'. These people are not confused or distracted or 'in shock'. They understand the extent of their injury and may touch the injured area or look at it. They just do not feel pain. Fifth, the analgesia has a limited time-course. By the next day, all these people are in pain. It is true that the relation of their pain to their injury is variable, but they are not pain-free. Sixth, the analgesia is localized to the injury. As we have seen, people may complain about an injection even though the more extensive injury does not hurt. The machine-shop foreman developed a painful cramp in his other leg while the stump of his amputated leg remained pain-free.

These characteristics are a challenge to any theory of pain. Simple explanations such as distraction of attention from the injury or the influence of the meaning of the situation may explain a few cases, but most of them cannot be explained satisfactorily. Conceivably, areas of the brain essential for pain experience and response may be engaged in other activities and are simply not accessible to the input, even when attention is focused on the injury. Whatever the explanation, situational analgesia highlights the variable link between injury and pain.

Pain without injury

In contrast to people who fail to feel pain at the time of injury, other people develop pain without apparent injury. Tension headache is a common form of pain which ranges in intensity from moderate to excruciating, yet there is no damage and no known explanation of the origin of the pain. It was widely believed that muscle tension was the cause, but no muscles have been found in contraction in spite of a very careful search (Olesen, 1986). Another common headache, migraine, was assumed to be caused by dilated blood vessels in the head, but recent research shows that the changes in blood vessels are more likely the result of the headache rather than its cause (Pikoff, 1984). A more rare but more severe pain of the head is trigeminal neuralgia, in which a light touch to a trigger point provokes an agonizing stab of pain, as though a knife had been jabbed into the face. Careful studies of the tissues and nerves of the face show them to be perfectly normal. A final example of such pains is the ubiquitous and crippling low back pain. Every structure in the region – muscles, nerves, joints, bone, tendons and discs – have been blamed for this condition and yet the best modern diagnostic techniques fail to find any responsible damage in 70 per cent of the cases (Loeser, 1994). In a later chapter, we shall discuss these pains as diseases which are caused by a failure in the function of central control mechanisms.

Pain disproportionate to severity of injury

Those who have experienced the passing of a kidney stone describe it as painful beyond any expectation that pain can reach such an intensity. The kidney may, under certain conditions, concentrate some components in the urine so that these compounds precipitate out and form small kidney stones (renal calculi). Small pieces of these stones break off and pass into the ureter that leads from the kidney to the bladder. In size, they are often not more than twice the size of the normal diameter of the ureter. Pressure of urine builds up behind the plug formed by the stone, tending to drive it into the ureter. As a result, the muscle in the ureter wall goes into localized strong contraction. This band of contraction moves down the ureter to produce peristaltic waves to drive the stone down. During this process, agonizing spasms of pain sweep over the patient so that the toughest and most stoical of characters usually collapses. The patient is pale, with a racing pulse, knees drawn up with a rigid abdominal wall and motionless. Even crying out is restrained because all movement exaggerates the pain. As the stone passes into the bladder, there is immediate and complete relief, leaving a dazed and exhausted patient. The reason for describing this condition here is that in mechanical terms it is a rather trivial event. Furthermore, it occurs in a structure which is poorly innervated when compared to any equal volume of skin. In spite of the minor nature of the actual event and the relatively small number of nerve impulses which are sent to the spinal cord, the effect in terms of pain is gigantic.

Pain after healing of an injury

Motorcycle accidents are typically associated with injuries of the head and shoulder. On hitting an obstruction, the rider is catapulted forwards and hits the road at high speed. Crash helmets have effectively decreased head injuries; but the next vulnerable point to hit the road is often the shoulder, which is violently wrenched down and back. The arm is supplied by a network of nerves – the brachial plexus – which leaves the spinal cord at the level of the lower neck and upper chest, and funnels into the arms. In the most severe of these injuries, the spinal roots are avulsed – that is, ripped out of the spinal cord – and no repair is possible.

C.A., aged twenty-five, an air-force pilot, suffered such an accident. After eight months he had completely recovered from the cuts, bruises and fractures of his accident. There had been no head injury and he was alert, intelligent and busy as a student shaping a new career for himself. His right arm was completely paralysed from the shoulder down and the muscles of the arm were thin. In addition, the limp arm was totally anaesthetic, so that he had no sensation of any stimuli applied to it. On being questioned, he stated that he could sense very clearly an entire arm, but it had no relationship to his real arm. This 'phantom' arm seemed to him to be placed across his chest while the real paralysed arm hung at his side. The phantom never moved and the fingers were tightly clenched in a cramped fist with the nails digging into the palm. The entire arm felt 'as though it was on fire'. Nothing has helped his condition and he finds that he can control the pain only by absorbing himself in his work.

Wynn Parry (1980) studied a hundred consecutive cases of this type of brachial plexus avulsion and found ninety-five to be in severe pain with very similar descriptions of their phantoms and their pain. We shall return to this subject later to consider the causes of the pain. It is introduced here to show that pain may persist long after all possible healing has occurred. Even the most damaging stimulation of the arm is incapable of producing pain, yet pain is constantly felt even though no injury is occurring.

Damage of peripheral nerves in the arms or legs, by gunshot wounds or other injuries, is also sometimes accompanied by excruciating pains that persist long after the tissues have healed. These pains may occur spontaneously for no apparent reason. They have many qualities, and may be described as burning, cramping or shooting. Sometimes they are triggered by innocuous stimuli such as gentle touches or even a puff of air. Spontaneous attacks of pain may take minutes or hours to subside, but may occur repeatedly each day for years after the injury. The frequency and intensity of the spontaneous pain-attacks may increase over the years, and the pain may even spread to distant areas of the body. The initial cause of these pains is sometimes far more subtle than peripheral nerve damage. Minor injuries may give rise to astonishingly severe pain. In these cases, Livingston (1943, p. 110) notes:

The onset of symptoms may follow the most commonplace of injuries. A bruise, a superficial cut, the prick of a thorn or a broken chicken-bone, a sprain or even a postoperative scar may act as the causative lesion. The event which precipitates the syndrome may appear both to the patient and the physician as of minor consequence, and both have every reason to anticipate the same prompt recovery that follows similar injuries. This anticipation is not realized and the symptoms tend to become progressively worse.

Pain: good and evil

These prolonged, agonizing pains inevitably force us to examine the purpose and value of pain. From the cases described so far, it is evident that pain can serve three purposes. First, the pain that occurs *before* serious injury, such as when we step on (or pick up) hot, sharp or otherwise potentially damaging objects, has real survival value. It produces immediate withdrawal or some other action that prevents further injury. Second, the pains that prevent further injury serve as the basis for learning to avoid injurious objects or situations which may occur at a later time. The larger the animal's brain, the more easily such learning occurs, and it generalizes to other situations. In man, the learning involves language and the use of other symbols, so that even people who are insensitive to pain can limit the extent of damage so that survival is possible. Third, pains due to damaged joints, abdominal infections, diseases or serious injuries set limits on activity and enforce inactivity and rest, which are often essential for the body's natural recuperative and disease-fighting mechanisms to ensure recovery and survival.

However, there are pains, such as those after brachial plexus avulsion or amputation of a limb, that serve no useful purpose. A person who has a leg removed because of a circulatory problem may suffer excruciating phantom limb pain for years, perhaps the remainder of his life, but gains nothing from the pain. Pain such as this now becomes a problem in its own right. It is no longer the symptom of a disease but becomes a serious medical syndrome that requires attention for its own sake. Chronic pain can even be detrimental to survival in man. The pain can be so terrible, so feared, that people would sooner die than continue living with it. Suicide among patients who suffer prolonged, unremitting pain is not uncommon. In cases such as these, the pain serves no biologically useful purpose. It is as though some normally adaptive mechanism has run amok and, like the dangerous criminal whose mind may be brilliant but warped, needs to be isolated, contained and treated. Leriche (1939, p. 23), a brilliant surgeon who spent much of his life attempting to relieve suffering, contemplated this aspect of pain:

Defence reaction? Fortunate warning? But as a matter of fact, the majority of diseases, even the most serious, attack us without warning. When pain develops . . . it is too late . . . The pain has only made more distressing and more sad a situation already long lost . . . In fact, pain is always a baleful gift, which reduces the subject of it, and makes him more ill than he would be without it.

The puzzle

The kinds of cases we have examined so far – ranging from the inability to feel pain in spite of injury to spontaneous pain in the absence of injurious stimulation – represent the extremes of the full spectrum of pain phenomena. They demonstrate that the link between pain and injury is often highly variable and unpredictable. We do not yet have a satisfactory explanation for either type of case. Instead we must resort to speculation and theory: the best possible guess on the basis of the available evidence.

It was once thought that the mechanisms that subserve pain would be entirely revealed if we applied noxious stimuli to the skin and then mapped the pathways taken by nerve impulses through the spinal cord and brain. Unfortunately, pain mechanisms are not as simple as this. When the skin is pinched or crushed, for example, it is true that receptors with very high thresholds are stimulated, but so are receptors with much lower thresholds which are ordinarily activated by gentle touch or vibration. The same is true for extreme heat, or cold, or any other noxious stimulus. Painful stimuli, in other words, are usually extremes of other natural stimuli, and they tend to activate receptors that may also be involved in eliciting other sensations such as tickle, touch, warmth or cold. The critical question is this: does the brain examine just a specific message ascending along specific fibres, or does it monitor *all* the input and make a decision on the basis of the activity in all fibres?

The answer to this question represents the key to the puzzle of pain. It therefore has profound implications for its treatment. It was long hoped that we need only find the pathways in the nervous system that send pain messages from the body to the brain, and pain could be eliminated simply by cutting the pathways. There are many forms of pain, however, that defy this simple solution. Attempts to stop spontaneous pains by cutting pathways in the spinal cord or the brain produce as many failures as successes (Sunderland, 1978). Other kinds of pain are more amenable to surgical treatment. Pain produced by cancer in the lower part of the body is totally relieved by spinal cord surgery in about fifty per cent of patients, and is partially relieved in another twenty-five per cent. But the remainder – about one out of four – continue to suffer (Nathan, 1963). Even those who are helped sometimes report that they now have intense 'girdle pains' at the level of the operation – pains which they did not have before (Noordenbos, 1959). In a few cases, the pain after surgery may be worse than the pain for which the patients were treated (Drake and McKenzie, 1953).

An important aim of pain research is the successful treatment of pathological pain. The clinical syndromes which result from peripheral nerve injury bewilder the scientist who tries to understand them. Still worse, the failure to solve the problems they present means prolonged suffering and tragedy to many patients. People who face death due to a malignant disease such as cancer also face the prospect of extreme pain. Those who sustain brain damage as a result of a stroke may suffer severe pain (often called 'central pain') for the rest of their lives. The pain may continue unabated until the end. Pain, then, is more than an intriguing puzzle. It is a terrible problem that faces all humanity and urgently demands a solution.

The field of pain research and theory has developed rapidly in recent years. These developments have come from many disciplines, including psychology, physiology and clinical medicine. As a result of this progress, exciting new techniques have been proposed for the treatment of pain. The purpose of this book is to describe the research and the theories, as well as the pursuit of new directions aimed at the control of pain.

2 The Psychology of Pain

Psychological and anthropological studies have shown that pain is not simply a function of the amount of bodily damage alone. Rather, the amount and quality of pain we feel are also determined by our previous experiences and how well we remember them, by our ability to understand the cause of the pain and to grasp its consequences. Even the culture in which we have been brought up plays an essential role in how we feel and respond to pain. Stimuli that produce intolerable pain in one person may be tolerated without a whimper by another. In some cultures, moreover, initiation rites and other rituals involve procedures that we associate with pain, yet observers report that these people appear to feel little or no pain. Pain perception, then, cannot be defined simply in terms of particular kinds of stimuli. Rather, it is a highly personal experience, depending on cultural learning, the meaning of the situation, and other factors that are unique to each individual.

Cultural determinants

Cultural values are known to play an important role in the way a person perceives and responds to pain. One of the most striking examples of the impact of cultural values on pain is the hook-swinging ritual still in practice in parts of India (Kosambi, 1967). The ceremony derives from an ancient practice in which a member of a social group is chosen to represent the power of the gods. The role of the chosen man (or 'celebrant') is to bless the children and crops in a series of neighbouring villages during a particular period of the year. What is remarkable about the ritual is that steel hooks, which are attached by strong ropes to the top of a special cart, are shoved under his skin and muscles on both sides of the back (Figure 1). The cart is then moved from village to village. Usually the man hangs on to the ropes as the cart is moved about. But at the climax of the ceremony in each village, he swings free, hanging only from

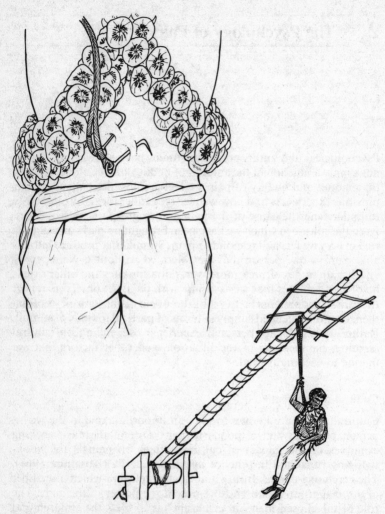

Figure 1. The annual hook-swinging ceremony practised in remote Indian villages. *Top* shows two steel hooks thrust into the small of the back of the 'celebrant', who is decked with garlands. The celebrant is later taken to a special cart which has upright timbers and a cross-beam. *Bottom* shows the celebrant hanging on to the ropes as the cart is moved to each village. After he blesses each child and farm field in a village, he swings free, suspended only by the hooks. The crowds cheer at each swing. The celebrant, during the ceremony, is in a state of exaltation and shows no sign of pain. (from Kosambi, 1967, p. 105)

the hooks embedded in his back, to bless the children and crops. Astonishingly, there is no evidence that the man is in pain during the ritual; rather, he appears to be in a 'state of exaltation'.

There are many examples of comparable procedures in other cultures. In East Africa, men and women undergo an operation – entirely without anaesthetics or pain-relieving drugs – called 'trepanation', in which the scalp and underlying muscles are cut in order to expose a large area of the skull. The skull is then scraped by the doktari as the man or woman sits calmly, without flinching or grimacing, holding a pan under the chin to catch the dripping blood. Films of this procedure are extraordinary to watch because of the discomfort they induce in the observers, which is in striking contrast to the apparent lack of discomfort in the people undergoing the operation. There is no reason to believe that these people are physiologically different in any way. Rather, the operation is accepted by their culture as a procedure that brings relief of chronic pain.

Pain thresholds

It is often asserted that variations in pain experience from person to person are due to different 'pain thresholds'. However, there are several thresholds related to pain and it is important to distinguish among them. Typically, thresholds are measured by applying a stimulus such as electric shock or radiant heat to a small area of skin and gradually increasing the intensity. Four thresholds can be measured by this technique: (a) sensation threshold (or lower threshold) – the lowest stimulus value at which a sensation such as tingling or warmth is first reported; (b) pain perception threshold – the lowest stimulus value at which the person reports that the stimulation feels painful; (c) pain tolerance (or upper threshold) – the lowest stimulus level at which the subject withdraws or asks to have the stimulation stopped; (d) encouraged pain tolerance – the same as (c) but the person is encouraged to tolerate higher levels of stimulation.

There is now evidence that the majority of people, regardless of cultural background, have a uniform *sensation threshold*. Sternbach and Tursky (1965) made careful measurements of sensation threshold, using electric shock as the stimulus, in American-born women belonging to four different ethnic groups: Italian, Jewish, Irish, and Old American. They found no differences among the groups in the level of shock that was first reported as producing a detectable sensation. The sensory conducting apparatus, in other words, appears to be essentially similar in all people so that a given critical level of input always elicits a sensation.

Cultural background, however, has a powerful effect on the *pain perception threshold*. For example, levels of radiant heat that are reported as painful by people of Mediterranean origin (such as Italians and Jews) are described merely as warmth by Northern Europeans (Hardy *et al.*, 1952). Similarly, Nepalese porters on a climbing expedition are much more stoical than the occidental visitors for whom they work: even though both groups are equally sensitive to changes in electric shock, the Nepalese porters require much higher intensities before they call them painful (Clark and Clark, 1980).

The most striking effect of cultural background, however, is on *pain tolerance levels*. Sternbach and Tursky (1965) report that the levels at which subjects refuse to tolerate electric shock, even when they are encouraged by the experimenters, depend, in part at least, on their ethnic origin. Women of Italian descent tolerate less shock than women of Old American or Jewish origin. In a similar experiment (Lambert *et al.*, 1960), in which Jewish and Protestant women served as subjects, the Jewish, but not the Protestant, women increased their tolerance levels after they were told that their religious group tolerated pain more poorly than others.

These differences in pain tolerance reflect different ethnic attitudes towards pain. Zborowski (1952) found that Old Americans have an accepting, matter-of-fact attitude towards pain and pain expression. They tend to withdraw when the pain is intense, and cry out or moan only when they are alone. Jews and Italians, on the other hand, tend to be vociferous in their complaints and openly seek support and sympathy. The underlying attitudes of the two groups, however, appear to be different. Jews tend to be concerned about the meaning and implications of the pain, while Italians usually express a desire for immediate pain relief.

However, not all differences are due to cultural factors. It has long been known that a small proportion of people suffer painless (or 'silent') heart attacks. They may survive several heart attacks without ever reporting pain in the chest. Because the pain of a heart attack (cardiac infarction) is usually severe, it forces the person to stop all ongoing activity and thereby decrease the heart's exertions. People with painless heart attacks may be unaware of their infarction (which can easily be detected with an electrocardiogram) and continue to be active, sometimes with fatal results. Studies of these people show that they have unusually high pain thresholds for electric shocks, heat pain and even arm-muscle cramp. Their pain-perception and pain-tolerance thresholds are significantly higher than those of patients who suffer pain during heart attacks (Procacci *et al.*, 1976; Droste *et al.*, 1986). There was no evidence that the two groups differed in nerve innervation of the heart or extent of diseased coronary vessels; nor did the body's 'natural opiates' appear to play a role. For reasons not understood, a small number of people feel pain less easily than others ('have higher pain thresholds') and may fail to feel chest pain during a major injury to the heart which is extremely painful to most people.

In contrast to these studies, which demonstrate *variability* in pain tolerance, other psychological experiments are aimed at revealing a precise mathematical relationship between the measured stimulus input and the intensity of sensation reported by the subject. Stevens *et al.* (1958) asked subjects to estimate the magnitudes of a series of electric shocks of varying intensity by assigning a number to each that expressed the subjective intensity of the shock. They found that the stimulus–sensation relationship is best described as a mathematical power function, a fact which has been confirmed by several other investigators. The actual value of the exponent, however, varies from study to study (Sternbach and Tursky, 1964). A similar orderly, psychophysical relationship between the intensity of electric shocks and the perceived intensity of the sensory and 'unpleasantness' components of pain has also recently been found, using verbal descriptors and hand-grip force to express the perceived intensities (Gracely, 1979).

Psychophysical studies that find a mathematical relationship between stimulus intensity and pain intensity are often cited (Mountcastle, 1980, 1986) as supporting evidence for the assumption that pain is a primary sensation subserved by a direct communication system from skin receptors to pain centre. A simple psychophysical function, however, does not necessarily reflect equally simple neural mechanisms. Activities in the central nervous system, such as memories of earlier cultural experience, may intervene between stimulus and sensation and invalidate any simple psychophysical 'law'. The use of laboratory conditions that minimize such activities or prevent them from ever coming into play reduces the functions of the nervous system to those of a fixed-gain transmission line. It is under these conditions that psychophysical functions prevail.

Past experience

The evidence that pain is influenced by cultural factors suggests that early experience influences adult behaviour related to pain. It is commonly accepted that children are affected by the attitudes of their parents towards pain. Some families make a great fuss about ordinary cuts and bruises, while others tend to show little sympathy towards even fairly serious injuries. There is reason to believe, on the basis of everyday observations, that attitudes towards pain acquired early in life are carried on into adulthood.

The influence of early experience on the perception of pain has also been demonstrated experimentally. Melzack and Scott (1957) raised Scottish terriers in isolation cages from infancy to maturity so that they were deprived of normal environmental stimuli, including the bodily knocks and scrapes that young animals get in the course of growing up. They were surprised to find that these dogs, at maturity, failed to respond normally to a variety of noxious stimuli. Many of them poked their noses repeatedly into a flaming match, and endured pinpricks with little evidence of pain. They invariably withdrew reflexively from the flame or pinprick and oriented to the stimuli, but few of them showed strong emotional arousal or behavioural withdrawal. In contrast, the litter-mates of these dogs that had been reared in a normal environment recognized potential harm so quickly that the experimenters were usually unable to touch them with the flame or pin more than once.

The abnormal behaviour of dogs raised in isolation appears to be due to a failure to attend selectively to noxious stimuli when they are presented in an unfamiliar environment in which all stimuli are equally attention-demanding (Melzack, 1965, 1969). The results suggest that young animals learn the significance – or meaning – of environmental stimuli during early life, and this plays an important role in later pain perception. It is important to note that heredity may determine the extent to which early experience influences behaviour. Beagles raised in isolation cages are not as severely disturbed as Scotties or mongrels and are capable of behaving more normally towards flaming matches and pinpricks (Melzack, 1965).

The role of early experience in determining pain perception and response is especially evident in studies of monkeys raised in isolation. In several experiments, infant monkeys were raised in individual cages that kept them isolated from the normal experience of encounters with damaging objects, or elders who slap or bite in the attempt to teach the youngsters how to live in a normal social environment. The resulting behaviour was disastrous. These monkeys, when released into a normal environment, often engaged in suicidal attacks against older and stronger monkeys. They also viciously bit their own limbs. These acts of self-destruction by the monkeys 'have on occasion resulted in broken bones and torn skin and blood vessels. After being repaired, many of these animals fail to profit from their experiences, continuing to bite themselves and to attack larger animals who inflict new wounds . . .' (Lichstein and Sackett, 1971, p. 340).

Meaning of the situation

The importance of the meaning associated with a pain-producing situation is made particularly clear in conditioning experiments carried out by Pavlov (1927, 1928). Dogs normally react violently when they are given strong electric shocks to one of the paws. Pavlov found, however, that if he consistently presented food to a dog after each shock, the dog developed an entirely new response. Immediately after a shock the dog would salivate, wag its tail and turn eagerly towards the food dish. The electric shock now failed to evoke any responses indicative of pain and became instead a signal meaning that food was on the way. This type of conditioned behaviour was observed as long as the same paw was shocked. If the shocks were applied to another paw, the dogs reacted violently. Pavlov reports that similar results were obtained in other experiments in which intense pressure or heat was used as the conditioned stimulus. This study shows convincingly that stimulation of the skin is localized, identified and evaluated *before* it produces perceptual experience and overt behaviour. The meaning of the stimulus acquired during earlier conditioning modulates the sensory input before it activates brain processes that underlie perception and response.

There are more familiar examples of the role played by personal evaluation of the situation. Abdominal sensations that are assumed to be gas cramps and are usually ignored may be felt as severe pain after learning that a friend or relative has stomach cancer. The pain may persist and get worse until a doctor assures the person that nothing is wrong. It may then vanish suddenly. Still another example is the frequent observation by dentists that patients who arrive early in the morning, complaining of a terrible toothache that kept them awake all night, sometimes report that the pain disappeared when they entered the dentist's office. They may even have difficulty remembering which tooth had hurt. The presence or absence of pain in these patients is clearly a function of the meaning of the situation: the pain was unbearable when help was unavailable, and diminished or vanished when relief was at hand.

Attention, anxiety and distraction

If a person's attention is focused on a potentially painful experience, pain will tend to be perceived more intensely than normal. Hall and Stride (1954) found that the simple appearance of the word 'pain' in a set of instructions made anxious subjects report as painful a level of electric shock they did not regard as painful when the word was absent from the instructions. Thus the mere anticipation of pain is sufficient to raise the level of anxiety and thereby the intensity of perceived pain. Similarly, Hill *et al.* (1952a and b) have shown that if anxiety is dispelled (by reassuring a subject that he has control over the pain-producing stimulus), a given level of electric shock or burning heat is perceived as significantly less painful than the same stimulus under conditions of high anxiety.

In contrast to the effects of attention on pain, it is well known that distraction of attention away from pain can diminish or abolish it. Distraction of attention may partly explain why boxers, football players and other athletes sometimes sustain severe injuries during the excitement of the sport without being aware that they have been hurt.

The common observation that pain is diminished when attention is wilfully directed towards other events, such as exciting games, books or films, has provided a simple 'home-made' remedy for pain. Every sufferer of chronic pain has learned to force himself to concentrate on activities that become so absorbing that pain is not felt or is greatly diminished. A well-known actress, for example, reports that her intense arthritic pain vanishes the moment her part begins on stage and returns as soon as it is over (Glyn, 1971). People who suffer severe pain after brachial plexus lesions (see Chapter 1) report that the most effective way to reduce their pain is to absorb themselves in their work (Wynn Parry, 1980).

A study of the effects of music and 'white noise' (a wide range of sound frequencies) on pain shows that people learn quickly to use the auditory inputs to decrease their pain. In this experiment (Melzack *et al.*, 1963b), the subjects had a hand immersed in ice-water, which produces a deep, aching, severe pain that few people can tolerate for more than a few minutes. However, when the subjects were given an opportunity to listen to music and white noise, they did not just passively sit back and listen to them. Instead, they tapped their feet, sang out, and continually turned the volume control buttons on the audio-apparatus in the attempt to distract their attention away from the pain.

Distraction of attention, however, is effective only if the pain is steady or rises slowly in intensity (Melzack *et al.*, 1963b). If radiant heat is focused on the skin, for example, the pain may rise so suddenly and sharply that subjects are unable to control it by distraction. But when the pain rises slowly, people may use auditory stimulation to distract their attention from it. They often find that the pain actually levels off or decreases *before* it reaches the anticipated intolerable level (Figure 2). Distraction strategies employing music and noise are used effectively by some people to control pain produced by dental drilling and extraction (Gardner and Licklider, 1959).

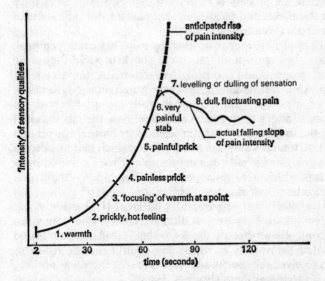

Figure 2. Idealized curve of sensory qualities produced by radiant heat, based on reports of subjective sensation. The subject anticipates a continuing rise in pain intensity which, instead, begins to fall after reaching a peak. Distraction stratagies enable people to tolerate the pain through level 6 on the curve, thereby prolonging their pain tolerance.
(from Melzack *et al.*, 1963b, p. 239)

Feelings of control over pain

In the course of growing up, we learn early in life that pain has a unique aspect to it: after an injury, such as a burned finger or a cut knee, the pain persists without possibility of escape. A severely burned patient can only scream out or weep as layers of dead skin are carefully removed (debridement) – an agonizing process. The procedure is repeated frequently and the patient dreads these horrible experiences. Yet there is no escape for the patient. It is possible to walk away from unpleasant sights, sounds or smells, but once the body is injured, there is no escape.

It is, of course, possible to avoid some kinds of pain. Touching a hot stove or stepping on a sharp stone often produces a sudden movement that may limit or prevent injury. It is also possible to change the level of pain by giving people the *feeling* that they have control over it even though, in fact, they do not. When burn patients are allowed to participate in the debridement of their burned tissues, they claim that the process is more bearable. Several studies have established the effects and conditions that play a role in the sense of control over pain (Weisenberg, 1994).

Rats, like people, are more disturbed by pain they cannot control. In one study, two groups of rats were shocked while they were eating. One group could 'control' (or terminate) the shock by jumping up, while the animals in the other group received the shock regardless of what they did. Although both groups received the same amount of shock during each testing session, the rats that had 'control' of the shock were less disturbed and ate more (Mowrer and Viek, 1948). A similar study showed that rats which had no control over the electric shocks had consistently greater rises in blood pressure than rats which *were* given 'control'. The input – the actual amount and intensity of shock – was the same for both groups, but the disruptive effects were significantly different (Hokanson *et al.*, 1971). In a comparable experiment, human subjects who were given a 'sense of control' over electric shocks, by being told how to respond to them, rated the shocks as much less painful than a group of people who received the shocks and were told that there was nothing they could do to avoid them (Bowers, 1968).

These laboratory studies have important implications for pain in real-life situations. It is now apparent that the severity of postsurgical pain is significantly reduced when patients are taught how to cope with their pain. Patients who were scheduled to undergo major surgery to remove the gall bladder, uterus or portions of the digestive tract were given detailed information about the pain they would feel after the operation and how they could best cope with it. They were told where they would feel pain, how severe it could be, how long it could last, and that such pain is normal after an operation. They were also shown how to relax by using breathing and relaxation strategies. Finally, they were told that total relaxation is difficult to achieve and that they should request medication if they were uncomfortable. The results showed that patients who received these instructions reported significantly less pain and asked for many fewer medications during recovery than a comparable group of patients who received no instructions (Egbert *et al.*, 1964).

It was originally thought that the information alone is sufficient psychological preparation to reduce the uncertainty and anxiety associated with major surgery. However, it is evident that know-ledge, in this case, may only increase the anxiety because of the certain expectation of pain and various discomforts. The essential ingredient is providing the patient with skills to cope with the pain and anxiety – at the very least, to provide the patient with a sense of control. Recent studies have shown that simply giving patients information about their pain tends to make them focus on the discomforting aspects of the experience, and their pain is magnified rather than reduced. However, when the patients are taught skills to cope with their pain, such as relaxation or distraction strategies, the pain is less severe (Langer *et al.*, 1975). Furthermore, control that is perceived as inadequate may be worse than not having any control (Weisenberg *et al.*, 1985).

Other studies have shown that the amount of post-surgical pain is profoundly influenced by the patient's personality. Taenzer *et al.* (1986) found that the patient's anxiety and fear evoked by the surgery were less important than the patient's personality traits of anxiety, neuroticism and extroversion. Post-operative pain was greater in patients who were typically predisposed to being emotional in threatening situations. These personality variables were prepotent in determining the effectiveness of coping strategies (Taenzer, 1983). Patients who expected complications and problems as a result of surgery ('catastrophizers') had more pain. However, patients who were taught special coping strategies, such as hypnosis, did not necessarily have less pain than patients in the 'control' group who were given standard nurses' information on simple stratagies to diminish pain. The results suggest that people who have the personal disposition to cope with life's stresses usually use any strategy available – and invent their own when necessary – to cope with specific threatening events such as surgery.

Suggestion and placebos

The power of suggestion on pain is clearly demonstrated by studies on placebos. Clinical investigators (Beecher, 1959) have found that severe pain, such as post-surgical pain, can often be relieved by giving patients a placebo (usually some non-analgesic substance such as a sugar or salt solution) in place of morphine or other analgesic drugs. About thirty-five per cent of the patients report marked relief of pain after being given a placebo. This is a strikingly high proportion because morphine, even in large doses, relieves severe pain in only about seventy per cent of patients.

Because suggestion, even in the subtlest form, may have a powerful effect on pain experience, the use of the 'double-blind' technique is essential in the evaluation of drugs. When this technique is used, both the experimental drug and the placebo are labelled in such a way that neither the patient nor the physician knows which one has been administered. Only then can the effect of the drug be evaluated in comparison with a physiologically neutral control chemical agent. The remarkably powerful effect of a placebo in no way implies that people who are helped by a placebo do not have real pain; no one will deny the reality of post-surgical pain. Rather, it illustrates the powerful contribution of suggestion to the perception of pain.

It is generally assumed that the suggestion itself is sufficient to produce the entire placebo effect. However, the placebo may also decrease anxiety because it makes the patient believe that something is being done to relieve the pain. Both effects probably always occur together. Whatever the explanation, it is clear that the physician may often relieve pain significantly by prescribing placebos to influence cognitive processes as well as by treating the injured areas of the body (Benson and Epstein, 1975; Wall, 1994).

A surprising recent discovery about placebos is that their effectiveness is always about fifty per cent of that of the drug with which they are being compared, even in double-blind experiments (Evans, 1985). That is, if the drug is a mild analgesic such as aspirin, then the pain relief produced by the placebo is half that of the aspirin. If it is a powerful drug such as morphine, the placebo has greater pain-relieving properties, again about fifty per cent of that of morphine. How is this possible? Anyone who has conducted a double-blind experiment quickly learns the answer. The experimenter has expectations of the power of the drug being tested and his enthusiasm is conveyed, implicitly or explicitly, to the subject. If the drug is new and especially effective, then certain patients are helped considerably at the beginning of the study, and the experimenter (or research assistant) is inevitably excited. Then, even though the 'double-blind' is maintained, the excitement is conveyed to the patient. The magnitude of the placebo effect, therefore, is about half the *assumed* strength of the analgesic drug being administered under double-blind conditions. This shows clearly that the psychological context – particularly the physician's and the patient's expectations of pain relief – contains powerful therapeutic value in its own right in addition to the effects of the drug itself (Evans, 1985).

There are large individual differences in susceptibility to placebos, and studies have been carried out to determine some of the factors that are involved (Evans, 1985). Placebos are more effective for severe pain than for mild pain, and are more effective when the patients are under great stress and anxiety than when they are not. Is it possible, then, that the placebo effect can simply be attributed to a reduction in anxiety? Experiments show that the reduction of anxiety may account for some – but not all – of the placebo effects (McGlashan *et al.*, 1969). Placebo-induced analgesia is not significantly related to suggestibility, hypnotic susceptibility, or anxiety induced specifically by pain or the therapeutic situation (which is known as 'state-anxiety'). However, placebo effects occur more powerfully in people who have chronic generalized anxiety (personality 'trait-anxiety'). Nevertheless, even in people with high trait-anxiety, placebos are effective when pain levels are high rather than low. Apart from trait-anxiety levels, no consistent differences have been found to distinguish between placebo reactors and non-reactors.

Several studies also show that placebo effects and medication effects interact and may be additive. One study (Lasagna *et al.*, 1954) demonstrated that a standard dose of morphine was only 54 per cent effective in placebo non-reactors but was 95 per cent effective in placebo reactors. Clearly, then, drug effects are dramatically enhanced in those people who are fortunate enough to be placebo reactors. The *kind* of pain is also an important factor. Most kinds of pain are relieved in 35 per cent of patients. However, 52 per cent of people suffering headaches are helped by placebos; it is possible that this may be due to a particularly strong role of anxiety in such sufferers. Clearly, the placebo effect is produced by suggestion, personality predispositions and other psychological factors. It is not due to any simple mechanism such as an outpouring of the body's 'natural opiates' (Gracely *et al.*, 1983).

There are other fascinating factors in the placebo response. Two placebo capsules, for example, are more effective than one capsule, and large capsules are better than small ones. A placebo is more effective when injected than when given by mouth, and is more potent when it is accompanied by strong suggestion that a powerful analgesic has been given. In short, the greater the implicit and explicit suggestion that pain will be relieved, the greater the relief obtained by the patient. Unfortunately, however, patients tend to get less and less relief from repeated administration of placebos.

It is clear, then, that placebo effects provide a remarkably powerful form of therapy for many medical problems. They are effective not only for pain but also for anxiety and depression as well as a variety of medical complaints in which psychological factors play a role. It is important to maximize these effects so that they contribute as much as possible to the relief of pain and suffering.

Hypnosis

The manipulation of attention together with strong suggestion are both part of the phenomenon of hypnosis. The hypnotic state eludes precise definition. But, loosely speaking, hypnosis is a trance state in which the subject's attention is focused intensely on the hypnotist while attention to other stimuli is markedly diminished. After people are hypnotized they can, with appropriate suggestion, be cut or burned yet report that they did not feel pain (Hilgard and Hilgard, 1986; Spanos *et al.*, 1994). They may say that they felt a sharp touch or strong heat, but they maintain that the sensations never welled up into pain. Evidently a small percentage of people can be hypnotized deeply enough to undergo major surgery entirely without anaesthesia. For a larger number of people hypnosis reduces the amount of pain-killing drug required to produce successful analgesia.

Self-hypnosis or auto-suggestion may be related to the state of meditation observed in mystics or other profoundly religious people. Deep meditation, or prolonged, intense focusing of attention on inner feelings, thoughts or images, may produce a state similar to hypnotic analgesia. Indian fakirs have frequently been observed to walk across beds of hot coals, or lie on a bed of nails or cactus thorns without evidence of pain. It is possible that the fakirs develop highly calloused skin. But this cannot be the whole explanation. It is more likely that they enter a trance-like state as a result of deep meditation.

An excellent study of a fakir who was able to pierce his body with swords and daggers showed that he required about two hours of intense concentration on one theme before he entered a phase of thinking about nothing (keeping his mind a blank) which he called his trance state (Larbig, 1982). During this state, the fakir's electro-encephalogram (EEG) showed a marked increase in theta activity, which is characteristic of intense mental activity, and heightened activity of the sympathetic nervous system, indicating it was geared for action, not relaxation. In this trance state, the fakir felt no pain and showed no bleeding as he repeatedly pierced his face, chest and abdomen with swords and knives.

Even though the precise nature of hypnosis remains a mystery, there are several features of it that are important in understanding the psychological contributions to pain. It is known, for example, that not all people can be hypnotized. About 30 per cent of people can reach a state of deep hypnosis, 30 per cent reach a moderate state, and another 30 per cent achieve a drowsy-light state. About 10 per cent of people are not susceptible at all. These figures are interesting because, broadly, they resemble the proportions of placebo reactors and non-reactors. However, there is strong evidence that the lack of responsiveness to pain in hypnotized subjects is more than a placebo effect. An elegantly designed experiment (McGlashan *et al.*, 1969) has shown that pain perception and pain tolerance levels are strikingly increased during hypnosis, but only the pain perception threshold is raised after administration of a placebo. In fact, this study demonstrated that the hypnotic procedure itself has a placebo effect, but also has an additional effect that raises pain threshold and tolerance still further.

The most exciting discovery about hypnotic analgesia in recent years is the phenomenon of the 'hidden observer'. Many highly hypnotizable people are able to respond to commands under hypnosis by 'automatic writing', in which one of the hands writes answers to specific questions but the person is not aware of it. In experiments on hypnotic analgesia, in which pain is produced by immersion of an arm and hand in ice-water, the subjects are told that there is a part of the mind of which they are unaware – metaphorically called the 'hidden observer' – which can communicate with the hypnotist by automatic writing by the other hand. Hilgard (1973, p. 398) describes the sequence of events:

We initially tried this procedure with a young woman highly experienced in hypnosis. In the normal non-hypnotic state, she found the experience of the circulating ice-water very painful and distressing. In the hypnotic analgesic state, she reported that she felt no pain and was totally unaware of her hand and arm in the ice-water; she was calm throughout. All the while that she was insisting verbally that she felt no pain in hypnotic analgesia, the dissociated part of herself was reporting through automatic writing that *she felt the pain just as in the normal non-hypnotic state*. Subsequent experiments with her and with additional subjects have similarly reported no conscious pain but some pain reported in automatic writing, at a level usually below that of the full pain in the normal non-hypnotic condition.

The results suggest that the intense cold evokes activity simultaneously in at least two areas for the brain. Hypnosis appears to be able to 'dissociate' one from the other, which implies that hypnotic suggestion given by the hypnotist is able to modify or suppress signals in one area but not in the other. It is not surprising, therefore, that hypnotized subjects who report no pain when a hand is immersed in ice-water, nevertheless show a rise in heart rate and blood pressure which is typical when pain is normally perceived.

While hypnosis is a fascinating research technique, it is important to recognize its limitations as a clinical therapy. Like the placebo, repeated hypnosis by a professional may become less and less effective, and exert its effects for shorter durations. Furthermore, only a small percentage of people can be deeply hypnotized (Perry, 1980). There are numerous anecdotal reports that hypnosis is effective in relieving severe clinical pains. However, although excellent studies of hypnotic analgesia have been carried out with experimentally induced pains (Hilgard and Hilgard, 1986), there is as yet no convincing evidence that hypnosis can be considered a useful tool for the control of any form of chronic clinical pain.

Psychogenic pain

When psychological factors appear to play a predominant role in a person's pain, the pain may be labelled as 'psychogenic'. That is, the person is presumed to be in pain because he needs or wants it. A typical case has been reported by Freeman and Watts (1950, pp. 354–5):

A woman of hysterical temperament began at the age of sixteen to complain of abdominal pain so persistently that she accumulated a series of twelve to eighteen abdominal operations, with what might be termed progressive evisceration. Following a trivial head injury, she complained so bitterly of pain in the head that a subtemporal decompression was performed. From 1934 to 1936 she was confined to bed because of agonizing pain in the back and limbs. Examination showed swollen knuckles, tender knee joints with contracture, and roentgenograms of the spine revealed lipping of the vertebrae. When we saw her for the first time, she appeared uneasy, would not give her history and began wincing and overbreathing before the bed covers were turned down. She lay constantly on her left side and cried out if any attempt was made to turn her on her back. She defended herself with her right hand from any examination of her back, and when the right hand was restrained and the region of the sacrum was gently stroked, she screamed and trembled violently. On account of exaggeration of the complaints with very little anatomic substrate, a diagnosis of conversion hysteria with polysurgical addiction was made.

The concluding sentence of this case history suggests that the patient suffered pain primarily because of psychological needs, and that she became addicted to multiple surgical operations as a way of satisfying her needs. This woman, Freeman and Watts (1950) report, then underwent a frontal lobotomy (to cut the neural connections between the frontal cortex and thalamus). The operation did not entirely relieve her pain, but she was not bothered by it as much and was able to live a useful life.

It is clear that we must recognize the psychological contribution to pain, but we must maintain a balanced view of it. The term 'psychogenic' assumes that medical diagnosis is so perfect that all organic causes of pain can be detected; regrettably, we are far from such infallibility. Even Freud (cited by Merskey and Spear, 1967) regarded pains with a major psychological basis as also having an organic substrate such as muscle tension. In such cases, the physical as well as the psychological symptoms require treatment.

Convincing evidence that chronic pain is usually the cause rather than the result of neurotic symptoms derives from studies of patients who are eventually relieved of their pain. Typically, these patients, while they are suffering chronic pain, show evidence of psychological disturbance on the Minnesota Multiphasic Personality Inventory (MMPI). In particular, they have elevated scores on the scales for hysteria, depression and hypochrondriasis. Some investigators have argued that these personality characteristics lead to chronic pain after minor injuries. However, the evidence points in the other direction: that pain produces the elevations in these emotional characteristics. Significant decreases in several key MMPI scales (hysteria, depression, hypochondriasis and anxiety) occur after successful treatment of chronic pain with a variety of therapies (Sternbach, 1974; Sternbach and Timmermans, 1975). Similarly, patients suffering several forms of chronic pain – including headache, colitis and abdominal pain – were found to have lower self-esteem than pain-free control groups. However, after these patients underwent several therapeutic procedures that significantly reduced their pain, they showed a striking improvement in their self-esteem ratings (Elton *et al.*, 1978).

It is evident from studies such as these that it is unreasonable to ascribe chronic pain to neurotic symptoms. The patients with the thick hospital charts are all too often prey to the physician's innuendoes that they are neurotic and that their neuroses are the cause of the pain. While psychological processes contribute to pain, they are only part of the activity in a complex nervous system. All too often, the diagnosis of neurosis as the cause of pain hides our ignorance of many aspects of pain mechanisms.

Implications of the psychological evidence

Taken together, the psychological data refute the concept of a one-to-one relationship between stimulus and sensation. The same injury can have different effects on different people or even on the same person at different times. Psychological variables may intervene between stimulus and perception and produce a high degree of variability between the two. In most instances, to be sure, a simple relationship holds: the harder the slam of a hammer on the thumb, the greater the pain is likely to be. The exceptions, however, illuminate the nature of the underlying mechanisms.

The psychological evidence strongly supports the view of pain as a perceptual experience whose quality and intensity are influenced by the unique past history of the individual, by the meaning he gives to the pain-producing situation and by his 'state of mind' at the moment. We believe that all these factors play a role in determining the actual patterns of nerve impulses that ascend from the body to the brain and travel within the brain itself. In this way pain becomes a function of the whole individual, including his present thoughts and fears as well as his hopes for the future.

The recognition that psychological processes influence pain has led to the development of psychological techniques to fight pain, which will be described in Chapter 12. These procedures produce some degree of pain relief in many people, and their use in combination with other therapies has led to increasing success in the battle against some of the most vicious forms of chronic pain.

3   The Varieties of Pain

The French novelist, Marcel Proust, noted that 'Illness is the doctor to whom we pay most heed: to kindness, to knowledge we make promises only: pain we obey.' Pain is by far the most common reason for a patient to seek help from a physician. When he first feels the pain, he may restrict his activity, waiting for it to pass. If the pain persists, common remedies may be tried, such as rubbing the painful area, applying heat or ice, or simply resting. These procedures are practised universally and are often effective.

If the pain rises to an intolerable level, or if it persists unabated, or keeps recurring, the sufferer goes to a physician. The doctor first listens to the patient, to the history of the development of the pain, and to the words used to describe and locate the pain. From his or her experience and training the doctor attempts to diagnose the cause of the pain and prescribes drugs or other therapy to relieve it.

In this simple, common consultation it is evident that there have been three quite separate processes. First, the patient has his reasons for seeking help. Second, the words used are aimed at convincing the doctor that the patient has pain and needs help. The pain may be particularly difficult to describe because the patient's ordinary language is rarely adequate to describe unusual sensations. Third, the doctor has an educated bias about how he expects his findings to match the patient's words. It can readily be seen that each of these three processes contains a multiplicity of possible variables so that the path from complaint to diagnosis and to treatment is always tortuous and needs to be followed with care and patience.

The time-course of pain

Transient pain

Pains of brief duration are usually recognized as having little consequence and rarely produce more than fleeting attention. A mild burn, a stubbed toe, the prick of a hypodermic, or a bang on the shin may produce pain for several seconds or minutes and then vanish. Little or no damage has been done and there is rarely any accompanying anxiety. The person may curse out loud, rub the area, and continue with whatever task occupied him before the injury or near-injury occurred. These momentary, transient pains are often felt as two pains. Anyone who has dropped a heavy book on his foot or accidentally put a hand on a hot stove usually feels a 'first' pain, which is relatively mild and well localized. From experience, however, we know that a 'second' pain will arrive shortly – and when it does, it wells up in our consciousness and obliterates all thought. It may rapidly decrease in intensity, or perhaps throb or feel like a series of shooting stabs for several minutes until it gradually fades away. All of these pains are characteristic of minor injuries.

When pain persists, however, we know that the injury was probably severe. The hot stove may actually have damaged the skin so that a blister will form. The book dropped on a toe may have broken it. The persistent abdominal pain may portend an inflamed appendix, an ulcer, or some other damage that we usually expect to remain, in varying degrees, until healing begins. These pains are generally known as *acute pains* – they are intense and usually diminish and disappear when healing is well under way. Sometimes, however, the pain persists even after healing is apparently complete. This may occur after injuries as innocuous as stabbing the finger on a rosebush-thorn or long after an operation which has proceeded without incident and all tissues appear to have healed normally. These persistent pains – *chronic pains* – often have tragic consequences.

Acute pain

The characteristics of acute pain are the combination of tissue damage, pain and anxiety. It is a transitional period between coping with the cause of the injury and preparing for recovery. There is obvious anxiety about the future consequences of the injury. Death or prolonged suffering are possibilities. The assessment of this threat and therefore the degree of anxiety will depend on such factors as personality and experience. Acute pain, then, encompasses the unpleasantness of past injury and the hope of future recovery. Once relative safety from the source of injury has been achieved, a new form of behaviour begins which is related to promoting recovery.

Pain initiates this behaviour and anxiety is directed at assuring safety from the original damage and the best conditions for treatment and recovery.

Chronic pain

One of the major advances in the field of pain in recent years has been the recognition that chronic, persistent pain is a distinct medical entity different from acute pain in many respects (Bonica, 1953, 1974a). Chronic pain, which persists after all possible healing has occurred or, at least, long after pain can serve any useful function, is no longer simply a symptom of injury or disease. It becomes a pain *syndrome* – a medical problem in its own right which requires urgent attention. Most important for diagnosis, treatment and prognosis is the recognition that treatments which are normally effective for most kinds of acute pain are not necessarily effective for chronic pain. Pain, which is normally associated with the search for treatment and optimal conditions for recovery, now becomes intractable. Patients are beset with a sense of helplessness, hopelessness and meaninglessness. The pain becomes evil – it is intolerable and serves no useful function. Recently, we have learned that chronic pain rarely has a single cause but is instead the result of multiple, interacting causes. A variety of subtle physical and psychological factors all interact and contribute to chronic pain. An understanding of chronic pain and new methods to relieve it are two of the salient challenges which provide the focus for most of this book (Craig, 1994).

The language of pain

Anyone who has suffered severe pain and tried to describe the experience to a friend or to the doctor often finds themself at a loss for words. Virginia Woolf, in her essay 'On Being Ill' touches on precisely this point: 'English,' she writes, 'which can express the thoughts of Hamlet and the tragedy of Lear, has no words for the shiver and the headache ... The merest schoolgirl, when she falls in love, has Shakespeare and Keats to speak for her; but let a sufferer try to describe a pain in his head to a doctor and language at once runs dry.'

The reason for this difficulty in expressing pain experience, actually, is not because the words do not exist. There is an abundance of appropriate words, but they are not words which we use often. There is another reason: the words may seem absurd. We may use descriptors such as splitting, shooting, gnawing, wrenching or stinging, but there are no 'outside', objective references for these words. If we talk about a blue pen or a yellow pencil we can point to an object and say 'that is what I mean by yellow' or 'the colour of the pen is blue'. But what can we point to to tell another person precisely what we mean by smarting, tingling, or rasping? A person who suffers terrible pain may say that the pain is burning and add that 'it feels as if someone is shoving a red-hot poker through my toes and slowly twisting it around'. These 'as if' statements are often essential to convey the qualities of the experience.

If the study of pain in people is to have a scientific foundation, it is essential to measure it. If we want to know how effective a new drug is, we need numbers to say that the pain decreased by some amount. Yet, while this is important to know, we also want to know whether the drug specifically decreased the burning quality of the pain, or if the tight, cramping feeling is gone. There is now a way to get this kind of information.

Until recently, the methods that were used for pain measurement treated pain as though it were a single, unique quality that varies only in intensity. The most common of these methods is the use of words such as 'mild', 'moderate', and 'severe', and subjects (or patients) are asked to choose the word that best describes the intensity of their pain. Another method consists of a five-point scale which ranges from 1 = mild pain to 5 = unbearable pain, and subjects are asked to choose the most appropriate number. In this way, some quantitative measure of pain is obtained. Still another method is the use of fractions, so that subjects who have received injections of analgesic drugs such as morphine are asked whether their pain is $\frac{1}{3}$, $\frac{1}{2}$, or $\frac{2}{3}$ of what it was before the injection. Yet another method is the 'visual analogue scale'. The patient or subject is presented with a line which is 10 centimetres long and has the numbers 0 and 10 at either end. He is told that one end represents no pain and the other represents the worst pain imaginable, and is then asked to make a mark on the line which represents the intensity of his pain. A ruler is then used to get a numerical measure of pain intensity, such as 7cm, or units of pain intensity. These simple methods have all been used effectively in hospital clinics, and have provided valuable information about the relative effectiveness of different drugs.

All of these methods specify only intensity. It is clear, however, that to describe pain solely in terms of intensity is like specifying the visual world only in terms of light flux without regard to pattern, colour, texture, and the many other dimensions of visual experience.

Clinical investigators have long recognized the varieties of pain experience. Descriptions of the burning qualities of pain after peripheral nerve injury, or the stabbing, cramping qualities of visceral pains frequently provide the key to diagnosis and may even suggest the course of therapy. The layman is equally aware of the many qualities and dimensions of pain. An evening of radio, television or newspaper commercials makes us aware of the splitting, pounding qualities of headaches, the gnawing, nagging pain of rheumatism and arthritis, the cramping, heavy qualities of menstrual pain, and the smarting, itching qualities apparently well known to sufferers of haemorrhoids. Despite the frequency of such descriptions, and the seemingly high agreement that such adjectives are valid descriptive words, studies of their use and meaning are relatively recent.

Melzack and Torgerson (1971) made a start towards the specification of the qualities of pain. In the first part of their study, subjects were asked to classify 102 words, obtained from patients and from articles on pain, into smaller groups that describe different aspects of the experience of pain. On the basis of the data, the words were categorized into three major classes and sixteen subclasses. The classes are:

1 Words that describe the *sensory qualities* of the experience in terms of temporal, spatial, pressure, thermal, and other properties.
2 Words that describe *affective qualities*, in terms of tension, fear, and autonomic properties that are part of the pain experience.
3 *Evaluative* words that describe the subjective overall intensity of the total pain experience.

Each subclass consists of a group of words that were considered by most subjects to be qualitatively similar. Some of these words are undoubtedly synonyms, others seem to be synonymous but vary in intensity, while many provide subtle differences or nuances (despite their similarities) that may be of importance to a patient who is trying desperately to communicate to a physician.

The second part of the study determined the pain intensities implied by the words within each subclass. Groups of doctors, patients and students were asked to assign an intensity value to each word, using a numerical scale ranging from least (or mild) pain to worst (or excruciating) pain. When this was done, it was apparent that several words in each subclass had the same relative intensity relationships in all three groups, despite their different backgrounds: for example, 'hot', 'burning', 'scalding' and 'searing'. Although the precise intensity values differed for the three groups, all three agreed on the positions of the words relative to each other.

The measurement of pain

The high degree of agreement on the intensity relationships among pain descriptors made it possible to develop a questionnaire (Figure 3) to determine the properties of different pain syndromes (Melzack, 1975a). In addition to the three major classes of pain descriptors, the questionnaire includes a fourth class of miscellaneous words arranged in four subclasses. It also contains the overall Present Pain Intensity (PPI). The PPI is recorded as a number from 0 to 5, in which each number is associated with the following words: 0, no pain; 1, mild; 2, discomforting; 3, distressing; 4, horrible; 5, excruciating. The average scale values of these words, which were chosen from the evaluative category, are approximately equally far apart, so that they represent equal scale intervals and thereby provide 'anchors' for the specification of overall pain intensity (Melzack and Torgerson, 1971).

The descriptor-lists of the McGill Pain Questionnaire are read to a patient with the explicit instruction that he choose *only* those words which describe his feelings and sensations at that moment. Two major indices are obtained. The first is the Pain Rating Index (PRI), which is the sum of the rank values of the words chosen, based on the positions of the words in each category or 'subclass' in Figure 3. The PRI score can be computed separately for the sensory (subclasses 1–10), affective (subclasses 11–15), evaluative (subclass 16), and miscellaneous (subclasses 17–20) words, in addition to providing a total score (subclasses 1–20). The second is the Present Pain Intensity (PPI) which measures overall pain intensity on a scale of 0 to 5.

The McGill Pain Questionnaire is now widely recognized as a valid, reliable instrument to measure pain experience (Melzack and Katz, 1994). It has been translated into many languages, and the existence of three major categories of pain experience – sensory, affective and evaluative – has been confirmed by several studies (Melzack and Katz, 1994). A short form of the questionnaire is now in use (Melzack, 1987); it requires less time to administer, yet is sensitive to different forms of therapy. The usefulness of the questionnaire in countless studies shows that pain can now be

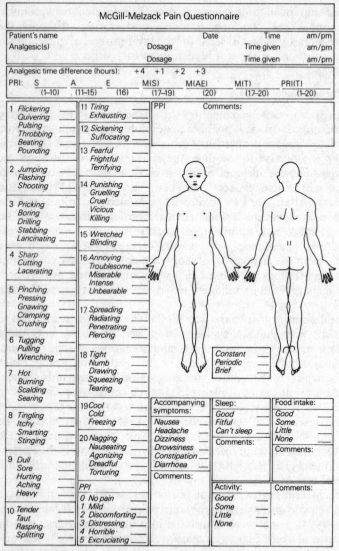

Figure. 3. McGill Pain Questionnaire, adapted for a study of narcotic drugs. Descriptors fall into four major groups: sensory, 1 to 10; affective, 11 to 15; evaluative, 16; and miscellaneous, 17 to 20. The rank value for each descriptor is based on its position in the word set. The sum of the rank values is the 'pain rating index' (PRI). The 'present pain intensity' (PPI) is based on a scale of 0 to 5. © R. Melzack, 1970.

accurately assessed in the clinic as well as in the laboratory (Melzack, 1983).

The varieties of pain experience

Because pain is a private, personal experience, it is impossible for us to know precisely what someone else's pain feels like. No man can possibly know what it is like to have menstrual cramps or labour pain. Nor can a psychologically healthy person know what a psychotic patient is feeling when he says he has excruciating pain (Veilleux and Melzack, 1976). But the McGill Pain Questionnaire provides us with an insight into the qualities that are experienced.

One of the most exciting discoveries made with the McGill Pain Questionnaire is that each kind of pain is characterized by a distinctive constellation of words (Dubuisson and Melzack, 1976). The questionnaire was administered to patients suffering from one of eight pain syndromes: post-herpetic neuralgia, phantom limb pain, metastatic carcinoma, toothache, degenerative disc disease, rheumatoid or osteoarthritis, labour pain, and menstrual pain. A statistical analysis of the data showed that each type of pain has unique qualities which are described by a distinctive set of words. Table 1 presents the words that characterize six of the syndromes – that is, words that were chosen by more than 33 per cent of the patients in each group. Later studies of pain due to tooth extraction (Van Buren and Kleinknecht, 1979), cancer (Graham *et al.*, 1980) and labour (Melzack *et al.*, 1981) have noted the remarkable consistency in the choice of words by patients suffering the same or similar pain syndromes.

The McGill Pain Questionnaire provides information about the intensity of pain as well as the qualities of the pain. Since the P R I total score provides an index of overall pain intensity, it is possible to compare the relative intensity (or severity) of pains on the basis of this measure. For example, Figure 4 shows the average pain intensity reported by patients with various forms of pain. While the data do not warrant strong statements that one pain is worse than another, they nevertheless provide an insight into the relative intensities of different kinds of pain.

Language and diagnosis

We have already noted that major kinds of pain are characterized by distinct constellations of words. Sometimes a few words can be

Table 1. Descriptions characteristic of clinical pain syndromes.

Menstrual pain (N = 25)	Arthritic pain (N = 16)	Labour pain (N = 11)	Disc disease pain (N = 10)	Toothache (N = 10)	Cancer pain (N = 8)
Sensory					
Cramping (44%)	Gnawing (38%)	Pounding (37%)	Throbbing (40%)	Throbbing (50%)	Shooting (50%)
Aching (44%)	Aching (50%)	Shooting (46%)	Shooting (50%)	Boring (40%)	Sharp (50%)
		Stabbing (37%)	Stabbing (40%)	Sharp (50%)	Gnawing (50%)
		Sharp (64%)	Sharp (60%)		Burning (50%)
		Cramping (82%)	Cramping (40%)		Heavy (50%)
		Aching (46%)	Aching (40%)		
			Heavy (40%)		
			Tender (50%)		
Affective					
Tiring (44%)	Exhausting (50%)	Tiring (37%)	Tiring (46%)	Sickening (40%)	Exhausting (50%)
Sickening (56%)		Exhausting (46%)	Exhausting (40%)		
		Fearful (36%)			
Evaluative					
	Annoying (38%)	Intense (46%)	Unbearable (40%)	Annoying (50%)	Unbearable (50%)
Temporal					
Constant (56%)	Constant (44%)	Rhythmic (91%)	Constant (80%)	Constant (60%)	Constant (100%)
	Rhythmic (56%)		Rhythmic (70%)	Rhythmic (40%)	Rhythmic (88%)

Note that only those words chosen by more than one third of the patients are listed, and the percentages of patients who chose each word are shown below the word. The word 'rhythmic' is one of three words 'rhythmic/periodic/intermittent' used in different versions of the McGill Pain Questionnaire (Melzack, 1975).

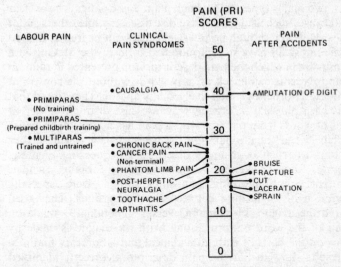

Figure 4. Comparison of pain scores, using the McGill Pain Questionnaire (from Melzack, 1984.

the basis of diagnosis by a physician. An eye specialist who is told by a patient on the telephone that the pain in his eye is a 'dull ache', may diagnose a serious condition which can produce blindness, and the ophthalmologist may ask the patient to see him immediately. A severe 'burning' pain in the chest may be the clue for a possible heart attack. A persistent 'gnawing' in the fingers may mean arthritis. It is not surprising, then, that the descriptors chosen by patients can be used for diagnosis. This kind of research has already begun, with the help of computers, and is extremely promising.

For example, the descriptors chosen by patients with one of eight different pain syndromes – six are shown in Table 1 – were fed into a computer which had to make a diagnosis on the basis of the words alone (Dubuisson and Melzack, 1976). The computer made a correct classification in seventy-seven per cent of the cases. When the sex of the patient and the location of the pain were also included, the classification was correct in one hundred per cent of the cases. It is evident, then, that there are appreciable and quantifiable differences in the way various types of pain are described, and that patients with the same disease or pain syndrome tend to use remarkably similar words to communicate what they feel.

Descriptor patterns can also provide the basis for discriminating between two major types of low back pain. Some patients have clear physical causes such as degenerative disc disease, while others suffer low back pain even though no physical causes can be found. Leavitt and Garron (1980) have used a modified form of the McGill Pain Questionnaire in which the pain descriptors are presented in random order and patients can check off any words without the constraint of the intensity order in which they usually appear. They found that patients with physical – 'organic' – causes use distinctly different patterns of words from patients whose pain has no detectable cause and is labelled as 'functional'. On the basis of their research, they found that a particular group of descriptors – squeezing, nagging, exhausting, dull, sickening, troublesome, throbbing, tender, intermittent, numb, shooting, punishing, tiring – were especially important in distinguishing between the two groups. They then compared the diagnosis – 'organic' versus 'functional' – made on the basis of the word patterns alone, with the diagnosis made by surgeons on the basis of elaborate clinical and laboratory findings. Their results showed that the pain descriptors correctly identified 220 out of 253 cases. This represents an accuracy rate of 87 per cent which, astonishingly, is higher than the success rates attained with the complex, highly respected Minnesota Multiphasic Personality Inventory (MMPI).

Specific verbal descriptors of the McGill Pain Questionnaire have also been shown recently to discriminate between reversible and irreversible damage of the nerve fibres in a tooth (Grushka and Sessle, 1984) as well as between trigeminal neuralgia and atypical facial pain (Melzack *et al.*, 1986). These results, taken together, point to the value of verbal descriptors in the measurement and diagnosis of different pain syndromes.

Towards a definition of pain

Despite the importance of pain in medicine and biology, it is astonishing to discover that the word 'pain' has never been defined satisfactorily. Consider three recent attempts at a definition. The first (Mountcastle, 1980, p. 391) states unequivocally that 'pain is that sensory experience evoked by stimuli that injure or threaten to destroy tissue, defined introspectively by every man as that which hurts'. This definition is unsatisfactory and misleading. No one can deny a link between pain and real or threatened tissue damage, but the link is so variable (as we have already seen) that pain cannot be defined exclusively in terms of tissue damage. Pain may occur in the absence of injury or long after an injury has healed. In several pain syndromes (which we will describe in the next chapter), severe pain is evoked by gentle stimulation of normal skin. The converse – the occurrence of injury without concomitant pain – is so common that it makes nonsense of definitions that rigidly link injury and pain. The definition also states that pain, introspectively, is 'that which hurts'. But this too makes no sense. If pain is a hurt, then how does one define a hurt? Presumably as a pain. The definition is circular and does not advance our knowledge of pain mechanisms. By designating tissue damage as the exclusive cause of pain, the definition ignores most of the clinical and psychological evidence on pain, and fails to incorporate the affective, motivational, and cognitive dimensions of pain as an integral part of the experience.

The second definition (Sternbach, 1968, p. 12) defines pain as an abstract concept that refers to '(1) a personal, private sensation of hurt; (2) a harmful stimulus which signals current or impending tissue damage; (3) a pattern of responses which operate to protect the organism from harm'. This definition is wrong on all three counts. To define pain as a 'sensation of hurt' is, as we have just seen, a circular argument that fails to advance our understanding. To define pain as 'a harmful stimulus' is equally wrong. It confuses the cause with the experience, the physical event with the complex psychological process. Finally, protective responses may occur without pain and pain may be experienced without protective responses. Multiple complex neural factors intervene between experience and response, and one cannot be defined in terms of the other.

The third definition is much better, but still falls short of being acceptable to all. Merskey *et al.* (1986) define pain as 'an unpleasant sensory and emotional experience associated with actual or potential tissue damage, or described in terms of such damage'. The great merits of this definition are its explicit recognition of the loose association between injury and pain, and its inclusion of the emotional dimension of pain experience in addition to its sensory dimension. The problem it encounters lies in the word 'unpleasant'. Pain, to be sure, is unpleasant; but it is much more. The unpleasant – or 'negative-affective' – dimension of pain is really comprised of multiple dimensions. It is the kind of 'unpleasantness' that makes people scream, fight, undergo crippling, disfiguring operations, or commit suicide. What is missing in the word 'unpleasant' is the misery, anguish, desperation and urgency that are part of some pain experiences. The qualities of 'unpleasantness' are complex and comprise multiple dimensions that have yet to be determined.

Pain research, it appears, has not yet advanced to the stage at which an accurate definition of pain can be formulated. However, the continuing debate on a definition of pain is a sign of the vigour, excitement and rapid development of the field. Even in the physical sciences, the basic concepts of 'matter' and 'energy' are still being continually re-defined, yet no one can deny the incredible advances of modern-day physics and chemistry.

The diversity of pain experiences explains why it has been impossible, so far, to achieve a satisfactory definition of pain. The word 'pain' represents a *category* of experiences, signifying a multitude of different, unique experiences having different causes, and characterized by different qualities varying along a number of sensory, affective and evaluative dimensions.

At present, we must be content with guidelines *toward* a definition rather than a definition itself. Too much remains to be learned about pain mechanisms before we can define pain with precision. In particular, not until we understand the perplexing phenomena of clinical pain syndromes can we hope to achieve a satisfactory definition.

4 Clinical Pains

The most compelling challenge of pain is to help the patient who is suffering pain. We learn a little about pain by subjecting ourselves or volunteers to painful stimuli in the laboratory. However, this situation differs from clinical pain in two important ways: (1) the subject can always call a halt to the pain, and (2) the subject knows that the experimental stimulus will not produce damage. These are the two points which distress the patient: the pain experienced is out of the patient's control and, furthermore, the patient is convinced that the pain signifies damage of the body. Worst of all, some pains are not only out of the patient's control, but are out of the doctor's control as well. These are the intractable pains, the vast majority of which have one of three causes: damage to deep tissue, damage to peripheral nerves, or damage to the sensory roots entering the spinal cord. We shall now describe a series of pains beginning with a simple scratch and then progress to more complex situations in order to define the nature of the challenge.

A scratch: an injury in two dimensions

We can learn a surprising amount from an injury as trivial as a scratch. Perhaps the best of all scientific traditions in matters of this kind is to be your own guinea pig. We propose that you – the reader – try one of the simplest experiments, one which was carried out long ago by Sir Thomas Lewis (1942), who asked simple questions that led to profound answers. To repeat Lewis's experiment, bare your forearm, and rest it comfortably on a table or your lap. Then press the edge of your thumbnail hard into the skin near your wrist and drag it hard and fast in a line toward the elbow.

The first observation is that the scratch produces a white line that persists for about 15 seconds. The white line occurs because the small blood vessels in the skin are sensitive to stretch and react by going into spasm. This is one of our mechanisms to prevent blood loss. While the damaged vessels are in spasm, substances are released which trigger the slower clotting mechanism, a much more powerful method of preventing blood loss.

Within a short time, the white line disappears as the spasm releases but the skin colour does not simply return to normal. It now becomes redder until the scratch line is red. This occurs because the blood vessels dilate (vasodilation) in the scratch region to a much wider diameter than normal. This remains for several minutes and is produced by chemicals which leak from the damaged cells. Until repair processes have restored the cells to normal, the vasodilation will remain. It will be noticed that the line may feel sore or itchy. If you have scratched rather gently or if you have tough skin, this may be all that happens.

However, if the scratch has been more severe, two further reactions will occur. The skin over the red line begins to swell and becomes pale; this is the weal. You may have to look quite carefully for this swelling. Now the vessels are so dilated that fluid leaks from the blood serum through the capillary walls into spaces between the tissue cells. Histological examination of such tissue shows that there are cell changes in progress. White blood cells invade and destroy broken cell debris. Soon special cells that form connective tissue begin to appear and there is evidence of growth of new tissue. At this stage, the line may ache or itch and feel sore if you move the arm. If you press gently on the line with a pencil tip, it will be clearly tender; that is, pressure which is felt as a light touch on normal skin is now sufficient to produce pain when it is applied to inflamed tissue.

So far, all reactions have been strictly limited to the area which received the scratch. However, it will soon be observed that an area of redness spreads on either side of the weal; this is the flare. Here, too, there is vasodilation, little or no swelling but quite clear tenderness. This sequence of events – white line, weal and flare – was called 'the triple response' by Lewis.

Before your eyes, then, in slow motion, you have observed the development of inflammation. This classically has four cardinal signs: redness, heat, swelling and pain. The redness is caused by vasodilation. The heat is produced locally by the presence of a large amount of hot blood close to the skin surface. The swelling, or oedema, is due to the leakage of fluids from blood vessels into the tissue. The cause of the pain is more complex (Levine and Taiup, 1994). The pressure on the swelling contributes to the pain but that is not a sufficient explanation for it. If the swelling is removed or prevented, the pain is still present.

A twisted ankle: an injury in three dimensions

This familiar experience is associated with a sequence of pains. As the injury occurs, there is a sharp, precisely localized pain which rises rapidly in intensity and then falls equally rapidly. After this pain, a second, quite different pain may be felt; it is deep, diffuse, poorly localized, steady and spreading. You, the reader, will also be aware that if the second pain is felt, you will be in trouble the next day and perhaps the next week. The nature of the trouble is not just pain and swelling in the region of the ankle, but tenderness over the lower leg and foot and an inability to use the leg. A twisted ankle is a minor injury to deep tissue and yet it results in widespread changes of the sensory and motor systems. A much more serious injury limited to skin hurts a great deal at the time but is not associated the next day with the widespread, long-lasting effects.

These common facts point to two areas we must explore further: 1) deep tissue damage differs from superficial damage, and 2) acute pain differs in its mechanisms and consequences from prolonged pains. These differences have been largely ignored until recently. By examining them, new dimensions of understanding of the physiological mechanisms of pain have been revealed to us. They have profound importance for our ability to diagnose and treat complex clinical pains that are now less mysterious than they were only a few years ago.

The sensitivity of different tissues

An opportunity to study the sensitivity of visceral tissue arose in the 1930s when a famous patient, Tom, drank burning-hot liquid that destroyed his oesophagus. Nowadays it is possible to replace the oesophagus by reconstructive plastic surgery, but this was not available at the time and the treatment was to make a permanent opening into the stomach through the abdominal wall (a gastrostomy). A liquid diet was then supplied by tube directly into the stomach. H. G. Wolff, one of the leading American pioneers of the study of pain, realized that Tom offered an unusual opportunity to study gastric function and sensitivity. Tom was a normal healthy man except for his gastrostomy, and Wolff arranged for him to be employed as janitor at a Medical School so that he could be observed. It was found that no sensation was evoked by touching, pinching or heating the stomach (Wolf and Wolff, 1943). This confirmed a great deal of evidence, obtained during abdominal surgery on lightly anaesthetized patients, that the gut does not evoke pain or spinal reflexes if it is manipulated, cut extensively, or even burned. However, pain is consistently evoked by stretching of the tissue by tugging, dilation or spasm. This principle holds true for the stomach as well as the small and large intestine (Blendis, 1994).

Nevertheless, Wolff discovered that if he artificially produced an area of intense vasodilation and secretion in the stomach, the area became exquisitely sensitive to pressure. The same happened when Tom went through a period of anxiety, which raised the stomach secretion of acid and made the lining become inflamed, red and sensitive. Visceral tissue, then, is remarkably different from normal skin. It is totally insensitive to extremely damaging stimuli such as cutting or burning and is highly sensitive to distension or stretch. Clearly, pain is profoundly influenced by the properties of the tissue which is injured (McMahon, 1994).

Viscera

It is evident, in considering deep structures, that we must examine at least three factors: (1) the degree of innervation and the location of nerve endings; (2) the type of stimulus which will fire the nerves; and (3) the state of the tissue. Normal gut, as we have seen, appears to evoke no sensation whatever unless it is stretched by tugging, dilation or spasm. We have already discussed the special case of the ureter, an organ which normally does not produce sensation unless it is greatly stretched. The urinary bladder, as we all know, is able to evoke sensation. If a normal bladder is filled slowly through a urethral catheter, the patient is unable to guess the degree of filling until it is about half full. As filling continues, there is the feeling of increasing fullness until, at some stage, discomfort and then pain begin to accompany the urgency to urinate. However, as those readers who have had an attack of cystitis know all too well, inflammation dramatically changes the situation. What may appear in cystoscopic examination to be a minor infection of the lining of the bladder is associated with a marked lowering of the filling level at which pain and urgency are triggered, so that the frequency of the need to urinate rises to socially embarrassing levels.

The gall bladder appears to follow similar rules and never, in the normal person, reaches the threshold of awareness but becomes a dominating feature of the patient's life if dilated or inflamed. The uterus has a double innervation. The body of the uterus is supplied by nerves which originate from the upper lumbar segments of the spinal cord (Figure 5) and gives rise to pain only if extensively dilated or infected, or is in strong contraction as in menstruation (in some women) and in labour. In contrast, the cervix is supplied by sensory nerves from the sacral segments of the spinal cord (Figure 5) and in the normal state evokes excruciating pain if the opening of the cervix (the os) is suddenly dilated by a few millimetres.

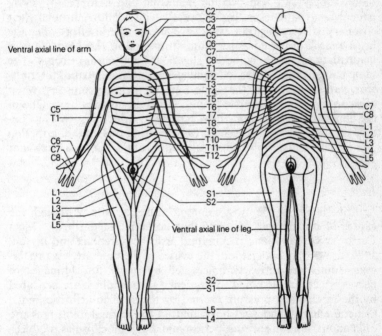

Figure 5. Distribution of dermatomes on the body surface. Each dermatome is the area of skin supplied by the dorsal roots of a given sensory nerve. The positions of the roots are labelled in terms of the level of the bones in the vertebral column. C: cervical; T: thoracic; L: lumbar; S: sacral. (from Keegan and Garrett, 1948)

Muscle

Muscles that move the limbs and torso (striated muscles) are heavily innervated by many types of sensory nerves but are rarely the source of pain – except in one special situation, in which muscle contraction occurs in the absence of an adequate blood supply (muscle ischaemia). Muscle cramps may occur during swimming in cold water when the muscles undergo strong contractions before an adequate blood supply can reach them. It is possible that some chemical substances may be released in this condition, but none have yet been discovered. (Experimentally, muscle ischaemia can be induced by blocking blood flow to an arm by means of a pressure cuff and asking the person to open and close the hand.)

Smooth muscle of the viscera that contracts without adequate blood supply can also become ischaemic and a source of severe pain. Many patients with deteriorating blood flow through their coronary arteries begin to experience angina due to effort when the heart muscle must contract more strongly and the blood flow is inadequate to supply sufficient sugars and oxygen for energy. The same patients may suffer the equivalent condition – called intermittent claudication – at the same time in their leg muscles, when exercise triggers unbearable pain in the main muscles used. One of the limits of prolonged maximal activity by athletes, such as racing cyclists, is set by their threshold for triggering this kind of crippling pain which results in their instantly falling out of the race (Newham *et al.*, 1994).

Joints

Arthritis is one of the most common causes of pain. Although the causes of the changes at joints that occur in osteoarthritis (MacCarthy *et al.*, 1994) and rheumatoid arthritis (Grennan and Jayson, 1994) are poorly understood, the causes of the pain are less mysterious. Joints are diffusely innervated by many fine branches of nerves which are assumed to fire when their endings are activated by the mechanical pressure exerted by the swollen arthritic joints. General clinical evidence shows that, in the normal joint, pressure on tendons, tendon sheaths, periosteum and joint capsules produces pain. The normal joint surface itself is not sensitive, but the tissue destruction and the associated inflammation that occur in arthritis produce a drop in thresholds of the innervating fibres. Minor changes of pressure produce great surges of pain because of changes in the central nervous system (as we shall see later) as well as in peripheral nerve endings.

The brain

Perhaps strangest of all the regions of our body which may be disturbed without producing pain is the brain. This astonishing fact allowed the development of modern neurosurgery. In some types of brain operations, it is desirable to operate on the brain under local anaesthesia so that the patient can communicate with the surgeon. After the scalp is anaesthetized, the surgeon cuts through it and exposes the skull. The surgeon then proceeds, without producing pain to the patient, to drill holes (trephination) through the skull and to saw between the holes in order to lift up a bone flap. The surgeon now faces the dura mater – which resembles thick, flexible cellophane – which is incised. Once the brain is exposed, the cerebral cortex itself may be cut into without the patient feeling any pain and, in most areas, without his feeling any sensation at all. Localized intense electrical stimulation in the depths of the brain has been frequently carried out in conscious man with no reports of pain unless the brainstem is entered.

The special case of cancer pain

Cancerous cells are made up of almost all the same chemical components as normal cells in the body. That is why cancer is so difficult to detect in its early stages, and also why the defence mechanisms of the body do not recognize it as foreign. Therefore, cancer does not induce the immune reactions which reject grafts. Furthermore, it does not even produce inflammation as a primary reaction. A crumb of bread accidentally breathed into the lungs sets off an immediate, painful violent coughing. A lung cancer may grow silently to the size of a grapefruit before any disorder is noticed. Yet cancer is rightly feared as a disease which is frequently painful in its last stages.

What, then, is the cause of pain if this silent enemy can infiltrate without disturbance? The answer is very largely mechanical and obeys the general principles we have already described. One of the commonest first signs of brain tumours is the appearance of severe, generalized headaches. Yet we have said that the brain itself is largely insensitive. The explanation is that the tumour has grown to sufficient size to begin to dam up the normal flow of cerebrospinal fluid which is generated in the ventricles of the brain. Since the fluid cannot escape, there is a rise of intracranial pressure so that brain tissue presses on innervated structures in the base of the skull and produces the headache. Any pharmacological or surgical manoeuvre which reduces this fluid pressure promptly relieves the headache although the cancer itself has in no way been changed.

Similarly, in abdominal cancer pains, by far the commonest cause is mechanical obstruction of one or another of the viscera, followed by dilation above the block. The blocks may occur in intestine, bile ducts, ureters and the bladder, producing the sequence of dilation and intense muscle contractions in the attempt to drive the contents of the structure past the blockade. Blood vessels and lymph ducts may become blocked in the same way. Since veins and lymph ducts contain fluid at a low pressure, they are easier to block than arteries and therefore swelling results from the build-up of pressure behind the block and may produce pain.

On occasion, the tumour may have directly painful effects by expanding and increasing the pressure on sensitive structures – such as a bone tumour which begins to involve the fibrous, vascular membrane that surrounds and nourishes the bone (the periosteum). However, tumours more commonly produce pain by the blocking effects of their mass. Tumours may send off secondary metastases which begin to grow in bone. Slowly the tumour grows at the expense of the bone which of course loses mechanical strength. Eventually the bone may collapse – a 'pathological' fracture. Tumours have a dominating, monopolizing character: they receive few blood vessels, push nerve fibres aside and are not themselves supplied by nerve fibres. Sometimes, therefore, these pathological fractures can be quite painless because all innervated tissue has been replaced by cancer. On other occasions, the long-range mechanical damage produced by the fracture involves normal tissue which is painful and undergoes normal inflammation. A common target for secondary bony metastases are the bones of the vertebral column of the back. When such a bone collapses, it is certain that there will be serious problems because the sensory nerve roots are damaged in the collapse. The other serious consequence is the crushing of the spinal cord in the collapse, which produces paraplegia. Finally, cancer can directly invade nerves and produce a form of painful nerve injury.

The mislocation of pain: referred pain

When the skin is jabbed with a pin, the pain is accurately localized and the eyes and hands move exactly to the point of injury. This ability to localize pain in the region of injury is limited to skin and does not apply when the source of the pain is in deep tissue. Visceral pain is often felt in bizarre locations. Here the doctor needs to know these patterns of pain or he, like the patient, may be misled as to where to search for the seat of the trouble. Fortunately, these strange mislocations usually have regular rules which are found repeatedly in patient after patient.

Inflammation of the diaphragm, for example, produces pain which the patient insists is located in his shoulder. The explanation for this strange referral is as follows. The diaphragm, which separates the chest (thorax) from the abdomen, originates in the embryo from muscle tissue which forms in the fifth cervical segment. This muscle migrates from the neck to the chest to form the diaphragm. Here it develops into our main respiratory muscle. During its migration from neck to thorax, the muscle carries with it its nerve supply which also originates from the fifth cervical segment. This is the phrenic nerve which runs down the lower neck and through the entire length of thorax to innervate the diaphragm. Apart from this special migration, the rest of the fifth cervical segment, like all other segments, forms local skin and muscle. The area of skin supplied by this segment, the dermatome, runs as a band from the midline of the back across the top of the shoulder blade and down the upper arm. As a result, pain triggered by nerve impulses arriving over the phrenic nerve is mistakenly interpreted as coming from the area of skin supplied by the rest of the spinal cord segment.

Appendicitis

The two commonest forms of referred pain are appendicitis and angina pectoris. The first signs of discomfort and pain from inflammation of the appendix seems to the patient to be located in the upper abdomen in the midline above the umbilicus. The appendix actually lies deep in the abdomen on the right side, nestled against the pelvis. In the embryo, the gut begins as a midline straight tube and then develops its coils and curves as the tube lengthens with growth. The overall pattern of sensory innervation is established early in embryonic life. The appendix grows at the junction of the small intestine as it enlarges to become the colon. Being a midline structure, it is innervated from both sides. The segments responsible for its nerve supply are in the lower thoracic part of the spinal cord which also develops into the lower ribs and upper abdominal wall. Thus, following the rule that the pain is referred to the segment of origin of the nerves, and since they come from both sides, the pain is first felt in the midline in the upper abdominal wall. As the appendicitis develops, the inflammation spreads and begins to involve the peritoneum – the membrane that covers the viscera – and the nearby abdominal wall. Now the rules change. When the abdominal wall is affected, it obeys rules like the skin, and the pain is correctly localized. Therefore, the classical course of events in appendicitis is a pain which is first felt in the midline above the navel, and which then shifts down to the right and is centred over the actual position of the appendix.

Angina pectoris

This condition is triggered by an inadequate blood supply to the heart. It feels to the patient as though a tight, broad belt is constricting his or her upper chest and then as the attack mounts, pains shoot down the left arm. The heart begins in the embryo as a midline structure innervated by the upper thoracic segments, so it is not surprising that the first pains should be felt in the upper chest wall. As the heart develops, the left side grows to a much greater mass since it is the left ventricle which does the major work of providing power for the entire arterial system except for the lung circulation. Therefore the left side of the spinal cord has more tissue to innervate and it is reasonable that the pain should be referred to the left. The uppermost thoracic segments also play a part in the development of the arms, so that some spinal cells receive converging signals from the heart as well as the arm. This convergence appears to be the reason why pain is referred to the left arm.

There is more to referred pain than just a mislocation by the patient. If you touch the left arm of a patient during an angina attack, you find that it is tender, although the right arm is not. This even applies when the patient is on the verge of having the attack. This is strange because there is no disease in his left arm. It is clear, then, that in addition to mislocation there is a summation of impulses from both sources. The tenderness of the arm suggests that nerve impulses from the heart and from the region where the pain is referred must converge and summate and thereby increase the pain. There is a very simple way of testing this idea. By using local anaesthesia it is possible to eliminate one of the sources of nerve impulses. In the case of the arm, it is possible to infiltrate the brachial plexus, the massed bundle of nerves at the root of the upper arm. If this is done, the arm becomes numb and it is found that the patient suffering from angina can do more exercise than normal before pain is triggered. This suggests that the pain is triggered by two sources of nerve impulses: a major one from the heart and a minor one from the arm. These two add together. If one source is removed, it becomes more difficult for the other to trigger the feeling of pain. This applies as a general rule to referred pains but even more universally it applies to all pains. It will be seen that summation – the excitatory effects of converging inputs – provides important clues to understanding the causes and treatment of these pains.

The onset of a heart attack and angina has often been observed in intensive care units where the condition of the heart is monitored. At the moment of block of a blood vessel, when the sensory afferent barrage rapidly reaches its maximum, some patients may report only a vague feeling of distress and fear. This may be all that is felt and is incorrectly called a 'silent' heart attack. It should be called a 'non-anginal' heart attack. The angina develops slowly during several minutes. Here, as with the twisted ankle, we witness two clearly separated phases of sensation (Procacci *et al.*, 1994).

Toothache

Sufferers and their dentists often have problems in locating the origin of a toothache, which is usually evoked by bacterial infection in the pulp of a tooth. Patients sometimes report that they have an earache when, in fact, the problem is not the ear but decay of the back upper teeth. In the case of front teeth, the patient frequently points to the wrong tooth, missing by one or two on either side of the culprit. The dentist knows he must search carefully. He therefore examines, probes, X-rays and adds local stimuli to each tooth to detect where he can add a stimulus and enhance the pain.

In some cases, if the tooth infection is neglected, the pain increases as the pulpitis gets worse. Eventually the infection may leak out of the root of the tooth and begin to affect the gum. Now there is an instant and dramatic change: the patient accurately points to the exact area of trouble. The damage now involves superficial tissue with its ability to signal the true location of the injury. We have here, in a small area, a repetition of the changes in pain during appendicitis. In the initial stages, damage is limited to deep tissue and is incorrectly located. Later, superficial structures become involved and then the area in which the pain is felt coincides with the location of the damage.

Low back pain

Low back pain is one of the most common types of pain, yet is poorly understood. It illustrates the complexity of interactions among different contributing factors and the need for multiple approaches in treatment (Cavanaugh and Weinstein, 1994).

The only definite causes of low back pain are herniation of discs and arthritis of vertebral joints. However, these conditions are not always found in patients with low back pain. As many as 60–78 per cent of patients who suffer low back pain have no apparent physical signs. That is, despite X-rays and thorough orthopaedic examination, there is no evidence of disc disease, arthritis, or any other symptoms that can be considered the cause of the pain (Loeser, 1980).

Even when there are clearcut physical and neurological signs of disc herniation (in which the disc pushes out of its space and presses against nerve roots), complete relief of back pain and related sciatic pain by surgery occurs in only about 60 per cent of cases. The rate of success in different reports ranges from 50 to 95 per cent. Removal of a disc is most likely to be effective in patients with clear evidence of nerve-root compression. However, in all cases, the evidence points to the great value of rest followed by progressive exercise. In fact, over half of the patients who suffer an episode of low back pain become symptom-free in a month or so without any health care intervention other than prolonged rest (Loeser, 1980; Watts, 1985).

There have been many promising therapies which have later turned out to be less exciting than the original expectation. The injection of papain, an enzyme, to dissolve the disc seemed at first to be a major advance but now turns out, in experimental studies, to be no more effective than an injection of an inert liquid (Martins *et al.*, 1978; Watts, 1985). Fusion of several vertebrae makes intuitive sense as a way to provide structural support to unstable vertebrae in people who suffer low back pain with evidence of a herniated lumber disc, but the results fail to show that fusion is beneficial. In fact it may be deleterious. Loeser (1994) and Sweet (1980) urge strongly against continuation of the procedure in cases of disc protrusion.

In short, even when physical causes are clearly present, low back pain remains a problem after surgery for a substantial number of patients. And we are still confronted with the high proportion of people who have no obvious physical signs and still suffer agony.

Low back pain usually has a particularly unpleasant quality. It is deep, aching and burning and sometimes immobilizes the patient who is terrified of moving and triggering a severe bout of pain. Often the pains radiate down the leg and are called sciatic pain because they follow the innervation pattern of the sciatic nerve. For patients with minor physical signs such as curvature of the spine, or 'normal' disc disease that occurs with aging, surgery is rarely effective. Such patients, then, in the desperate search for relief of their pain, sometimes prevail on surgeons to carry out successive operations. The greatest danger for patients in rich countries is to have repeated operations which are demoralizing failures.

A variety of forms of physical therapy may help low back pain. The most effective is a regimen of special exercises that develop the back muscles. Transcutaneous electrical nerve stimulation, ice massage, and acupuncture may all help some patients. Injections of trigger points may be effective as well. Recently, it has been shown (Brena *et al.*, 1980) that injection of a long-lasting anaesthetic (bupivacaine) into the sympathetic ganglia relieves pain in a substantial number of people. But so does injection of saline, indicating that the mere stimulation of the ganglia can bring about changes in the nervous system.

It is possible that the major culprit in many cases of low back pain is abnormal activity in nerve-root fibres due to minor changes in the surrounding vertebrae and tissues. The roots may be affected by compression caused by degenerated disc material (which commonly occurs during normal ageing), interference with the blood supply, stress on ligaments and joints that surround the nerve, and so forth. These 'minor' irritations may be cumulative and eventually produce symptoms of 'low back sprain' (Gunn and Milbrandt, 1978). This can be the beginning of a 'vicious circle', because later pain would enhance the autonomic effects, produce spasm, pain, and progressive deterioration of a situation that began 'harmlessly' with normal aging processes (or possibly due to relatively minor physical trauma in younger people.) Whatever the reason, the ensuing mechanisms are complex.

The actual neural mechanisms that are involved in back pain, even when disc herniation has occurred, are not clear. Evidently, either an increase or a decrease in input may be the basis of pain. Howe *et al.* (1977) found that chronically scarred axons tend to fire repetitively after mechanical compression and thereby produce an abnormal, high-frequency input through the dorsal roots, which could be the basis of low back pain and sciatica. On the other hand, prolonged compression of a nerve root may have the opposite effect – it may produce a marked decrease (rather than the expected increase) in firing in the root fibres (Wall *et al.*, 1974). The decrease could, of course, remove inhibitory influences and produce hyperactive spinal cells, which would tend to 'open the gate' and produce more pain.

As a result of the persistence of low back pain despite orthopaedic surgery, neurosurgery and countless drugs – most fail to work and some, such as tranquillizers, increase depression – it is not surprising that psychological therapy has become an important new approach to the problem. Indeed, anti-depressants (such as the tricyclic drugs) are sometimes remarkably effective in relieving the pain as well as the patient's depression. The various kinds of therapy that are effective are behaviour modification, progressive relaxation, hypnosis, biofeedback to help learn to relax muscles, and so forth. All of these, it has been shown, help *some* patients. But no one of them is more effective than the others. In fact, clinics that employ several procedures at the same time get the best results. One group (Swanson *et al.*, 1976) found that patients with several syndromes, but mostly low back pain, were helped by a combination of techniques; about 80 per cent of patients received marked to moderate improvement after treatment, and 50 per cent claimed they were still improved 3 to 6 months later. Interestingly, most patients reported that the pain was unchanged but they were able to work, to live with their pain, and led more normal lives. Another study, specifically on chronic low back pain (Gottlieb *et al.*, 1977), also used a battery of techniques and found that about 60 per cent of patients were able to resume a normal life style. The therapy in this study, it should be noted, required an average hospitalization period of 45 days. At 6 months after the programme, about 80 per cent of the successful patients contacted still reported that they were living a normal life style.

The evidence on low back pain permits two important conclusions: (1) low back pain is not a single syndrome produced by a single causal agent; and (2) the most effective approach to pain relief and return to a normal life style is to use multiple convergent procedures.

It has been seen that disc disease and vertebral arthritis play a role in only a relatively small proportion of patients. However, other physical factors may play a role. Many patients with low back pain have tense muscles and many have clearcut trigger points which evoke severe pain when they are mechanically activated. Furthermore, many patients become depressed by their disability, lose their self-esteem, become obsessed with their health and are anxious. Finally, it has become clear that in a proportion of patients, low back pain is referred as a result of disease in another part of the body, especially in the pelvis (Loeser, 1994). Pain may be referred to the lower back as a result of a variety of visceral diseases that have gone undetected. Jones (1938), in a remarkable study, showed that inflating a balloon at various levels of the digestive system sometimes produces pain felt in the back. In other people, the pain is felt at the site of a scar of an earlier operation. Surgery of the back, then, can leave a scar that may potentially become the site of referred pain.

Therapists must look for trigger points, evidence of excessive sympathetic and muscle activity, and other physical contributions which can be helped by any one of the variety of sensory-modulation procedures. In addition, psychological assessment is essential to determine the psychological contributions – tension, anxiety, fear, and especially depression. The psychological methods described above can all potentially help to some degree. Finally, the patient, who has been terrorized by the pain and sometimes victimized unintentionally by health care professionals who do not understand the complexity of the problem, must be guided back to a normal life style. Behaviour modification methods, particularly those that recognize the patients' capacity to understand the problem and their need for satisfactory coping strategies, appear to be useful. The studies which report impressive relief of low back pain (Swanson *et al.*, 1976; Gottlieb *et al.*, 1977) have utilized virtually all of the above procedures at the same time.

Phantom limb pain

Phantom limb pain is one of the most terrible and fascinating of all clinical pain syndromes. Its description by Ambroise Paré in 1552 captures the sense of awe and mystery it evokes in people who hear about it for the first time:

Verily it is a thing wonderous strange and prodigious, which will scarce be credited, unless by such as have seen with their eyes, and heard with their ears, the patients who have many months after the cutting away of the leg, grievously complained that they yet felt exceeding great pain of that leg so cut off.

The proportion of amputees with phantom limb pain is astonishingly high. The most careful investigation (Jensen *et al.*, 1983, 1985) found that 72 per cent of amputees had phantom limb pain 8 days after amputation, and 65 per cent had it 6 months later. Two years later, phantom limb pain was reported by about 60 per cent, and even 7 years later (Krebs *et al.*, 1984) 60 per cent still continued to complain of pain. These percentages are consistent with those of other studies (67 per cent: Carlin *et al.*, 1978; 78 per cent: Sherman *et al.*, 1984). The only heartening aspect of this story is that the painful attacks decrease in frequency. Despite attempts to relieve pain by using one or more of 40 types of therapy which are used for phantom limb pain (Sherman *et al.*, 1980), not more than 15 per cent of patients are totally relieved of their pain. This pathetically low success-rate reflects the extent of our ignorance about the mechanisms that underlie phantom limb pain (Jensen and Rasmussen, 1994).

There is a dangerous tendency to subdivide patients according to a presumed origin of the pain, such as stump versus phantom, spinal versus brain, or psychiatric versus organic. While these may be felt necessary for practical clinical situations, it is wrong to accept these categories as implying mutually exclusive origins of the pain. It is more likely that all of these phenomena contribute in varying degrees. The most sensible approach for the scientist in this situation is to stand back without joining a particular diagnostic or therapeutic school, and to describe the phenomena as seen in man and animals.

The painless phantom

Amputees report feeling a phantom limb almost immediately after amputation of an arm or leg (Simmel, 1956). The phantom limb is usually described as having a tingling feeling and a definite shape that resembles the real limb before amputation. It is reported to move through space in much the same way as the normal limb would move when the person walks, sits down, or stretches out on a bed. At first, the phantom limb feels perfectly normal in size and shape – so much so that the amputee may reach out for objects with the phantom hand, or try to get out of bed by stepping on to the floor with the phantom leg. As time passes, however, the phantom limb begins to change shape. The arm or leg becomes less distinct and may fade away altogether, so that the phantom hand or foot seems to be hanging in mid-air. Sometimes, the limb is slowly 'telescoped' into the stump until only the hand or foot remain at the stump tip.

Amputation of a limb, however, is not essential for the occurrence of a phantom. A painless phantom is often reported by subjects or patients who have a local anaesthestic block of a sufficiently large part of the body. This has been described in detail by Simmel (1962) for patients who received a block of the lower spinal cord and by

Melzack and Bromage (1973) for patients who received a block of the brachial plexus, which blocks the nerves from the arm to the spinal cord. We have all experienced a version of this in dental anaesthesia when we notice that the anaesthetic lip is apparently swollen and attracts our attention so that we may touch the lip repeatedly and inspect it in the mirror. One of us experienced a phantom arm after a block of the brachial plexus (Melzack and Bromage, 1973), and the other experienced a phantom hand when his radial, ulnar and median nerves were blocked at the wrist (Wall, *et al.*, 1973). In both cases, the hand felt enlarged as though it were a boxing glove and the feeling was so vivid that it held the centre of attention until the anaesthetic wore off. It is wrong to imagine that the patient's initial phantom is a vague sensation; it appears as a startling reality. This phantom, which occurs after an anaesthetic nerve block, implies that the central nervous system produces the phantom in response to the lack of normal input.

After a brachial plexus block, the phantom arm is felt as having a strong tingling or pins-and-needles feeling, in which the hand and fingers are felt especially vividly, and as occupying a definite position in space. Yet when the subject looks at the real arm, which may be distant from the perceived phantom arm, the phantom instantly 'fuses' with the real anaesthetized arm. When the eyes are then closed, the phantom usually assumes its previous position (Melzack and Bromage, 1973; Bromage and Melzack, 1974). These phenomena suggest that the phantom limb is produced by brain activities which normally underlie the body schema – the neural substrate of our perception of the position of the body during movement or rest (Head, 1920). Normally, the body schema is guided by sensory inputs from skin, muscles and joints. But when these inputs are reduced below a critical level, the body schema is felt in positions that are totally unrelated (in the absence of visual cues) to the position of the real limbs.

The painful phantom

The distinction between a painless and a painful phantom is not a rigid one. Some amputees have so little pain or feel it so infrequently that they deny having any. Others suffer pains periodically, ranging from several bouts a day to one each week or two. Still others have continuous pains which vary in quality and intensity. The pain is described as cramping, shooting, burning or crushing. It may start immediately after amputation, but sometimes appears weeks, months, even years later. The pain is felt in definite parts of the phantom limb (Livingston, 1943). A common complaint, for example, is that the phantom hand is clenched, fingers bent over the thumb and digging into the palm, so that the whole hand is tired and painful.

If the pain persists for long periods of time, other regions of the body may become sensitized so that merely touching these new 'trigger zones' will evoke spasms of severe pain in the phantom limb (Cronholm, 1951). Pain, moreover, is often triggered by visceral inputs produced by urination and defecation (Henderson and Smyth, 1948). Even emotional upsets such as an argument with a friend may sharply increase the pain. Still worse, the conventional surgical procedures (Figure 6) often fail to bring permanent relief, so that these patients may undergo a series of such operations without any decrease in the severity of the pain.

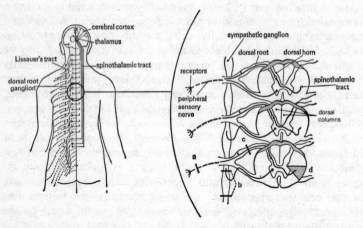

Figure 6. Traditional concept of pain and several conventional surgical procedures. *Left* is Larsell's (1951) diagram of the pain pathway: pain fibres from each dermatome enter the spinal cord, ascend a few segments (in Lissauer's tract), and connect with fibres that cross the cord and form the spinothalamic tract to the thalamus. Fibres from the thalamus project to the cortex. *Right* is a diagram of spinal cord cross sections and adjacent sympathetic ganglia, showing several neurosurgical procedures to relieve pain. a: neurectomy; b: sympathectomy; c: rhizotomy; and d: cordotomy.

Properties of phantom limb pain

Phantom limb pain is characterized by four major properties:

1 The pain may endure long after the healing of the injured tissues. While the pain is transient in many patients, it may persist for years or decades in others (Sunderland, 1978), even though the original area of damage seems completely healed. Sometimes, the pain may resemble, in both quality and location, the pain that was present before amputation (Bailey and Moersch, 1941; White and Sweet, 1969). Thus, a patient who was suffering from a wood sliver jammed under a fingernail, and at that time lost his hand in an accident, subsequently reported a painful sliver under the fingernail of his phantom hand. Similarly, lower limb amputees may report pain in particular toes or parts of the phantom foot that were ulcerated or diseased prior to amputation. As long as two years after amputation, 45 per cent of patients reported that the phantom limb pain was in the same location, and 35 per cent said it had the same qualities as the pain in the intact limb the day before amputation (Jensen *et al.*, 1985). Similar observations and their underlying mechanisms are described by Katz and Melzack (1990) and Coderre *et al.* (1993).

2 Trigger zones may spread to healthy areas on the same or opposite side of the body (Cronholm, 1951). Gentle pressure or pinprick on another limb or on the head (Figure 7) may trigger terrible pain in the phantom limb. There is also evidence that pain at a site distant from the stump may evoke pain in the phantom limb. Thus, amputees who develop anginal pain as long as twenty-five years after amputation may suffer severe pain in a phantom arm during each bout of anginal pain, although phantom limb pain may never before have been experienced (Cohen, 1944).

3 Prolonged relief of pain may occur after temporary *decreases* of somatic input. The most obvious therapy for phantom limb pain is to decrease the input by injecting a local anaesthetic at sensitive spots or nerves in the stump. Astonishingly, these blocks may stop the pain for days, weeks, sometimes permanently, even though the anaesthesia wears off within hours (Livingston, 1943). Successive blocks may produce increasingly longer periods of relief. Similarly, an anaesthetic injected into the lower-back interspinous tissue in leg amputees produces a progressive numbness of part of the phantom limb and prolonged, sometimes permanent, relief of pain in all or part of it (Feinstein *et al.*, 1954).

4 Prolonged relief of pain may occur after *increases* of the sensory input. Injection of small amounts of hypertonic saline into the interspinous tissue of amputees (Figure 8) produces a sharp,

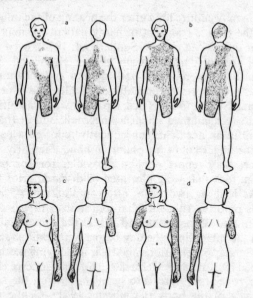

Figure 7. Cronholm's (1951) observations on stimulation sites which evoke pain sensation in the phantom limb. *Top* shows a 59-year-old man who received compound fractures of the lower left leg at the age of twenty-one; amputation was four months later. Pressure (A) or pinpricks (B) were applied to the skin. Stimulation of effective sites (crosshatched areas) produced severe shooting pains and other sensations in the phantom limb. *Bottom* shows a 34-year-old woman: amputation was at the age of fourteen. Pressure (C) or pinpricks (D) were applied to the skin. Stimulation of effective sites (crosshatched areas) produced sensations of a diffuse, unpleasant 'irritation' in the phantom hand.

localized pain that radiates into the phantom limb, lasts only about ten minutes, yet may produce dramatic partial or total relief of pain for hours, weeks, sometimes indefinitely (Feinstein *et al.*, 1954). Vigorous vibration of the stump may also produce relief of phantom limb pain (Russell and Spalding, 1950). The most recent of these techniques (Wall and Sweet, 1967) applies electrical stimulation to the stump and has become an established method for the control of pain in the phantom limb and stump (Krainick *et al.*, 1980). In a related technique, the electrodes may be placed surgically on to the dorsal columns of the spinal cord (Figure 6). This procedure has become the most successful of the surgical therapies for phantom limb pain (Sherman *et al.*, 1980; Krainick *et al.*, 1980).

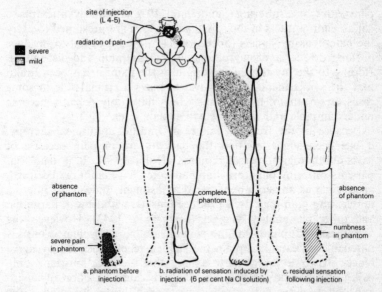

severe
mild

site of injection
(L 4-5)

radiation of pain

absence
of phantom

complete
phantom

absence
of phantom

numbness
in phantom

severe pain
in phantom

a. phantom before
injection

b. radiation of sensation induced by
injection (6 per cent Na Cl solution)

c. residual sensation
following injection

Figure 8. Observations by Feinstein *et al.* (1954) on the effect of hypertonic saline injection into lumbar (L4–L5) interspinous tissues on phantom limb pain. The saline injection, in this case, produced a radiation of pain to the right hip and thigh, and sudden detailed awareness of the complete phantom limb. After injection, numbness was felt in the previously painful area. Pain relief, after this procedure, may last for days, weeks, sometimes permanently.

The search for causal mechanisms

The mechanisms underlying phantom limb pain have been the basis of bitter controversy. The crux of the problem has been the attempt to discover a single factor as the whole explanation. Historically, the search for *the* causal mechanism has progressed from the periphery to the central nervous system, each site on the way leading to a proposed mechanism and a particular therapy to relieve pain (Figure 6, p. 64). The earliest treatment was to surgically remove the neuromas (small nodules of tangled, regenerated nerve fibres) which form after a major nerve is cut and prevented from regenerating normally. However, this procedure generally fails to relieve phantom limb pain. The next treatment was to cut the sensory roots that lead from the nerves of the stump to the spinal cord (operation C in Figure 6); yet this surgery usually fails, often replacing the original pain with worse suffering (Sunderland, 1978). Similarly, attempts to cut ascending tracts in the spinal cord which are presumed to carry the pain-evoking signals (operation D in Figure 6) fail to produce prolonged relief and may ultimately increase pain and discomfort. Adding to the mystery of the origin of the pain, it has been found that the sympathetic nervous system plays a crucial role in some cases, by means of mechanisms which have only recently become understandable and which we will explain later.

Because of the frequent failure of traditional surgical therapy, it has been suggested that the patients are in pain because of psychopathological personal needs (Kolb, 1954). It is true that patients suffering phantom limb pain often have emotional disturbances such as anxiety about social adjustment. Indeed the intense, unrelenting pain may itself produce marked withdrawal, paranoia, and other personality changes (Livingston, 1943). However, the hypothesis that phantom limb pain always has a psychiatric basis is untenable. It cannot explain the sudden relief produced by nerve blocks. It would be wrong to assume that the injections have only psychotherapeutic (or placebo) value, because injection of an inappropriate nerve fails to relieve pain, even though injection of the appropriate nerve in the same patient is effective (Livingston, 1943). Moreover, statistical analysis of the data presented by Ewalt *et al.* (1947) indicates that patients with phantom limb pain do not have a greater incidence of neuroses than those without pain in the phantom limb. Emotional factors undoubtedly contribute to the pain but are not the major cause.

In summary, these data, taken together, indicate that phantom limb pain cannot be satisfactorily explained by any single mechanism such as peripheral nerve irritation, abnormal sympathetic activity, or psychopathology. All contribute to the pain in some way. The question is: how? Later, we will describe the cascade of changes after nerve injury that alters the normal functions of the periphery and the central nervous system.

Phantom body pain in paraplegics

Paraplegia refers to the total loss of sensation and voluntary motor activity that occurs after severe damage of the spinal cord. Immediately after a serious automobile or shooting accident, a person may report that he or she has no sensation below a certain level of the body – the level of the spinal damage. Sometimes the legs feel as though they are up in the air with the toes over the head even though they are stretched out straight on the bed.

Three kinds of pain are reported by paraplegic patients: (1) *root pain* (or 'girdle pain') localized at or near the level of the cord lesion; (2) *visceral pain* which usually accompanies a distended bladder or bowel; and (3) *phantom body pain* which is felt in the areas of complete sensory loss. Because many earlier studies fail to distinguish among the three kinds of pain, the frequency of occurrence of each is difficult to determine. On the basis of the available data, however, it is estimated that five to ten per cent of paraplegic patients suffer severe phantom body pains. The patients complain of burning, tingling pains in segments of the body below the level of the lesion in which there is a complete loss of sensation to sensory stimuli. These pains are sometimes replaced by 'severe, crushing pressure, by vice-like pinching sensations, by streams of fire running down the legs into the feet and out the toes, or by a pain produced by the pressure of a knife being buried in the tissue, twisted around rapidly and finally withdrawn all at the same time' (Davis and Martin, 1947, p. 486). The onset of pain may be immediate, but may also occur months or years after injury. In the most severe cases, the pain may persist for years without abating (Botterell *et al.*, 1954). The severity of pain in these patients has often led to multiple operations: rhizotomies, cordotomies and sympathectomies (Figure 6). Although claims of success have been made for one or another procedure, most operations fail to provide lasting relief.

The most striking feature of phantom body pain in paraplegics is its presence even when the spinal cord is known to be totally transected. Melzack and Loeser (1978) have recently reviewed these cases, of which the following is typical:

D. G. sustained a fracture of the upper spine in an automobile accident and was subsequently paraplegic. Although he had some muscle spasms during the first few weeks, he did not complain of significant pain. When he was seen one year later, he complained of muscle spasms in his legs, knife-like pains in the chest, burning pain in his hips and cramping pains in his abdomen. He had no sensation or voluntary motor activity below the mid-chest level. Anaesthetic blocks at the level of the spinal lesion eliminated the muscle spasms but did not change his pain. The following year, the patient was seen again and complained of three types of pain: crushing, knife-like pain in the chest; cramping pain in the abdomen; and burning pain in the hips and legs. A neurosurgical operation was then carried out to cut the pathways (cordotomy, Figure 6) that are traditionally held to carry pain signals. The cordotomies were performed on both sides above the level of spinal lesion, but the pains were unchanged. Several drugs were tried but they failed to relieve the pain. Four months later, anaesthetic blocks of the sympathetic system were performed on both sides but instead of helping, they increased the abdominal cramping and burning hip pain. New analgesic drugs were tried but they had no effect. Finally, the decision was made to remove an entire segment of spinal cord – an operation known as a cordectomy which is rarely carried out. After complete removal of about an inch of spinal cord above the level of the lesion, the patient reported that the operation relieved his back pain and some of his chest pain but did not alter his cramping abdominal pain, the burning pain in his hip or the tingling and burning pain in his legs. Eight months after the operation, the patient reported that most of his chest pain had returned, and his abdominal and leg pains were not altered. When last seen he persistently complained of cramping pain in the lower abdomen and burning, tingling pain in the hips and legs.

Paraplegic patients present a remarkable puzzle: they feel pain in specific areas of the trunk or the limbs below the level of a complete spinal transection. The surgical removal of a segment of spinal cord precludes any possibility of transmission from peripheral receptors to the brain through spinal cord pathways. Furthermore, although these patients are often depressed, there is no evidence that the pain is produced by psychological factors. The cause of the pain must lie in the neural changes that are a result of the massive loss of sensory input from the body to the brain.

Causalgia

The classic description of causalgia was recorded by Mitchell (1872, pp. 292–6) after the American Civil War. He describes the case of Joseph Corliss, who was shot in the left arm by a bullet that entered just above the elbow, penetrated without touching the artery, and emerged through the belly of the biceps.

On the second day the pain began. It was burning and darting. He states that at this time sensation was lost or lessened in the limb, and that paralysis of motion came on in the hand and forearm. The pain was so severe that a touch anywhere, or shaking the bed, or a heavy step, caused it to increase.

The pain persisted despite healing of the wound, so that two years after the injury:

He keeps his hand wrapped in a rag, wetted with cold water, and covered with oiled silk, and even tucks the rag carefully under the flexed finger tips.

Moisture is more essential than cold. Friction outside of the clothes, at any point of the entire surface, 'shoots' into the hand, increasing the burning (pain) . . . Deep pressure on the muscles has a like effect, and he will allow no one to touch his skin, save with a wetted hand, and even then is careful to exact careful manipulation. He keeps a bottle of water about him, and carries a sponge in the right hand. This hand he wets before he handles anything; used dry, it hurts the other limb. At one time, when the suffering was severe, he poured water into his boots, he says, to lessen the pain which dry touch of friction causes in the injured hand . . . He thus describes the pain at its height: 'It is as if a rough bar of iron were thrust to and fro through the knuckles, a red-hot iron placed at the junction of the palm and (thumb), with a heavy weight on it, and the skin was being rasped off my finger ends.'

The debilitating effects of such prolonged pain have been described by Mitchell (pp. 196–7):

Perhaps few persons who are not physicians can realize the influence which long-continued and unendurable pain may have upon both body and mind. The older books are full of cases in which, after lancet wounds, the most terrible pain and local spasms resulted. When these had lasted for days or weeks, the whole surface became hyperaesthetic, and the senses grew to be only avenues for fresh and increasing tortures, until every vibration, every change or light, and even . . . the effort to read brought on new agony. Under such torments the temper changes, the most amiable grow irritable, the soldier becomes a coward, and the strongest man is scarcely less nervous than the most hysterical girl.

Causalgia is characterized by an intense burning pain in the area served by a damaged nerve. This area is slightly less sensitive than normal skin but once a sensation is evoked, it is extremely unpleasant. The horrible sensation is often delayed after a stimulus is applied, and usually long outlasts the stimulus. The condition was first described as being produced by bullets (Mitchell, 1872) and later writers concentrated on military casualties (Livingston, 1943; White and Sweet, 1969; Sunderland, 1978). However, it is now evident that causalgic pain can occur after any type of peripheral nerve injury, including damage caused by bone fractures, and cancerous invasion of nerves, and it even occurs in diseases such as multiple sclerosis which are limited to the central nervous system (Noordenbos, 1959; Schott, 1986). Fortunately, this terrible type of pain occurs in only a small percentage of patients with nerve injuries.

The onset of causalgic pain may occur immediately after a nerve injury or after delays of weeks or months. Once established, the area of abnormal sensitivity spreads to involve skin far removed from the area supplied by the damaged nerve. Sensitivity of the skin increases so that small movements or even vibrations produced by loud noises may trigger the pains. The sight of a patient guarding a limb which is wrapped in wet towels is often sufficient to make the diagnosis.

It is known that gentle, innocuous stimuli applied to the skin can trigger causalgic pain and that local anaesthesia distal to the area of damage can relieve it, sometimes for long durations (Livingston, 1943). It is also known that the sympathetic nervous system plays a role in the abnormal triggering events since inactivation of the sympathetic system by surgery (Leriche, 1939) or chemical guanethidine (Hannington-Kiff, 1994) may relieve the pain, even if the original disease was limited to the central nervous system (Loh *et al.*, 1980, 1981; Blumberg and Janig, 1994). However, it is clear that the sequence of events moves from the periphery into the spinal cord. Noordenbos and Wall (1981) found that meticulous nerve grafts to repair an injured nerve produces, at first, complete anaesthesia, followed, tragically, by the reappearance of the original causalgic pain after the new nerves have regenerated into the periphery.

The neuralgias

There are several pain syndromes associated with peripheral nerve damage that are generally categorized as neuralgic pain. Their properties are essentially similar to those of phantom limb pain and causalgia, and are characterized by severe, unremitting pain which is difficult to treat by surgical or other traditional methods. The causes of neuralgic pain include viral infections of nerves, nerve degeneration associated with diabetes, poor circulation in the limbs, vitamin deficiencies and ingestion of poisonous substances such as arsenic. In brief, almost any infection or disease that produces damage to peripheral nerves, particularly the large nerve fibres, may be the cause of pain that is labelled as neuralgic (Bennett, 1994; Fields, 1994; Scadding, 1994).

Post-herpetic neuralgia

Infection by the virus *herpes zoster* (which is related to the virus that causes chicken pox) produces inflammation of one or more sensory nerves. The inflammation, which is painful, is associated with eruptions (or 'shingles') at the skin at the termination of the nerve.

The herpetic attack is itself painful, but the pain usually subsides. In a small number of people, however, the post-herpetic pain persists and may become worse. Noordenbos (1959) notes that neuralgic skin areas are not only the site of spontaneous pain (in the absence of stimulation), but are extremely hyperaesthetic, so that the pain is aggravated by any cutaneous stimuli applied to them. Even the friction of clothes is highly unpleasant and contact is avoided as much as possible. The pain may also be intensified by noise in the immediate vicinity or by emotional stress. This condition may last for many months or even years, and is extremely resistant to most forms of therapy including surgical treatment.

Noordenbos (1959) describes two major characteristics of post-herpetic pain. The first is the remarkable summation of stimulation. One of the stimuli Noordenbos used was a test-tube containing hot water. When the hot tube was applied to normal skin, the patient reported that it felt hot but tolerated it without discomfort for long periods of time. When it was then placed on the neuralgic skin area, an entirely different sequence of events occurred. There was no sensation of temperature for the first few seconds. The tube was then gradually felt as warm or tingling, slowly becoming hotter. If stimulation was continued, the patient stated that it began to burn and finally he cried out with pain and pushed the examiner's hand away. This whole sequence took from twenty seconds to as long as a full minute or longer. Noordenbos notes that if a larger surface of the hot tube was applied to the skin the entire sequence was accelerated, starting as indifferent and rapidly going through all the intermediate sensations to end in unbearable pain. Thus the speed of summation of input was dependent on the size of the area that was stimulated.

The second characteristic is a marked delay in the onset of pain after stimulation. This was apparent in the sequence of events Noordenbos observed after application of the hot test-tube. It was especially clear when he applied multiple gentle pinpricks to the affected skin areas. After a distinct delay following onset of the pinpricks, the patients reported feeling intense pain that spread over large areas and then wore off slowly. The onset of pain was 'very sudden, almost explosive in character, and had an extremely unpleasant quality that differed markedly from the pain evoked in normal skin with the same stimulus' (Noordenbos, 1959, p. 8).

This disease has a combination of pathologies. A substantial number of nerve fibres are destroyed and the fibre loss presumably produces a state of raised excitability in neurons in the spinal cord.

The activity of these cells is assumed to produce a deep ongoing pain which is influenced by peripheral manipulation. This combination of peripheral and central pathology produces a mixture of raised thresholds, abnormal unpleasant evoked sensations, and ongoing pain.

Trigeminal neuralgia

Trigeminal neuralgia, also known as tic douloureux, is a striking example of an apparently simple condition with no known anatomical pathology. In this pain syndrome, which tends to be found in older people, gentle stimulation of the face or mouth provokes a massive, stabbing pain which inevitably produces a cry of anguish and brings tears to the eyes. The trigeminal nerve is the obvious target of suspicion because the disease is restricted to the territory it innervates and because local anaesthesia of the trigger zone abolishes the disease until the anaesthesia wears off. Meticulous studies of the anatomy of the nerve, from the periphery to the pons and medulla, have failed to identify any abnormality. Even more surprising, Kugelberg and Lindblom (1959) showed that, unlike the other neuralgias, there is no change of threshold for detecting stimuli even though a normally innocuous stimulus (such as a gentle touch) is responsible for triggering the pain. Since the disease disappears if the normal input is temporarily blocked, great ingenuity has been shown by surgeons in the attempt to interrupt transmission along the nerve by cutting it, or by massaging, decompressing, poisoning, burning or freezing it. All of these procedures work temporarily but the disease recurs.

This leads to the possibility that the abnormality lies in the trigeminal nuclei (in the brainstem), which are unable to handle a normal input without an explosive, massive response. This explanation, in terms of a mechanism in the central nervous system, is supported by the fact that many cases respond well to the antiepileptic drug, carbamazepine (tegretol), which has no known effect on peripheral nerves but does limit the explosive firing responses of central cells. Furthermore, some cases of trigeminal neuralgia occur when multiple sclerosis destroys brain tissue near the trigeminal nuclei but does not affect the peripheral nerves. It is evident that there are serious, localized pains for which no pathology has yet been found. Careful studies of anatomical, physiological and biochemical mechanisms have so far failed to reveal the culprit and the cause remains a mystery. But we must resist the tendency to leap to a psychiatric explanation. New research techniques and concepts will ultimately reveal the mechanisms that now elude us. As diagnoses and understanding improve, there is a decrease in the number of cases attributed to hysteria (Loeser, 1994).

Migraine

Among the 20 per cent of the population who suffer migraine in its various forms (classic migraine, common migraine and cluster headache), no one doubts the reality and severity of the pain. There is no evidence that anxiety and tension are the ultimate cause although they may, on occasion, enhance the pain. The underlying cause of migraine remains unknown. Experts suspect several possible structures – blood vessels, muscles, joints, meninges, nerves and the brain – but there is no cogent evidence to identify any of them as a cause of the pain (Olesen, 1986). Migraine, which has been intensively studied with the most advanced neurological techniques, still awaits a good concept to explain it and a good therapy to cure it.

Implications of the clinical evidence

The implications of the pathological pain syndromes described above are the following:

Summation
Gentle touch, warmth, and other non-noxious somatic stimuli can trigger excruciating pain. The fact that repetitive or prolonged stimulation is usually necessary to elicit pain, together with the fact that referred pain can often be triggered by mild stimulation of normal skin, makes it unlikely that the pain can be explained by postulating hypersensitive 'pain receptors'. A more reasonable explanation is that abnormal information processing in the central nervous system allows these remarkable summation phenomena to occur.

Multiple contributions
The pain, in these syndromes, cannot be attributed to any single cause. There are, instead, multiple contributions. The cutaneous input from the affected part of the body obviously plays an important role. However, inputs that result from sympathetic activity are also important. So too are inputs from the auditory and visual systems. All of these inputs appear to act on structures in the central nervous system that summate the total activity to produce nerve

impulse patterns that ultimately give rise to pain. Anxiety, emotional disturbance, anticipation and other cognitive activities of the brain also contribute to the neural processes underlying these pains. They may facilitate or inhibit the afferent input and thereby modulate the quality and severity of perceived pain.

Delays

Pain from hyperalgesic skin areas often occurs after long delays and continues long after removal of the stimulus. Gentle rubbing, repeated pinpricks, or the application of a warm test-tube may produce sudden, severe pain after delays as long as forty-five seconds. Such delays cannot be attributed simply to conduction in slowly conducting fibres; rather, they imply a remarkable temporal and spatial summation of inputs in the production of these pain states.

Persistence

The durations of these pain states often exceed the time taken for tissues to heal or for injured nerve fibres to regenerate. Causalgia tends to disappear as regeneration occurs, but sometimes it persists for years, as does neuralgic or phantom limb pain. Furthermore, in all of these syndromes pain may occur spontaneously for long periods without any apparent stimulus. These considerations – together with the observation that pain in the phantom limb frequently occurs at the same site as it occurred in the diseased limb prior to amputation – suggest the possibility of a memory-like mechanism in pain.

Spread

The pains and trigger zones may spread to unrelated parts of the body where no pathology exists. This is further evidence that the central neural mechanisms involved in pain receive inputs from multiple sources. The organization of these mechanisms does not reflect the precise dermatomal (or segmental) innervation of the body by the somatic nerves. (This is immediately evident when Figures 6 and 7 on pp. 64 and 66 are compared.) Instead, the mechanisms appear to be more widespread and receive inputs from all parts of the body.

Resistance to surgical control

The widespread distribution of the neural mechanisms associated with these pain states is also indicated by the frequent failure to abolish pain by surgical methods. Surgical lesions of the peripheral and central nervous systems have been singularly unsuccessful in abolishing these pains permanently, although the lesions have been made at almost every level from receptors to sensory cortex. Even after such operations, pain can often still be elicited by stimulation below the level of section and may be more severe than before the operation.

Evolution
Neither diseases nor the pain mechanisms that accompany them are stationary processes. Rather, dynamic, continuous changes occur in both as time progresses. During the first few seconds after a peripheral injury, the associated pain is obviously triggered by nerve impulses from the periphery. In the minutes, days and weeks after the initial period, the needs of the body change from avoidance of further injury to recovery of healthy function. The pain mechanisms also change so that the major procedures to control the pain shift from the periphery to the central nervous system. This evolution of need and mechanism calls for a *sequence of therapies* to prevent and to cure pains.

These properties and their implications provide valuable clues towards an understanding of pain. They represent parts of a puzzle which, together with those obtained from psychology and physiology, will ultimately reveal the solutions to perplexing, urgent problems. Any satisfactory theory of pain must be able to explain the properties of these syndromes. If our theories do not lead eventually to effective treatment, they have failed, no matter how elegant or compelling they may seem. The clinical problems of pain, in other words, represent the ultimate test of our knowledge.

Part Two
The Physiology of Pain

'I was brought up in a medical generation in which . . . pain was [considered to be] a primary sensation dependent upon the stimulation of a specific sensory ending by a stimulus of a certain intensity, and conducted along a fixed pathway to ring a special bell in consciousness. Pain was as simple as that . . . The idea that anything might happen to sensory impulses within the central nervous system to alter their character, destination, or the sensation they registered in consciousness was utterly foreign to my concept. But in practice I found that it was incredibly difficult to make this concept consistent with clinical observations.'

William K. Livingston, 1943

5   Peripheral Nerve and Spinal Mechanisms

The psychological and clinical phenomena of pain provide a framework for the physiological problems we will now consider. Two terms are especially critical in our attempts to understand the physiology of pain: *specificity* and *specialization*. *Specificity* implies that a receptor, fibre, or other component of a sensory system subserves only a single specific modality (or quality) of experience; it assumes a rigid, fixed relationship between a neural structure and a psychological experience. *Specialization* implies that receptors, fibres, or other components of a sensory system are highly specialized so that particular types and ranges of physical energy evoke characteristic patterns of neural signals, and that these patterns can be modulated by other sensory inputs or by cognitive processes to produce more than one quality of experience or even none at all. It is the latter approach – specialization of function – that provides the conceptual framework for this chapter.

It is customary to describe the somatosensory system by proceeding from the peripheral receptors to the transmission routes that carry nerve impulses to areas in the brain. However, it is essential to remember that stimulation of receptors does not mark the beginning of the pain process. Rather, stimulation produces neural signals that enter an active nervous system that (in the adult organism) is already the substrate of past experience, culture, anticipation, anxiety and so forth. These brain processes actively participate in the selection, abstraction and synthesis of information from the total sensory input. Because sensory physiological processes are complex, a brief outline of the somatic sensory system will be provided first, and each step will then be examined in more detail. Only later, when we analyse the contemporary theories of pain, will we try to choose the data that seem most relevant and put them together in a way that is consistent with the psychological and clinical data.

Outline of somatic sensory mechanisms

We may ask at this point: what is the nature of the sensory nerve signals or messages that travel to the brain after injury? Let us say a person has burned a finger; what is the sequence of events that follows in the nervous system? To begin with, the intense heat energy is converted into a code of electrical nerve impulses. These energy conversions occur in nerve endings in the skin called receptors, of which there are many different types. It was once popular to identify one of these types as the specific 'pain receptors'. We now believe that receptor mechanisms are more complicated. There is general agreement that the receptors which respond to noxious stimulation are widely branching, bushy networks of fibres that penetrate the layers of the skin in such a way that their receptive fields overlap extensively with one another (Figure 9). Thus damage at any point on the skin will activate at least two or more of these networks and initiate the transmission of trains of nerve impulses along sensory nerve fibres that run from the finger into the spinal cord. What enters the spinal cord of the central nervous system is a coded pattern of nerve impulses, travelling along many fibres and moving at different speeds and with different frequencies.

Before the nerve-impulse pattern can begin its ascent to the brain, a portion of it must first pass through a region of short, densely packed nerve fibres that are diffusely interconnected. This region, found throughout the length of the spinal cord on each side, is called the substantia gelatinosa (Figure 9). It is in the course of transmission from the sensory fibres to the ascending spinal cord neurons that the pattern may be modified.

Once the sensory pattern has been transmitted to the spinal cord neurons, it projects to the brain along nerve fibres – some of which occupy the anterolateral (front and side) portions of the spinal cord. Some of these fibres continue to the thalamus, forming the spinothalamic tract. The majority of the fibres, however, penetrate a tangled thicket of short, diffusely interconnected nerve fibres that form the central core of the lower part of the brain (Figure 9). This part of the brain is called the reticular formation, and it contains several highly specialized systems which play a key role in pain processes. From the reticular formation, there emerges a series of pathways, so that sensory patterns now stream along multiple routes to the limbic system, which is involved in emotion and motivation, and to the cortex. We now know that the cortex is not a final destination (or 'pain centre') but that it processes the information it

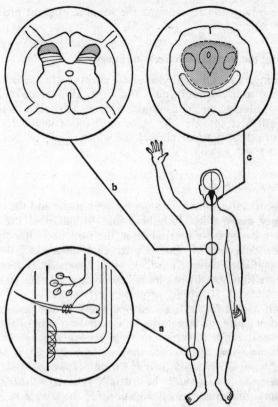

Figure 9. Schematic representation of the receptors and projection pathways of the somatic sensory system. A: The diagram of the skin shows widely branching free nerve endings (which produce overlapping receptive fields) as well as some specialized end-organs. The fibres project to the spinal cord. B: The cross section of the spinal cord shows the laminae (layers) of cells in the dorsal horns which receive sensory fibres and project their axons toward the brain. The crosshatched area represents the substantia gelatinosa (laminae 1 and 2). C: The brainstem (lower part of the brain) receives a large somatosensory input, and projects to higher as well as lower areas of the central nervous system. The crosshatched area represents the reticular formation. Below it on each side is the medial lemniscus. The spinothalamic projections – which are shown within the reticular formation – lie above the lemniscal tracts.

receives and transmits it to deeper portions of the brain. In short, the afferent process from skin to cortex marks only the beginning of prolonged, interacting activities.

We are now ready to examine the somatic afferent processes in greater detail.

Acute pain: the immediate effects of injury

A sudden injury produces physiological effects within seconds. Then, as pain evolves in the hours, days and weeks after tissue is damaged, the pain-producing mechanisms also evolve and change as time goes by. We will first consider the basic mechanism which comes into action abruptly with sudden injury and which results in acute sudden pain.

Receptor mechanisms

The receptor is the point of contact between tissue and the ending of the sensory nerve fibre. It is here that the state of the tissue – determined by pressure exerted on it, the surrounding temperature and its chemical content – initiates nerve impulses which then travel to the spinal cord (Meyer *et al.*, 1994). This specially sensitive tip of the nerve fibre usually nestles naked among the cells whose state is being detected. However, in particularly sensitive and exposed areas such as the finger tips and lips many of the sensory nerve fibres end in elaborate structures. In the smooth skin of the human hand, several types of structure were recognized by nineteenth-century histologists, after whom they are named, such as Meissner, Merkel, Pacini, Golgi-Mazzoni and Ruffini. However, these specialized nerve-endings can hardly be crucially necessary for the perception of particular qualities of sensation for the simple reason that they are not present in the ear lobe (Sinclair, 1982), and yet it is obvious that stimulation here can evoke distinct sensations of warmth, cold, touch, tickle, itch, pain and erotic sensations.

Nerve fibres

The major nerves, with names such as the sciatic nerve or the ulnar nerve, are large structures surrounded by their own sheath of connective tissue and special blood vessels (Figure 10). They are divided into bundles, surrounded by sheets of connective tissue, which are visible to the naked eye. The individual bundles are routinely dissected out by surgeons using low-power dissecting microscopes. Each bundle contains huge numbers of the real working units, the nerve fibres, each of which is composed of a cell body, an axon and dendrites.

Each cell sends out a long cylindrical process called an axon (Figure 10). This is the basic structure which carries the nerve impulse and can also transport chemicals along its entire length. An adult human has tens of thousands of these to supply the foot alone, and the tubular axons run all the way from the spinal cord to the foot – a distance of about one metre – without interruption. If the axon is more than 1 micron in diameter, it is covered by cuffs of

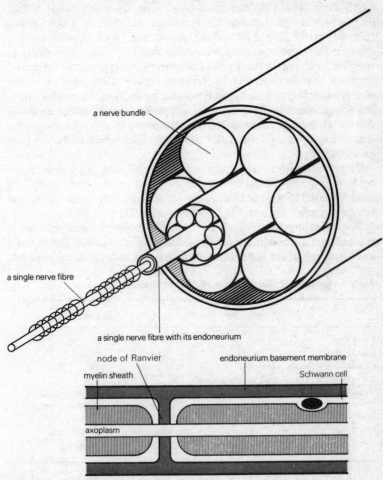

Figure 10. *Top:* drawing of the component parts of a peripheral nerve – with its sheath. *Bottom:* drawing of the detailed components of a single nerve fibre.

myelin, a laminated fat-protein insulating material. The cuffs are one to two millimetres in length and there is a gap between them where they meet along the axon. The gaps are called 'nodes of Ranvier' and it is here that ions can pass in and out of the axon to generate the nerve impulses. The entire axon lies embedded within its own special type of cell, the Schwann cell, and, for the large axons, one such cell lies between each node of Ranvier. Many small fibres which do not have the myelin layer can nestle within one Schwann cell. Outside the Schwann cell there is a continuous tube of material, the basement membrane, and outside that, a connective tissue tube, the endoneurium. The axons therefore, in their entire distance from spinal cord to periphery, run in their own personal tubular channels. Each major nerve is a mixed nerve – that is, it contains three functional types of axons: (1) motor axons whose impulses cause muscle to contract; (2) sensory axons whose impulses deliver afferent signals to the spinal cord; (3) sympathetic axons whose impulses control such 'autonomic' activities as blood flow and sweating.

The sensory fibres are traditionally divided into three groups: A-beta or large myelinated, A-delta or small myelinated, and C or unmyelinated fibres. About sixty to seventy per cent of all the sensory afferents are in the C group (table 2).

We must understand clearly exactly how physiologists have studied and classified these nerve fibres. They isolate single units and then search for the type of stimulus to which the fibre responds

Table 2. Properties of different types of afferent fibres.

	Myelinated		Unmyelinated
Fibre type	A-beta	A-delta	C
Diameter	5–15 μm	1–5μm	0.25–1.5μm
Conduction velocity	30–100 m/sec	6–30 m/sec	1.0–2.5 m/sec
Receptor type	specialized & free	free	free
Respond to *a*	light pressure	1 light pressure	1 light pressure
		2 heavy pressure	2 heavy pressure
		3 heat (45°C+)	3 heat (45°C+)
		4 chemicals	4 chemicals
		5 cooling	5 warmth

a Each fibre in the A-delta and C group may respond to only one or to more than one of the types of stimuli; for example, there are C 'polymodal fibres' that respond to heavy pressure, heat and chemicals.

best: hair movement, skin indentation, skin crushing, warming, cooling, chemicals, and so on. Of course, not all fibres can be tested with all stimuli but it does appear that some fibres are exquisitely sensitive to specific stimuli. For example, there are four types of fast A-beta nerve fibres in the human fingertips which respond to light pressure (Sinclair, 1982): Type F A I: 43 per cent of all fibres, responds if the skin is indented 10 micra, attached to Meissner corpuscles, sensitive to low frequency vibrations. Type F A II: 13 per cent of all fibres, responds if the skin is indented 8 micra, attached to Pacini and to Golgi–Mazzoni receptors, sensitive to high frequency vibration. Type S A I: 25 per cent of all fibres, responds if the skin is indented by 50 micra, attached to Merkel discs, fires continuously in the presence of an edge pressed on the skin. Type S A II: 19 per cent of all fibres, responds if skin is indented 200 micra, attached to Ruffini endings, fires continuously to lateral stretch of the skin.

These fibres are finely tuned to begin firing nerve impulses when a particular event occurs at a very low intensity in the region of their terminals. Similarly, there are A-delta fibres which commence firing when the skin is cooled by a fraction of a degree. Some A-delta and C fibres respond to temperature increases. For the detection of large increases which threaten tissue, there are A-delta fibres and huge numbers of C fibres. The A-delta fibres may respond to intense pressure, to temperatures above 45°C or to destructive chemicals. All of the C fibres in humans respond to all three noxious events.

The classical writers made a straightforward guess that activity in each of these specialized classes of fibres should evoke a distinct sensation: A-beta activity was assumed to produce touch; A-delta fibres activated by cooling were supposed to evoke a cold sensation; A-delta and C fibres stimulated by warming were held to be responsible for the sensation of warmth; and pain was presumed to be evoked by A-delta and C fibre activity. Now we no longer have to guess the relationship between fibre activity and perceived sensation, thanks to the technique of inserting microelectrodes into human nerves (Vallbo and Hagbarth, 1968). This technique of *neuronography* permits the recording of nerve impulses in all the different types of sensory afferent in conscious people who can simultaneously report what they are feeling. The results, reviewed by Wall and McMahon (1985), show a very different result from the classical expectation of a fixed relation between the sensation perceived and the onset of activity in a specialized type of fibre.

It might be expected that the onset of firing of one of the types of high-threshold fibres would coincide with the onset of the sensation of pain. This is not observed. Furthermore, different painful stimuli, chemicals, pressure, heat and cold provoke firing in different groups of sensory fibres but, surprisingly, people cannot differentiate between the pains produced by these stimuli (Chery Croze and Duclaux, 1980; Ong *et al.*, 1980). A particularly interesting example to show that the type of peripheral nerve fibre does not determine the modality of sensation is seen in a study by van Hees and Gybels (1981). Since C fibres respond to pressure, heat and chemicals, they were able to relate the onset of pain produced by these three stimuli to the firing of the nerve fibres. Pressure stimuli had to evoke firing rates of more than 10 hertz (Hz) before pain occurred, while chemicals produced pain with accompanying firing rates of 3–6Hz and intense heat evoked pain when firing rates were 0.4Hz. These observations refute the idea of a simple relationship between fibre-type and quality of sensation. Instead they support the concept of interactions among fibres proposed in the gate-control theory (Melzack and Wall, 1965).

High-pressure stimuli necessarily co-activate both low- and high-threshold afferents, and the low-threshold afferents inhibit the central excitation produced by the high-threshold input. It is therefore necessary to obtain a higher frequency of input with a pressure stimulus in order to produce the same effect as that produced by the low-frequency, heat-induced barrage, because the latter does not co-activate the inhibitory afferents. Furthermore, not only is the modality of sensation unrelated to the firing of one type of fibre, but the time-course of the sensation is very poorly correlated with the time-course of the afferent barrage.

Other physiological observations fail to support the concept of rigid, straight-through transmission lines which carry specific sensations from specific receptors and fibres. For example, it was observed about a century ago that the ability to perceive stimuli is not evenly distributed on the surface of the skin but occurs in spots. This observation led to the proposal that each spot is innervated by a special type of nerve fibre which could evoke only one sensation. This cannot be true for four reasons:

1 *Spots move.* Many spots fail to produce a sensation after successive stimulation, while new ones appear (Dallenbach, 1927). The spots fluctuate in location from one examination to another

(Waterston, 1933) and sensitive areas fragment and coalesce (Melzack *et al.*, 1962).

2 *Spots do not overlie special end-organs.* The prediction that particular corpuscles would be found under particular spots has been tested at least twelve times and all tests failed to support such a correlation.

3 *The number of receptors and nerve fibres exceeds the number of spots.* Johansson and Vallbo (1979) estimate the density of low-threshold mechanoreceptors at the tip of the human finger to be 241 per square centimetre, and Bruce and Sinclair (1965) find 2000 Meissner corpuscles in that same area. In contrast, there are many fewer spots than receptors or the large fibres that innervate them. Moreover, the number of afferent C fibres in skin is even larger than the number of A fibres (McLachlan and Janig, 1983).

4 *Stimulus area and skin gradients determine spot modality.* Spots do not show a true picture of the distribution of sensitivity since testing with stimuli of different sizes shows that a particular sensation is extracted from continuous gradients of sensitivity, where highly sensitive areas are surrounded by regions of decreasing sensitivity (Jenkins, 1941).

The modality of a stimulus is generated not from specific spots of elementary sensation, but from a synthesis of a complex afferent barrage, and factors other than fibre type are likely to be important. For instance, a temperature probe at 43°C with a variable diameter of 1 to 20mm rested on the human back produces a pricking pain at 1mm, stinging pain at 2 to 5mm and pleasant warmth at 20mm (Melzack *et al.*, 1962). The creation of a perceived pain spot out of an afferent barrage which involves a wide variety of afferent fibres can be observed by pressing a sharp pencil into a fingertip. A highly localized point of pain is felt. A wide cone of indentation of skin at least 1mm deep is seen to exist on the fingertip. We have seen that such a stimulus activates the full range of mechanoreceptors in an area of many square millimetres and yet we perceive only a localised point.

In summary, the results of neuronography show clearly that modality, time-course, intensity and localization are not the unique properties of specialized types of nerve fibre. Those fibres transmit messages as a distributed pattern and the central nervous system determines the meaning of the message by unravelling that pattern. That process begins in the spinal cord to which we now turn.

Spinal cord mechanisms in acute pain

The spinal cord has a strikingly similar appearance in all vertebrates. Cell bodies lie in the middle of the cord and form the grey matter with its characteristic butterfly shape (see Figure 9, p. 83). Around this grey matter, the white matter consists of axons running up and down the cord bringing messages to and from the cord and the brain. The arriving afferent fibres from the body comprise the dorsal roots and terminate on cells in the dorsal horn. The output cells to the skeletal (or 'striped') muscle all lie in the ventral horn, and the output cells to the viscera, smooth muscle, sweat glands, and other structures under autonomic control tend to concentrate in the lateral horn. The trigeminal nerve which supplies the face has an equivalent central apparatus in the medulla with the same components as those seen in each spinal segment.

The cross-sectional size of the spinal cord varies in a quite predictable way (Figure 11). The nerves to the arms have grown out of the lower cervical and upper thoracic segments and so these segments are large, forming the cervical enlargement, which supplies a lot of sensitive skin as well as many muscles capable of fine control. Similarly, there is a lumbar enlargement for the legs. Since the body surface between the arms and legs consists of relatively insensitive skin and little muscle, the horns are quite small in these segments but there is a lot of white matter carrying ascending and descending information. The pelvis contains many visceral organs which need to be controlled, and so in the sacral segments one finds particularly large and elaborate visceral (autonomic) mechanisms. The overall plan is identical throughout the spinal cord, and each segment includes a self-contained mechanism for the reception and control of the particular structures which grew from that segment in embryo. While this is the basic pattern, all nervous system components are integrated and therefore the segments must co-ordinate with each other and must consult with the brain – which gains increasing control over the segmental circuits in higher animals.

The cells in the grey matter

Thanks to the Swedish anatomist, Bror Rexed (1952), we now recognize that the cells of the spinal cord are arranged in laminae (or layers) in a dorsal-ventral direction and that these laminae run the entire length of the spinal cord. The dorsal horn contains six laminae (Figure 12 and Table 3). Laminae 1 and 2 form a clear zone visible to the naked eye and are called the substantia gelatinosa Rolandi.

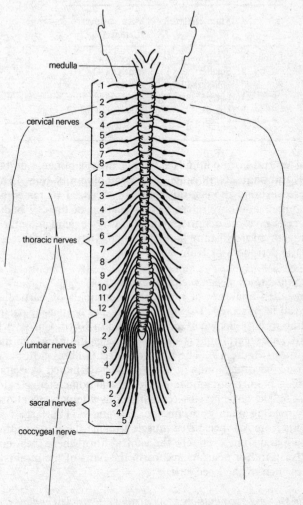

medulla

cervical nerves
1
2
3
4
5
6
7
8

thoracic nerves
1
2
3
4
5
6
7
8
9
10
11
12

lumbar nerves
1
2
3
4
5

sacral nerves
1
2
3
4
5

coccygeal nerve

Figure 11. Schematic diagram of the spinal cord, showing the entering sensory nerves, the ganglia that contain the cell bodies of the nerve fibres, and the roots entering the cord. Cervical nerves 5 to 8 and thoracic 1 aggregate on each side to form the brachial plexus which innervates each arm. Similarly, lumbar and sacral nerves form the complex lumbosacral plexus which sends nerves to the pelvis and leg. Not shown are the vertebral bones or the chain of sympathetic ganglia that lie just outside the vertebral column on each side.

Table 3. The dorsal horn laminae.

	Main cell size	Main sensory afferents
Lamina 1	Small and large	A-delta and C
2	Small	A-delta and C
3	Small and large	A-beta
4	Large	A-beta
5	Large	A-beta and delta
6	Large	Muscle afferents

The ventral horn contains a further three laminae, numbers 7, 8 and 9, and finally there is an intriguing column of cells, lamina 10, clustered around the central canal. It is crucial to remember that this laminar anatomy refers to the location of the cell bodies, but these cells give off dendrites which always extend into the neighbouring or more distant laminae where they may contact axons from the periphery or from other cells.

The terminations of peripheral afferents

The detailed anatomy of the central terminals of particular fibre types can be observed. This careful work has been done particularly in Edinburgh by Brown *et al.* (1978) and in North Carolina by Perl (1980). The general rule is that the thicker the fibre, the deeper it penetrates (Figure 13). The unmyelinated C fibres do not seem to penetrate beyond lamina 2. The small myelinated A-delta fibres terminate mainly in laminae 1 and 2, and some struggle down to lamina 5. The large myelinated cutaneous afferents penetrate more deeply, ending mainly in laminae 3, 4 and 5. The largest sensory afferents from the specialized muscle stretch afferents penetrate into lamina 6 and some even into the ventral horn where they terminate directly on motor neurons and form the basis of the monosynaptic reflexes such as the knee jerk.

The origin and termination of control systems descending from the brain

The general rule is that nerve fibres descending in the white matter penetrate into the grey matter and innervate the cells nearest their tract in the white matter. The dorsolateral white matter is therefore well situated to send axons into the most dorsal laminae and does so. It contains fibres from the brainstem, particularly from the raphe

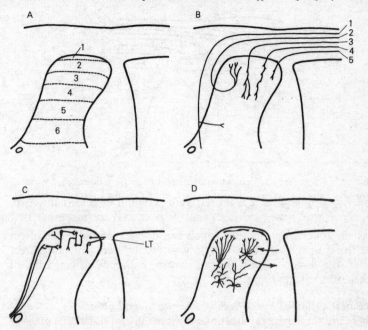

Figure 12. A cross section of lumbar dorsal quadrant of spinal cord.

A: The Rexed laminae into which cell bodies are divided, Laminae 1 and 2 are the substantia gelatinosa. Laminae 1, 2 and 3 contain small cells. Laminae 1, 4, 5 and 6 contain large cells.

B: The pattern of arriving peripheral nerve afferents: 1, represents the course of a large proprioceptive axon which terminates in lamina 6 and the ventral horn; 2, a hair follicle afferent with recurrent terminal arborizations in laminae 3 and 4; 3, a touch afferent; 4, a small delta myelinated afferent; 5, an unmyelinated C afferent.

C: The small cells in substantia gelatinosa (SG) end on each other and perhaps on afferents and the dendrites of deeper cells. These send some axons into the Lissauer tract (LT) and back into (SG). They also send axons to the opposite (SG) by way of the dorsal commissure.

D: Large cells in laminae 1, 4 and 5 and their dendrites. Descending fibres from the brainstem.

nuclei, the locus coeruleus, the large cell region of the reticular formation and from the hypothalamus. Slightly more central, there is the pyramidal tract from the cortex and, although this is classically thought to be a motor system, it floods into the dorsal laminae as well and affects cell groups in laminae 3–6. More ventrally still, there are massive descending pathways from the vestibular system

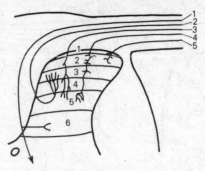

Figure 13. The course and destination of afferent fibres from dorsal root to dorsal horn containing six laminae. Afferent fibres: 1, muscle spindle afferent; 2, hair afferent; 3, touch corpuscle afferent; 4, δ afferent; 5, C afferent.

and the reticular formation which can directly or indirectly affect the firing of sensory cells. While we describe here only the direct input, the direct systems are, of course, indirectly affected by all other parts of the brain.

The destination of fibres from cells in the dorsal horn

There are three general locations to which dorsal horn cells project: (1) cells in the same segment; (2) cells in other segments (the propriospinal system); and (3) cells in the brain (by way of the long running tracts). The local segmental circuits undoubtedly make up the bulk of the connections and, among other functions, form the reflex pathways by which arriving sensory signals produce motor outputs.

The small cells in substantia gelatinosa (Figure 14) seem to have predominantly intrasegmental effects; they project on to nearby laminae, although some of the axons project up and down the cord by way of a tiny tract on the surface of the cord named after Lissauer. The short, intersegmental propriospinal fibres run in the grey matter and in white-matter bundles close to the grey matter, and end in nearby segments on both sides of the cord. It is obvious that these short connections could link with each other and eventually deliver messages to the brain.

However, attention has naturally focused on the large, long-running tracts which project directly to various brain structures. The furthest penetration into the brain is by way of a fibre system – the spinothalamic tract – which ends in the thalamus, and an inordinate amount of attention is paid to it in spite of the fact that, in

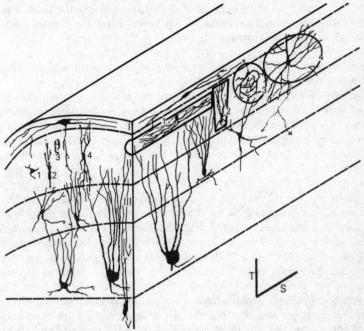

Figure 14. The arrangement of the various cell types found in the upper dorsal horn of the human spinal cord. The cell shapes are shown in the transverse plane T and in the sagittal plane S. The Rexed laminae I–IV are shown, see Figure 12 – A. The cell types in lamina II are: 1, islet cells; 2, filamentous cells; 3, stalk cells; 4, stellate cells. Axons of the cells are indicated by the dotted lines.
(from Schoenen, 1980)

man, it contains only about a thousand fibres. Adding to the fascination of the spinothalamic tract is the fact that it runs in the ventrolateral white matter which, if cut, leads to analgesia. In spite of the fact that the tract represents less than one per cent of the fibres that are cut, the operation is often called a spinothalamic tractotomy. Each of the six dorsal laminae, except for lamina 2, reports its state of activity to the brain. The destination of these fibres includes the reticular formation, the thalamus and the cerebellum, and are described in detail by Yaksh (1986).

Finally, we must mention a special pathway – the dorsal columns – which contains primary afferent fibres. The large A-beta cutaneous afferents divide on entering the cord and send terminals into the nearby grey matter and a long branch which ends in the dorsal column nuclei at the entry point of the spinal cord into the skull. This pathway also contains fibres which come from the dorsal horn, particularly from lamina 5.

The response of cells in the dorsal horn of the spinal cord: when the brain is unable to influence the spinal cord
Excitation. If the spinal cord has been cut across, as in paraplegia, the cord below the level of the lesion retains its local organization and can produce reflexes. The cells in the dorsal horn are very excitable, particularly in response to skin stimuli. It is possible to record from three types of cells in the dorsal horn. The simplest respond only to light touch on the skin and they are found particularly in laminae 3 and 4 where the low-threshold A-beta fibres terminate. The second type is rare and responds only to intense stimuli. The third and by far the largest category responds to light touch and increases its firing rate steadily as the stimulus rises into the noxious range. These cells, identified by Wall (1967) and Mendell (1966), are often called 'wide dynamic range' (WDR) cells and are excited by all types of fibre and by all types of stimuli. A very important group of cells is that which receives its input from the viscera by way of small afferent fibres. These cells are all in the WDR category and, surprisingly, are also excited by low-threshold afferents from the skin (Pomeranz *et al.*, 1968). We find here, at the first central synapse, the mechanism for referred pain in which deep damage is incorrectly located and appears to originate in superficial tissue.

There has naturally been a vigorous debate on which category of cell is associated with pain (Woolf, 1994). Those who follow the classical specificity approach naturally guess that the cells which begin firing only when stimuli are intense are responsible for pain. Just as the firing of particular categories of peripheral fibre can be examined in relation to perceived sensation, so too the firing of dorsal horn cells can be examined in animals in relation to the animals' ability to detect and avoid noxious events. There is now strong evidence that it is the WDR cells which contain the information used to discriminate pain (Dubner *et al.*, 1981). In other words, pain is associated with a certain level of firing, not with the sudden appearance of activity in a specia ized set of spinal transmission cells.

Inhibition. Even an isolated segment of spinal cord contains mechanisms to decrease firing. Spinal inhibitory cells determine which of the arriving afferents can excite spinal cells which transmit to higher levels. This means that they control the area of peripheral tissue (the receptive field) and the type of afferents which can excite the spinal cells. The most powerful of these inhibitions in the isolated cord is produced by an afferent input in the large A-beta, low-threshold mechanoreceptors. Thus, gentle brushing or rubbing of the skin or low-level electrical stimulation of a peripheral nerve produces a shrinkage of receptive fields and limits the firing rate of cells that respond to intense stimuli (Hillman and Wall, 1969). Part of this inhibition is produced by a feedback on to the terminals of the arriving sensory fibres. This presynaptic inhibition prevents the messages from entering the cord while other postsynaptic inhibitions control the orderly, co-ordinated and integrated distribution of the impulses to their subsequent stations.

The response of cells in the dorsal horn of the spinal cord: when the brain and spinal cord are connected
Excitation. It is astonishing that spinal cells in the awake, moving animal are much quieter and less excitable than cells in the isolated spinal cord (Wall *et al.*, 1967). Even if the whole forebrain has been removed, the remaining midbrain, pons and medulla maintain a steady inhibition on dorsal horn cells (Hillman and Wall, 1969; Wall, 1967). Receptive fields are small and the dynamic range of response is narrow. The type of stimulation to which the cell responds may differ so that cells in lamina 6, which normally respond only to muscle-stretch, respond solely to cutaneous stimuli if the brain is not functional. This does not mean that the brain is working poorly. It means that the intact system is precise and controlled. Furthermore, as we shall see, these controls rapidly switch on and off so that the brain allows those messages which are relevant to the situation to be received and transmitted. The brain is not the slave of its input and it begins the process of control by permitting specified cells in the spinal cord to transmit while it silences others.

Inhibition. Inhibition is much more powerful and elaborate in the intact nervous system than when the spinal cord is cut. A steady inhibition descends from the medullary reticular formation. The inhibition produced from the periphery is much more effective. In addition to the local circuits close to the entry point of arriving nerve impulses, some messages travel to the brain and there trigger descending inhibitory messages from the pons and medulla, which decrease traffic still further (Le Bars *et al.*, 1983). The long descending fibres originate from the reticular formation, the raphe nuclei and the locus coeruleus (Basbaum and Fields, 1978). Even descending motor systems, such as the pyramidal tract, have a powerful control over dorsal horn sensory cells so that there is simultaneous control over motor movement and the sensory input associated with it (Fetz, 1968).

The dorsal horns: the gate-control system

In 1965, we brought together the facts known at the time to propose the existence of a fast-acting spinal gate-control system with three stages. First, nerve impulses arriving from injured tissue excite dorsal horn neurons – transmission (T) cells – which transmit to reflex circuits and to the brain. Second, low-threshold afferents excite inhibitory interneurons which decrease the injury-evoked discharge of the T cells. Third, ongoing and evoked activity in long descending pathways excites inhibitory interneurons which can further limit the firing of T cells.

Since 1965, these three components have been described in considerable detail (Yaksh, 1986). The subtlety of the control, which goes far beyond a simple gain control, is now emerging. For example, Fields and his colleagues have described steadily active cells in the brainstem which continuously inhibit spinal withdrawal reflexes. In specified circumstances, these cells stop firing. This does not produce movement but instead permits the spinal circuits to generate the withdrawal reflex. This descending control does not generate orders; it grants permission to a reflex circuit to operate if the local conditions require withdrawal.

An even more subtle example comes from the work of Dubner *et al.* (1981) who recorded from first central cells in a monkey while the animal was learning a game in which it was rewarded with orange juice if it reached out and turned off a heat stimulus applied to its skin. Before training, the cells simply signal the stimulus as expected. After training, many of these cells emit a burst when the monkey receives a signal that the game is about to begin. Then they respond a second time very precisely and strikingly when the test stimulus is applied. In other words, the controls at the entry point in a trained animal generate, first, a test sample of the expected signal, followed by the real signal. The first central cells report the state of the peripheral tissue in a context affected by attention, expectation and many factors which affect sensation in addition to the simple presence or absence of the stimulus.

The rapid excitation of nerve cells in the spinal cord is probably produced by the release from the afferent terminals of simple amino acids such as taurine. This presents a problem for the control of these impulses by systemic drugs because these amino acids are so widespread and important that it is unlikely that antagonistic drugs would counteract their action without serious side-effects. The local inhibitory cells emit fast-acting compounds such as gamma-aminobutyric acid (GABA). Here there is hope that drugs may exaggerate this inhibition since the diazepams used as tranquillizers increase GABA action. The third component of the gate, the long descending inhibitory pathways, operate by emitting serotonin (5-hydroxytryptamine), noradrenaline, dopamine and other compounds.

These well-known compounds are associated with an extensive pharmacology so that it is possible to exaggerate the effect of descending control by the use of drugs. For example, the use of anti-depressant drugs in pain treatment is in part justified by their ability to increase the central catecholamines and thereby exaggerate the inhibitory effect of central control systems.

Pain mechanisms minutes and hours after injury

An acute injury, such as a twisted ankle, produces a familiar sequence of pains. The moment of injury is usually associated with a sharp, rapidly rising pain that is precisely localized, and this form of pain decreases in seconds. It is replaced by a deep, spreading, sickening pain which is hard to localize. When this second type of pain is felt, it augurs poorly for the ensuing days and weeks. Not only is the ankle painful but there is widespread tenderness and it is difficult to move the leg. We will now analyse what happens. It is reasonable at first to search the periphery for an explanation, but we will show that part of the problem is transferred by the peripheral nerves from the region of injury to the spinal cord. Here we discover a special role for the slowly conducting, unmyelinated C fibres, which change the organization of the cord from the acute state to one suitable for protection and recovery of the wounded part.

Changes in the periphery

Direct action on nerve terminals
Once nerve endings have been stimulated by some major event, it is not too surprising that they do not return immediately to normal. Some endings become very much more sensitive than before, while

others become less sensitive. Even in the case of a minor burn where there is little damage to the skin, previously high-threshold A-delta fibres may become very sensitive and this may explain some of the tenderness where a normally innocuous stimulus produces pain (allodynia).

Tissue breakdown and inflammatory products
The destruction of tissue releases chemicals into the fluid which bathes the nerve endings. This in turn disrupts other particularly fragile cells, the mast cells, which release further pain-producing and inflammation-producing chemicals into the area. These chemicals include bradykinin, histamine, prostaglandins, leukotrienes, peptides and proteolytic enzymes, all of which either produce pain by themselves or sensitize the nerve endings. The leukotrienes and the prostaglandins are the breakdown products of fatty acids. The accumulation of prostaglandins is particularly important and is prevented by aspirin and its related compounds. These not only produce pain but play a role in the other aspects of inflammation, redness and swelling. They dilate the blood vessels and make them leaky to produce the swelling. They also play a role in attracting the leucocytes which enter the area of damage to begin their scavenging, and in directing the fibroblasts which arrive to replace damaged tissue with scar tissue.

Chemicals released from stimulated C fibres: the axon reflex
The description of a scratch on pp. 47–8 showed that part of the reaction to injury depends on the presence of unmyelinated sensory fibres in the tissue. As these fibres are stimulated by the injury, they leak chemicals into the area of damage. These include substance P, neurokinins A and B, and other peptides. They spread and further extend the area of sensitization, vasodilation and the leaking of blood vessels (neurogenic oedema).

Chemicals released from sympathetic fibres
In healthy tissue, the activities of the sympathetic nervous system have little effect on sensation except indirectly – producing goose bumps, chills, flushing and sweating – by their action on smooth muscle, blood vessels and sweat glands. However, in the presence of damage, their role becomes increasingly important with the release of noradrenaline, adenosine, acetylcholine and peptides. The sympathetic nervous system begins to play a new role within minutes of damage and contributes not only to pain but to the other aspects of inflammatory processes.

Changes induced in the central nervous system

When we proposed the gate-control theory of pain in 1965, there were many examples of clinical and experimental pain in which the pain long outlasted the peripheral injury and sometimes spread far beyond the area involved in the damage. The physiology of the time did not provide a convincing mechanism for this spread in time and space and we therefore limited ourselves to a discussion of acute pain.

Recent physiological studies point to a mechanism that produces these phenomena – the unmyelinated fibres which were long known to be involved in pain, but which had no clear function. It has long been a mystery why A-delta fibres *and* C fibres seem both to be responsible for carrying information about an injury. A valuable clue was discovered by Mendell and Wall (1965), who found that introducing C fibre activity on top of A-delta activity led to a long-term increase of activity which they called the 'wind-up' effect. This led to new questions about the role of C fibres.

The mystery of C fibre function

The first mystery is the huge number of C fibres. In every mammal and in every tissue, C fibres outnumber all the myelinated sensory fibres. The second is that the C fibres conduct their impulses slowly so that it takes more than a second for the nerve impulses to inform the spinal cord that a foot is injured, while the myelinated fibres have delivered the same information long before. The third is that the C fibres are not as finely tuned to the characteristics of the injurious agent – such as pressure, thermal or chemical – while the A-delta fibres have the properties to carry such information with precision. The mystery deepens on the discovery that the C fibres and not the A fibres contain a specific family of chemicals, the peptides. Furthermore, they terminate in a specific destination in the spinal cord in laminae 1 and outer 2. Even more surprising, their terminations form a very precise map of the skin from which they originate. This map of the body surface within the spinal cord is much more precise than the map formed by the myelinated afferent terminals.

The time has clearly come to seek the functions of C fibres and the cells on which they end, which are not simply poor imitations of the function of A fibres. Even the idea that they produce a 'second pain' which sometimes echoes a 'first pain' is not well supported (Sinclair,

1982). Could it be that they are responsible for the changes which follow injury while the A fibres produce the immediate reaction? We will start by examining the sequence of changes which occur in the flexion reflex after injury.

The evolution of the flexion reflex after injury

A pinch of the foot of a person or a rat produces a brisk withdrawal. Only A fibres need to be stimulated to produce such a reaction. If the pinch is repeated several times, the withdrawal reflex fades. However, if the injury is serious, and particularly if it involves deep tissue, as in a twisted ankle, the sensory and reflex changes grow and persist. Furthermore, there is tenderness and difficulty in moving. Some of this persistent change is undoubtedly due to the progressive changes in the region of the damaged tissue which we described earlier. However, Woolf (1983) showed that even in a decerebrate and spinal rat, the flexion reflex to an injury remained changed for a long time (hours) even if the injured region was anaesthetized. This was a crucial experiment in a number of ways. It provided a way in which the long-term spinal consequences of injury could be studied in an ethically acceptable way, since the rat's brain was removed so that it felt no pain. Furthermore, the experiment showed that injury produced long-term changes even when only the spinal cord remained functional. More surprising was Woolf's (1983) demonstration that the enhanced excitability persisted when the injured area no longer provided an input to the spinal cord. This has led to a series of experiments and questions.

What is the long-term central effect of C fibre stimulation?

By electrical stimulation of isolated nerves, it is possible to deliver a message to the spinal cord without actual injury of skin or other tissue so that the incoming message stops as soon as stimulation ceases. Knowing that deep tissue injuries produce much longer-lasting, chronic disturbance than superficial injuries, Wall and Woolf (1984) compared the effect of identical messages from skin nerves and from muscle-joint nerves. They watched the long-term result of twenty stimuli to each type of nerve at 1Hz. Of course, each stimulus resulted in a reflex which was subject to the gate-control mechanism. Wall and Woolf were interested in what would happen after they stopped the stimulation. When they stimulated a cutaneous nerve and delivered an A and C fibre volley to the spinal cord, the flexion reflex was exaggerated for about 3 minutes; but if they stimulated a muscle nerve once a second for 20 seconds, the reflex was affected for 90 minutes.

Now they had a phenomenon reminiscent of human pain states which they could analyse in the laboratory. They knew that it was produced by C fibres because it occurred only if they raised the electrical stimulus to a level sufficient to excite C fibres. Furthermore, they used a substance – capsaicin – which poisons C fibres and inactivates the central effect of C fibres. This substance, the hot principle of paprika, initially stimulates C fibres but then inactivates them. If a nerve is soaked in capsaicin, the central effect of C fibres is abolished. Wall and Woolf found that if they stimulated a peripheral nerve after capsaicin treatment, the long-term effects of C fibre stimulation failed to occur.

What is the long-term effect of tissue stimulation?
Wall and Woolf (1984) now wished to move from the artificial stimulation of whole nerves to specific stimuli which would prolong sensory inputs limited to C afferents. Fortunately, mustard oil stimulates only C fibres for about 5 minutes. They therefore examined the effect of the application of small doses of mustard oil to joint, periarticular tissue, bladder, muscle and skin. The effect on the flexion reflex of this stimulation of the joint lasted more than two hours, while the same stimulus produced shorter effects when the oil was applied to the various tissues, down to a few minutes when it was applied to skin.

The results showed clearly that the effect of joint stimulation by mustard oil long outlasted the afferent barrage from the joint. The prolonged effect was also shown by the fact that anaesthesia of the joint 20 minutes after the stimulus (and the resultant enhancement of the reflex) did not abolish the enhancement. Evidently the afferent barrage had triggered a change in the spinal cord but some central mechanism now maintained the enhancement with no further input.

What is the effect of injury?
Wall and Woolf used this model of the chronic decerebrate spinal rat and its flexion reflex to move from the artificial and perhaps misleading effects of electrical stimuli or chemicals to conditions which imitate real diseases, such as cramp, arthritis, cystitis and muscle tendon rupture. In each condition, the spinal cord is informed by the C fibres that a disease exists in the periphery and that a

reorganization of central circuits is appropriate. Now the question arises, how can C fibres deliver such information?

What are the C fibre messages?

The usual answer to this question is that nerve messages consist of nerve impulses which emit a special neurotransmitter at the central terminal. Furthermore, the arrival of impulses in the spinal cord is followed by a rapid burst of impulses in spinal cord cells, which can probably be attributed to the release of amino acid neurotransmitters. However, there is a problem because these same fibres contain neuropeptides which are also released and which have marked postsynaptic effects. These peptides include substance P, neurokinins A and B, cholycystokinin, calcitonin gene-related peptide, vasoactive intestinal peptide and many others. Not only do the amino acids and particular peptides co-exist, but many cells contain more than one peptide. The peptide make-up of the C fibres depends on which tissue they innervate. Crossing nerves from one tissue to another changes the peptide content. Here we have a new kind of multiple signalling system.

What is the relation among the various messages in the same fibre? It is possible that these messages signal separate fast and slow events and produce fast and slow effects. Evidence for this is provided by nerve damage, which we will describe shortly. Here we will present only one experiment. If a nerve is cut, the anatomy of the nerve fibres central to the cut is maintained and the nerve fibres can still carry nerve impulses. The immediate central effect of the arrival of these nerve impulses in both A and C fibres is, if anything, exaggerated for reasons we shall discuss in the next chapter. However, the chemistry of the C fibres is grossly changed by a peripheral cut – most of the peptides disappear from the central terminals. We may now ask, what is the immediate and long-term effect of nerve impulses arriving in the spinal cord in C fibres which have lost their peptides? The answer is that the immediate effects are exaggerated and the long-term effects disappear. This suggests that it may be the peptides released from C afferents which produce the long-term effects. This is supported by evidence that soaking the spinal cord in particular peptides can convert the brief cutaneous effect to the prolonged muscle effect. The most interesting result relates to the effect of narcotics.

Although the analgesic effects of morphine and its related compounds have been known for two thousand years, it was not until the 1970s that it was discovered that there are receptors for narcotics on the endings of primary afferents in the spinal cord. Furthermore, it was found that there are cells in layers 1 and 2 which generate endogenous narcotics. These narcotics are of two kinds: the enkephalins (short-chain peptides) and the dynorphins (longer-chain peptides). Duggan *et al.* (1977) showed that localized infusion of narcotics into layers 1 and 2 inhibited the response of deeper cells to noxious inputs. Yaksh (1986) showed that local application of narcotics on the surface of the cord produced an analgesia in the bathed segments, and this has led to the exciting new procedure of injecting narcotics on to spinal cord segments ('epidural morphine') in patients with severe pain; this produces localized analgesia without the psychedelic effects of narcotics.

Could it be that the arrival of impulses in C fibres releases peptides which affect a peptide-sensitive chain of neurons which in turn influence the circuitry of the spinal cord? There is a paradox in the use of narcotics in animal experiments. In man, narcotics produce excellent relief of prolonged pain and tenderness but are not analgesics in the sense that they abolish the pain of an acute injury, such as a pinprick. Animal tests, in contrast, have usually used very high doses of narcotics to eliminate reactions to sudden injurious stimuli. Wall and Woolf (1986) therefore used very low doses of narcotics to see if they would prevent the development of the long-term effects of a C fibre input. They found that such doses have no effect on the acute immediate reaction but totally abolish the long-term effect.

It is evident, then, that the short-term and long-term effects of an afferent barrage are completely dissociated by the origin of the impulses, the chemistry of the C fibres and the pharmacology of the particular type of injury. We can now turn to the response of the cells in the spinal cord in the acute and delayed states.

Prolonged changes produced in spinal cord cells after injury

We have thus far discussed the prolonged change in a complete reflex circuit. Now we can search for the component which is responsible.

Is the change located in the sensory afferents?
Sensory nerve fibres in the region of damage may well show long-term changes and play a part in the tenderness of the sick region – that is, show the signs of primary hyperalgesia. However, the tenderness can spread to distant regions, including the opposite side of the body, so that there is no known way in which these afferents could be affected. Careful investigation of these afferents, from the

periphery to their central terminals in the spinal cord, shows them to be unchanged. This means that normal afferent impulses delivered to the spinal cord over normal fibres produce an abnormal effect since the spinal cord has been changed. This produces secondary hyperalgesia.

Is the change in reflexes located in the motor neurons?

Since muscle contraction is lively and exaggerated after injury, it might reasonably be proposed that the motor neurons are the source of the hyperexcitability. Surprisingly, recordings show that these cells, like the afferents, are completely unchanged. This strongly suggests that it must be the interneurons which link the input to the output that are generating the abnormal messages.

Afferents produce prolonged changes in dorsal horn cells

There is evidence that, even without damage, the receptive fields of cells in the substantia gelatinosa are unstable. The area of tissue which excites them expands, contracts and shows shifts in its boundaries. First, Dubuisson (1981) and then McMahon and Wall (1984) noticed that punctate injuries act as a magnet so that the receptive fields of substantia gelatinosa cells tend to expand in order to incorporate the area of injury. Most recently, Cook *et al.* (1986a,b) have shown that the arrival at spinal cord cells of a brief burst of impulses in C fibres from muscle, leads to a vast expansion of receptive fields. Cells which, in their normal state, responded to touch and pressure only, expanded their receptive fields to respond to half the leg. Cells which had previously responded only to a strong pinch now responded to light touch. Cells took about 10 minutes after the brief input to develop their full excitability and then returned to normal in 90 minutes.

The significance of the slow changes

Prolonged pains almost invariably involve tenderness. The pain is not continuous because the patient can often find some comfortable position. The problem is that normally innocuous movement or touch generates intolerable pain. We have demonstrated a spinal cord readjustment of sensitivity which is triggered by afferent impulses but is maintained by a central mechanism. The slow onset is reminiscent of a number of clinical states. The most dramatic of these is the onset of pain observed in intensive care units. The sudden occlusion of a coronary artery results in an instantaneous massive afferent barrage in C fibres. The patient at this time reports a strong general sense of unease which slowly evolves into the classical angina with pain referred to the chest wall and arm. The area to which the pain is referred is extremely tender and movement is not tolerated. Now we can understand that the initial volley slowly activates the interneurons which receive inputs from the skin, and the end result is pain and tenderness. The most dramatic way to generate a massive afferent barrage is to cut a nerve. On occasion such accidents result in extensive pain and tenderness which tend to persist. Then the question is why the state of tenderness normally disappears. Early evidence suggests that it does not simply fade away but is positively turned off by restorative control mechanisms. A failure in the activation of such controls would produce a steady continuation of the disease.

We have reviewed evidence that prolonged tender states are produced by the massive release of peptides on to substantia gelatinosa cells. It has now been discovered that such compounds can produce striking changes of slow onset and very long duration, so that ionic channels in the nerve cell membrane and enzymes within the cytoplasm are changed.

These prolonged changes have profound implications for our understanding of the clinical phenomena of pain. The nervous system which handles acute pain has its circuitry radically changed into a new state to cope with the biologically important situation of having been injured (Dubner and Basbaum, 1994). The new state has the function of greatly diminishing movement or manipulation. This state, even though it may be annoying, is the optimal condition to speed recovery from deep injury. Sometimes the state persists long after any usefulness and long after apparent recovery from the injury. The physician then searches, with cautious optimism, for drug therapy that might prevent or cure the new state, since it is triggered by particular chemicals and maintained by chemical change within the cells.

6 The Physiology of Prolonged Pain after Nerve Injury

Some of the most terrible and most intractable pains are associated with injury or disease of the nervous system itself. There are three sites of such injury with somewhat different mechanisms: the peripheral nerves, the sensory dorsal roots and the spinal cord and brain. To understand the effects of nerve injuries, we must describe a second method of signalling in the nervous system which complements the messages represented by nerve impulses.

Chemical transport as a second signalling system

A nerve cell consists of the cell body region, which contains the nucleus, and the long axonal extensions which reach out to make contact with the other cells. The cell body contains the DNA and RNA complex which is the site of synthesis of all the proteins, enzymes, peptides and neurotransmitters used to make the structure of the whole cell and to allow it to function. The axon and the dendrites contain no such synthetic apparatus. Therefore a transport system must exist to carry the necessary chemicals from their place of manufacture to the places where they are used. If an axon is cut, the portion still connected to the cell body survives while the distant part of the axon is cut off from its supply of essential chemicals and dies.

The chemicals are transported along tubules within the axon and move at slow rates of 1-240mm per day, in contrast to nerve impulses that move at much faster speeds of 1-100 metres per second. The neurotubules are made of special proteins which are mechanically fragile and sensitive to poisons.

At the terminal end of axons, the nerve affects other cells by emitting small vesicles which contain the neurotransmitters. This is not a one-way traffic, since vesicles are reabsorbed into the axon end and can therefore bring in samples of large and small molecules which are present in the tissue fluid surrounding the nerve end. In this way the nerve end is both secreting its special compounds and absorbing the chemicals which surround it.

So far, we have written only about the orthograde transport system from the cell body down along the axon. However, the mechanism is like a continuous two-way conveyer belt and includes retrograde transport from the periphery to the cell body. For example, the cell bodies of sensory nerves are in the dorsal root ganglia and axons grow out of the cell bodies in the embryo to reach and innervate peripheral tissue. The dorsal root ganglion cells make the proteins necessary for that growth and for the maintenance of the fibre. They also make the easily identified peptides, such as substance P, which then move down the axon. If a nerve is ligated, these substances pile up central to the point where the flow is dammed. This is only the beginning of the story, since the nerve is also picking up substances, particularly if it is cut, and transporting them back to the cell body. This constitutes a chemical message which tells the cell body the nature of the tissue with which the axon is in contact. If an easily identified marker protein, such as the enzyme horseradish peroxidase, is placed around the nerve end, it is transported from the nerve end to the cell body. This is now the most common technique used to identify the destination of axons. Because the transported chemicals represent messages about the state of the periphery, the cell body 'knows' that the axon has been cut and changes its chemistry. The first reaction of the cell body is an attempt to regenerate the axon by providing new building material. If this fails and the axon cannot reach the normal supply of messenger chemicals on which the cell body depends, some cell bodies sicken and die.

The importance of these retrograde messages is matched by an equally crucial role of orthograde transport. The axon is totally dependent on this transport, but what happens to the cell which the axon contacts? Muscle cut off from its motor nerves undergoes rapid atrophy. This is partly because it no longer receives nerve impulses which make it contract, and partly because it no longer receives crucial chemicals on which it is dependent. Changes are also seen in nerve cells which lose their input. The normal structure and function of nerves is dependent on their receiving both nerve impulses and chemical messages. Both types of message are changed by nerve damage and we will now follow the consequences.

Peripheral nerve injury

Immediate effects

If a nerve is cut, all types of nerve fibres fire at their maximal frequency, producing the 'injury discharge'. It is conceivable that the arrival of this massive, abnormal volley in the spinal cord may produce damage through the excessive discharge of central cells. After only seconds of this intense activity, all the damaged nerve fibres fall silent.

Nerve fibres may be silenced without the initial injury discharge by means of local anaesthetics or the slow application of pressure. When the nerves fall silent, whether after a block or a cut, a phantom of the denervated area is sensed in man. In animals, it has been found that blocking of the normal input to cells in the central nervous system may be followed immediately by the appearance of alternative effective inputs. An example of this is shown in figures 15 and 16, where cells in the dorsal column nuclei undergo changes and respond to a distant area when their normal afferents are blocked. Since this occurs at early stages of the transmission pathway, it is inevitable that many similar changes occur in the sensory areas of the cerebral cortex. Here we have an example of the continuous action of 'gate-control' at the synapse so that failure of one input immediately unmasks the presence of inputs which are being continually suppressed by inhibitory mechanisms. Evidently, the central effects of a peripheral block are not just a failure of excitation of cells from the silent nerve but are also the release of normally ineffective inputs.

Later local changes

A cut axon is an open tube with cytoplasm exposed. Within an hour, a membrane forms over the end and establishes again the continuity of the nerve membrane over the whole surface of the cell. Very soon the sealed end begins to emit sprouts which probe into adjacent tissue in an attempt to regenerate. They especially seek the Schwann cells, on which the nerve sprouts grow with great vigour at the rate of about 1mm per day. If the distal nerve has been lost, as in an amputation, the sprouts probe out into the scar tissue which is forming, extend for a few millimetres and then stop. The end result is a tangled mass of nerve sprouts and scar tissue called a neuroma. If the nerve has been cut in an accident and the missing gap is only a few millimetres, or if the cut ends have been reunited by surgical

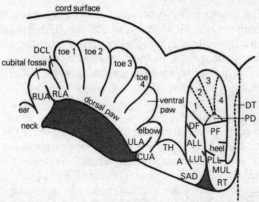

Figure 15. A 'felinculus' of the body surface representation within the gracile and cuneate nuclei. Abbreviations from left to right: RUA, rostral upper arm; RLA, rostral lower arm; DCL, dew claw; ULA, ulnar lower arm; CUA, caudal upper arm; TH, thorax; A, abdomen; SAD, saddle and lumbar back; LUL, lateral upper leg; ALL, anterior lower leg; DF, dorsal foot; PD, foot pad; PF, plantar foot; PLL, posterior lower leg; MUL, medial upper leg; RT, root of tail; DT, distal tail. Cross-hatching indicates areas where deep pressure is necessary to fire the cells. (from Millar and Basbaum, 1976)

sutures, many of the outgrowing sprouts will encounter a tube with Schwann cells and will be able to grow out towards their original target. The optimum situation for regeneration is a crush injury in

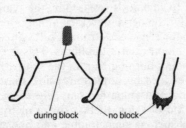

Figure 16. An example of how the input to some cells can change as soon as the normal input is blocked. Here a single cell was being studied in the foot area of the gracile nucleus (see Figure 15). It responded only to pressure on the toes – 'no block'. Then all input from the leg was blocked by cooling the lumbar spinal cord. As soon as the leg input was blocked, the cell began to respond to touch on an area of the flank – 'during block'. When the block was removed by rewarming the lumbar cord, the receptive field of the cell returned to the foot and the responsive area on the flank disappeared. (from Dostrovsky *et al.*, 1975)

which the basement membrane tubes around the axon (Figure 10, p. 85) remain intact. Here the sprouts are guided back to their original Schwann cell tube, rapidly encounter a medium in which to grow and are guided back to their original target.

The sprouts that grow into an area of damage differ from their parent axon in at least five important ways.

Mechanical sensitivity

Normal nerve fibres require a sharp heavy blow before they generate nerve impulses. When we hit our 'funny bone', we actually hit the ulnar nerve that lies above the humerus. The term 'funny bone' comes from the 'funny' feeling generated by ulnar stimulation. Outgrowing sprouts can be detected in man by gentle tapping along the course of a damaged nerve. The gentle taps stimulate the sprouts which produce a 'funny feeling', known as the Tinel sign.

Spontaneous activity

Most normal fibres are silent unless stimulated. Many of the out-growing sprouts become so excitable that they produce nerve impulses without any obvious stimulation. The patient feels tingling, 'pins and needles' and other unusual sensations – paraesthesias – which may become so intense as to be painful (Devor, 1994).

Sensitivity to sympathetic system activity

An important abnormality of damaged nerve membrane is that it becomes sensitive to chemicals released by the sympathetic nervous system. Specifically, the nerve develops alpha adrenergic receptors so that noradrenaline released from local sympathetic fibres or adrenaline in the blood excites the fibres. This is one of the mechanisms of the ongoing burning pain in the sympathetic dystrophies and of the pains evoked by sudden arousing stimuli. It is also the basis of treatment by sympathectomy either by surgery or by chemical destruction of sympathetic ganglia or by the use of anti-sympathetic drugs such as guanethidine and phenoxybenzamine.

Ephapses

It was long ago proposed that artificial synapses might develop between damaged nerve fibres so that efferent impulses, especially in the sympathetic system, might jump and excite the damaged sensory fibres and generate a pain-producing input. Some ephapses have been found but they are very rare and take many weeks to develop and none have been found between the sympathetic output and the sensory input. This attractively simple idea now seems unlikely to be the cause of pain.

Absorption of abnormal chemicals

Not only are the sprouts abnormal but they are in an abnormal chemical environment, particularly if they have failed to find Schwann cells to envelop them. Such sprouts will absorb marker chemicals, such as horseradish peroxidase (HRP), which have been intentionally placed around them and naturally occurring compounds such as serum albumin with which they would not normally be in contact. In addition to abnormal chemicals, the outgrowing sprouts are not in contact with the chemicals normally generated by their target tissue, such as nerve growth factor (NGF). Fitzgerald *et al*. (1985) have shown that the injection of a supply of NGF in the region of outgrowing sprouts prevents many of the distant effects of nerve lesions, which we discuss below. There is now strong evidence that nerve fibres, particularly C fibres, are continually 'tasting' the tissue in which they end and changing their chemistry accordingly. This change, in turn, affects the central cells on which they end. Therefore, when a nerve end finds itself in damaged tissue, the transported chemicals are changed. Some substances which are normally present tend to disappear while other unusual molecules appear. These changed chemical patterns comprise messages that are received at a distance.

Later distant changes

A cascade of changes occurs at a distance from the site of a nerve injury:

Dorsal root ganglion cells

By way of the slowly transported chemical message, the dorsal root ganglion cells 'know' that their axons are damaged. The RNA is reorganized, and many of the peptides and enzymes that are normally synthesized no longer appear. At the same time, physiological changes are in progress in which the dorsal root ganglion cell membrane changes in ways similar to the alteration of the sprouts in the periphery. They become exquisitely sensitive to mechanical pressure, are spontaneously active and are excited by sympathetic amines (such as noradrenaline). In this way the damaged nerve generates abnormal nerve impulses from two abnormal (ectopic) locations in the same cell. The two locations are the outgrowing sprout and the cell body.

The spinal cord terminations of the sensory fibres

A single axon is protruded from the normal dorsal root ganglion cells, but, after a short run, it splits at a T junction into two branches. One branch runs towards the periphery to make up the sensory axons of the peripheral nerves. The other branch runs centrally in the dorsal roots to terminate in the spinal cord. Impulses generated in the periphery sweep past the junction to end in the dorsal horn of the spinal cord. Chemicals manufactured in the dorsal root ganglion cell are distributed to both branches of the axon. Therefore, when a peripheral nerve is cut and the ganglion cell changes its metabolism, chemical consequences are apparent in the spinal terminals of the afferent fibres. The afferent C fibres contain a number of peptides, such as substance P, somatostatin, calcitonin gene related peptide (CGRP), vasoactive intestinal peptide (VIP) and certain specific enzymes. When the peripheral branch of the axon is cut, synthesis changes in the cell. Therefore, the chemistry of the spinal cord terminals also changes. After some days, the concentration of all but one of the chemicals listed above decreases in the central terminals, only VIP increases. With some lesions, even the morphology of the terminals changes as a result of shrinkage, even though the fibres still carry impulses.

Spinal inhibitions

Presynaptic inhibitions. If this cascade of changes reaches the afferent terminals after peripheral nerve section, do changes also extend to the spinal cord cells on which the changed afferents end? In the normal spinal cord, postsynaptic cells release gamma-amino-butyric acid (GABA) after the arrival of an incoming volley. This affects the afferent terminals which have carried the incoming volley. The effect of this feedback is to de-polarize the terminals and to decrease the excitatory effect of subsequent arriving impulses. This presynaptic inhibition is one of the modulating 'gate-control' mechanisms that limit the central effect of arriving impulses and produce a prolonged dorsal root potential. If axons are cut in the periphery and the central ends are stimulated several days later, impulses still arrive at the spinal cord and fire peripheral spinal cells. However the feedback on to the afferents fails to occur after peripheral nerve section. Thus, a normal inhibitory mechanism has failed.

Postsynaptic inhibitions. In addition to presynaptic inhibitory mechanisms there are also postsynaptic inhibitions in which spinal cord cells inhibit other spinal cord cells as part of the normal integrative process. That is, the excitation of some cells is accompanied by an inhibition of others. Furthermore, once a cell starts firing, its excitation is normally halted by turn-off inhibitory mechanisms. Woolf and Wall (1982) therefore examined these inhibitions and found that they too are greatly reduced after a nerve injury. The surprising consequence of the loss of these inhibitions is that if the nerve which has been cut is electrically stimulated central to the cut, it produces larger and more prolonged firing in the spinal cord. This occurs because the central ends of the peripheral nerve fibres are intact and can deliver their normal nerve impulses to the cells in the spinal cord. However, as a result of the injury, normal inhibitory mechanisms are weakened and excessive excitation occurs due to the absence of the inhibitory processes which normally counteract excitation and hold it in check.

The consequences on central nerve cells

The terminations of nerve fibres in the spinal cord and the cells on which they terminate are arranged in a precise, orderly way. Each of the six laminae of the dorsal horns (described in Chapter 5) contains a map of the body surface. Distant parts of the body are represented medially, and nearby proximal parts project to the lateral part of the spinal cord. Each dorsal root receives fibres from a strip of skin – the dermatome (Figure 5, p. 51). The whole body surface is served by these overlapping strips which feed into their own segmental dorsal roots from the coccygeal segments to the upper cervical segments. The face is similarly served by its special sensory nerve: the trigeminal nerve. Thus, if you were able to look into the spinal cord from the back you would see a representation of the whole body surface with the toes, abdomen and hands represented medially, and the thighs, back and arms represented laterally. Within this overall map, each cell has its special territory called its receptive field which comprises a fraction of the dermatome. Cells in the medial part of the lower lumbar dorsal horn have their receptive fields on the toes, while those in the lateral part have their fields on the upper leg.

Prolonged effects of injury of the nervous system

Peripheral nerve injury

Now let us consider what happens if the nerves to the foot are completely severed or if the lower leg is amputated. Clearly, the medial dorsal horn cells lose their normal input. The immediate effect is that no stimuli applied to the periphery will make them fire. Their receptive fields have lost their ability to send them messages. However, we have seen that this is not the end of the story because the failure of the normal nerve impulses and the chemical messages to arrive, triggers a cascade of changes which sweep centrally. Those changes include the disappearance of inhibitions and a consequent rise of central excitability. Inevitably the cells' properties change in three ways: (1) ongoing activity rises and some cells fire sudden bursts; (2) if the cut nerve is stimulated central to the cut, the cells fire more than usually; (3) the receptive fields expand. If the receptive field grows large enough, the cell gains functional contact with intact nerves and once again the cell responds to peripheral stimuli. For example, if the foot of a rat is made completely anaesthetic by cutting all of its nerves, the immediate effect is to leave the medial dorsal horn cells cut off from their input, and therefore without receptive fields. As days and weeks pass, some of these cells begin to respond in the upper leg.

Let us consider the sensory consequences of this in an amputee some time after injury which caused loss of the leg below the knee. A stimulus given to the knee produces a normal excitation of the normal nerves supplying the knee. These arrive in the spinal cord and excite the 'knee' cells. However, because the nearby 'foot' cells have become so excitable, some of the foot cells also respond. In sensory terms, this means that the stimulus is felt in the knee as well as the foot of the phantom, and gives the impression that the nonexistent lower leg and foot have also been stimulated. The presence of deafferented central cells, with their raised excitability, produces an incorrect localization of the stimulus and also increases the overall activity produced by an innocuous stimulus. If the level of excitability increases sufficiently, it produces not only ongoing flashes of pain but an excessive sensitivity of the stump.

These expanded receptive fields in the spinal cord have now been observed in a number of laboratories, and they also occur in the trigeminal nucleus serving the face. Apart from the spinal cord, the other destination of some arriving afferent fibres is the dorsal column nuclei (Figure 15, p. 111), which contain a precise map of the body surface. Here too, partial denervation is followed by an expansion of receptive fields so that cells begin to respond to inappropriate and unusual areas of skin which are still innervated. It is inevitable that if the response of spinal and trigeminal cells is disturbed by denervation, there will be disturbances in the deeper brain structures activated by the first central cells. Many such examples have now been observed in midbrain, thalamus and cortex.

Mechanisms of long-term central effects of nerve injury

There are two routes by which the periphery can affect the central nervous system. One is by way of nerve impulses and the other is by chemical transport. The loss of the normal input pattern of nerve impulses after peripheral nerve section certainly produces some immediate central effects. However, there is reason to believe that the long latency, prolonged central effects described above are not produced by nerve impulses. By applying tetrodotoxin to nerves, which blocks nerve impulses, without affecting axon transport, the central changes which are so apparent when a nerve is cut do not occur. Furthermore, crushing a nerve, which produces complete peripheral degeneration and regenerating sprouts, also fails to produce the central changes. Therefore, it seems likely that the message which triggers the central reorganization is a change of chemicals which are transported when sprouts of damaged nerve enter an abnormal environment, as in a neuroma. This conclusion is demonstrated by an experiment in which the transported chemicals are manipulated by continuous perfusion of nerve growth factor (NGF) around the cut end of a nerve. The result was a striking reduction in the changes of inhibitions and receptive field size. This not only supports the role of axon transport but gives some promise of therapy for the terrible pa... that may occur after peripheral nerve damage.

So far, we have dealt with damage to a peripheral nerve without asking which fibres in the nerve are responsible for the changes in inhibition and receptive field size. To test which nerve fibres might be involved, capsaicin (the hot substance in paprika) was used, since soaking a nerve in capsaicin inactivates C fibres, while apparently leaving all the myelinated fibres intact. The results showed that capsaicin abolishes the postsynaptic inhibitions and expands receptive fields (Wall *et al.*, 1982). In other words, blocking C fibres is all that is necessary to imitate the most important prolonged central effects of peripheral nerve damage. This applies both to the prolonged effects of arriving nerve impulses (discussed in Chapter 5) and the effect of nerve section on transported chemicals. These two actions of C fibres, which are distinct from those of myelinated fibres, indicate that they are not just another group of fibres, but are responsible for slow modulation of the pathways over which A fibre impulses travel.

An additional study examined the central effect of C fibre blockade in the periphery on the organization of cerebral cortex (Nussbaumer and Wall, 1985). The most striking example of somatotopic mapping is found in the mouse cortex where special anatomical and physiological areas exist, one for each whisker. Barrels of cells group together in the sensory cortex in rows and careful anatomical and embryological studies have shown that each one is connected to a single whisker. Single cells in each barrel respond to movement of a single long hair or sometimes to two neighbours. If the nerve which supplies the whiskers is treated with capsaicin, the A fibres which innervate each whisker and respond to the smallest vibration are unaffected but most cortical cells now respond to more than one whisker. As a result of the selective destruction of C fibres by capsaicin, the receptive fields of the cortical cells expand and the normal precise map becomes distorted.

What, then, is the exact nature of the alteration in central organization which allows the expansion of receptive fields? Careful studies have shown that it is not due to sprouting of the central terminals into the territory of the nerves which had been cut. If no new anatomical connections are made, it follows that pathways exist which are normally ineffective and which are unmasked in abnormal conditions. Relatively ineffective synapses are known to exist in normal central cells and form the basis of the subliminal fringe around each receptive field. If afferents are activated from outside the normal receptive field under conditions of exaggerated excitability or optimal synaptic transmission, the normal receptive field can be made to spread artificially. We still do not know exactly how the ineffective synapses are normally kept out of action and then become effective after peripheral lesions. The likely possibilities are either abolition of steady presynaptic inhibition, abolition of postsynaptic inhibition or some subtle morphological change.

In summary, the presence of peripheral nerve damage is signalled rapidly by nerve impulses and slowly by chemical transport. The long-term end result is that central cells whose input has been cut in the periphery increase their excitability and expand their receptive fields. This can be seen as an example of a homeostatic mechanism. The nervous system specializes in maintaining stability in systems by sensing the physiological state of tissue and then, when conditions are altered, producing actions that re-set the state to a required level. The duty of sensory cells is to receive incoming information.

When cut off from the source of their information, the cells react by increasing their excitability to such an extent that they begin to fire both spontaneously and to distant, inappropriate inputs.

Dorsal root injury

When dorsal roots are damaged, due to brachial plexus avulsion, herpes zoster, arachnoiditis or other diseases, sensory axons are destroyed and the central end is now isolated from the cell body in the dorsal root ganglion (Dubuisson, 1994). Consequently, the central end of the axon degenerates so that the cells on which they end in the spinal cord are denervated. Unfortunately, dorsal root axons are unable to regenerate, and the changes which now take place are permanent and uninfluenced by events in the periphery.

It is well known that peripheral structures, such as smooth muscle, striped muscle or sympathetic ganglia, become hyperexcitable ('denervation hypersensitivity') when they lose their innervation. It may be that the same changes occur in dorsal horn cells when the dorsal root is cut. The cells which receive afferents have not only lost their normal supply of nerve impulses and chemical transport, but the inhibitory mechanisms normally activated by some sensory afferents also fail. Therefore these cells dramatically undergo the three changes described following peripheral nerve lesions: (1) increased excitability; (2) spontaneous firing; (3) expanded receptive fields.

The local inhibitory mechanisms are inactivated and afferent impulses with inhibitory effects no longer penetrate into the hyperexcitable region. Only some of the segmental and long-range inhibitory systems in the brainstem survive. Therefore, the pains generated by root lesions are peculiarly unpleasant and intractable.

Injury of the central nervous system

Diseases which intrude on the dorsal horn or the trigeminal nuclei can disrupt the balance of excitatory-inhibitory mechanisms in the same way that peripheral nerve or dorsal root lesions do. These diseases include multiple sclerosis and syringomyelia. They mimic the effects of peripheral nerve or dorsal root damage and thus provide additional evidence that some of the prolonged pains following peripheral injury are in fact caused by the transfer of the disease from the periphery to the central nervous system.

Pain is also associated with damage of the long tracts of the spinal cord. The most tragic of these occurs after section of the ventral lateral spinal cord for the treatment of pain. This operation produces a profound analgesia on the side opposite to the cut. However, the patients frequently begin to experience unpleasant sensations in the area of the analgesia, and the pain which was abolished tends to return. There are no studies of the origin of these pains but it is reasonable to expect that cells in the brainstem, thalamus and cortex undergo the same changes after denervation which we have described in deafferented dorsal horn cells.

Central pain also occurs after damage in the forebrain and may be produced by strokes. This pain is called the 'thalamic syndrome' even though there is no evidence that the thalamus is involved. It is associated with peculiarly unpleasant dysesthesias which the patient finds difficult to describe. Nothing is known of the mechanism although it is assumed that denervation hyper-sensitivity plays a part. Although the origin of this disorder is certainly in the forebrain, changes extend as far as the peripheral nerves. This emphasizes the interrelationships among all parts of the nervous system. We have noted that the pathological processes which underlie pain may move from the periphery to the central nervous system. In the 'thalamic syndrome', movement appears to be directed from the brain to the spinal cord and the periphery.

Summary and an answer to the puzzle of the C fibres

Nerve impulses produced by injury are conducted rapidly to the central nervous system by the small myelinated A-delta afferents. Why then are there unmyelinated C afferents? They exist in all mammals and in all innervated tissue in larger numbers than myelinated afferents. They conduct impulses slowly and the great majority require intense stimuli before they respond. The old explanation that they represent a back-up, redundant second system in case of injury to the myelinated afferents is hardly credible. The research described in this chapter indicates that these C fibres have two unique properties which they do not share with the A fibres, and which are crucial for pain mechanisms. First, we showed in Chapter 5 that the arrival of C fibre impulses at the cord is followed after some time by a very long-lasting increase of excitability, which is the best candidate to explain tenderness. In this chapter, we have shown that the C fibres have a second function based on their slow chemical transport. This signalling system is the basis for the long-lasting changes which follow nerve damage. It might reasonably be maintained that such an elaborate transport system is unlikely to have evolved just to detect the unlikely accident of nerve injury. Therefore, we need to propose a less dramatic, more subtle function for C fibres in addition to their role in nerve injury. A clue to such a role came from the surprising observation that the signals which travelled from the periphery to the central nervous system could differentiate between a cut and a crush, as we have seen. Furthermore, we found that C fibres with similar physiological properties had markedly differing chemical features depending on the tissue they innervated. Peptides in C fibres from the skin are different from peptides in C fibres from muscle even though they are all mainly high-threshold, polymodal nociceptors. The crucial experiment was carried out by McMahon and Gibson (1987) who cut adult skin and muscle nerves, crossed them, and allowed skin nerve to grow into muscle and vice versa. The chemistry of the nerves changed and became appropriate to the target. Furthermore, it was found that once the target is changed and the C fibres have changed their chemistry, the long-term central effect is appropriate to the target tissue and not to the peripheral nerves which innervate them. In summary, it now seems likely that C fibres are literally tasting, absorbing and signalling the chemical nature of the tissue with which they are in contact. Furthermore, they transmit this information to their cell bodies and to the central terminals so that the relevant changes take place in the spinal cord. C fibres, therefore, may play a role in shaping the central nervous system to respond to the dramatic necessities of gross injury and may also respond to minor abnormalities and the shifting needs of normal tissue.

7 Brain Mechanisms

Studies of the organization of the spinal cord, described in Chapter 5, show clearly that signals which trigger pain are transmitted to the brain by multiple pathways and that the information processed in the dorsal horns is controlled by descending systems. Brain processes related to pain are even more complex; the old concept of a 'pain centre' is obviously nonsense. Many areas of the brain are involved in pain processes and they interact extensively. We will first outline the basic anatomical organization of the brain and then look at the mechanisms related to pain.

Basic organization of the brain

The spinal cord begins to enlarge and change shape as it enters the skull. This marks the transition from the spinal cord to the brainstem. In the lowest part of the brainstem, some nuclei (groups of cell bodies) receive fibres from the dorsal columns and spino-cervical tract. This area also contains the nerve cells which receive fibres from the trigeminal nerve, which is the sensory nerve of the face. As we move forward (rostrally), the brainstem becomes larger until it terminates in the large group of nuclei that form the thalamus. On the basis of anatomical landmarks, portions of the brainstem up to the thalamus are designated as the medulla, the pons, and the midbrain (Figure 17). The pons – an enlarged portion of the brainstem – is the level of origin of the cerebellum, which carries out complex functions related to movement. The midbrain lies between the pons and the thalamus, which is the major relay station of the forebrain (or cerebrum).

The structure of the brainstem is basically the same in all vertebrate species. Knowledge of the groundplan in one species allows relatively easy identification of comparable (homologous) structures in other species. (However, although structurally similar, their functions are not necessarily the same in all species.) If a cross-

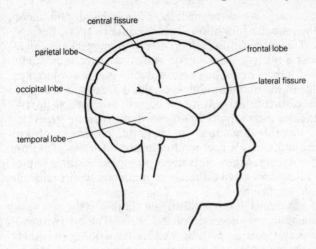

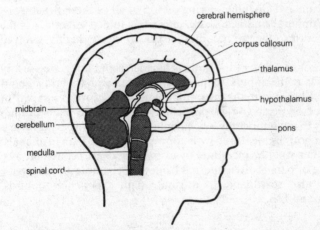

Figure 17. Schematic diagrams of the brain. *Top:* the major lobes and fissures. *Bottom:* a cross-section through the centre of the brain revealing the major components of the brainstem and other structures.

section of the medulla or midbrain of the rat, for example, is compared to a homologous cross-section in the human brain, the similarities are striking. The naked eye can easily see the medial lemniscus on each side, which consists of a large bundle of myelinated fibres that project to the posterior (back) part of the thalamus. These posterior nuclei send most of their axons to the somatosensory cortex. In the central core of the medulla, pons and midbrain, there is an area – the reticular formation – which contains small, densely packed cells. The reticular formation is not homogeneous, and, examined under a microscope, consists of distinct structures, some easily identified, others not. The periaqueductal grey, for example, is highly visible in the midbrain, but specialized areas within it and below it can be distinguished only on the basis of microscopic differences. The reticular formation is a particularly fascinating structure because it is superbly organized to integrate information from diverse sources and exerts a profound influence on sensory, motor and autonomic activity. Many of its fibres project back down to the spinal cord while others extend directly or indirectly to virtually all the areas of the cerebrum.

A 'ring' of structures – often called the 'limbic system' – surrounds the thalamus on each side of the brain. These structures, which play a major role in pain as well as virtually every other kind of behaviour, include the hypothalamus, hippocampus, amygdala, septum and cingulum. Lying on top of all of these structures – and enveloping them like a thick, intricately folded 'mantle' – is the cerebral cortex, which becomes larger in more highly evolved animals.

The major function of the brain is to receive and integrate sensory inputs, relate the inputs to past experience, and to bring about purposeful behaviour that is optimally adapted to the survival of the animal or person in its particular environment. Pain in man comprises two components – behaviour and conscious experience – which can both be measured with appropriate tools. Pain in animals, however, can only be measured by examining overt behaviour. The experience of pain is often inferred from the behaviour of mammals, and it is also reasonable to attribute pain experience to birds, amphibia and fish.

Ascending systems

Embryological and anatomical studies of fish, amphibians, and reptiles reveal that, even in the lowest vertebrates, reflexes are created by internuncial cells that link the sensory input to the motor output. During embryological development in these species, behaviour becomes increasingly a function of earlier sensory inputs as a result of the memory traces they have etched into the neural connections. Behaviour, then, is not merely the expression of a response to a stimulus, but a dynamic process comprising multiple interacting factors. Coghill (1929) was first to propound this principle, based on his brilliant neuroembryological-behavioural studies of salamanders, which has been substantially confirmed by later investigators. Given this fundamental principle – that organisms are not passive receivers manipulated by environmental inputs but act dynamically on those inputs so that behaviour becomes variable, unique and creative – the remainder of evolution becomes comprehensible as a gradual development of mechanisms that make each new species increasingly independent of the push-and-pull of environmental circumstances.

One of the most striking discoveries in the 1950s was the fact that injury signals are transmitted to the brain by multiple ascending pathways, each with distinctive conduction velocities and terminations in the brain (Kerr *et al.*, 1955; Bowsher and Albe-Fessard, 1965; Guilbaud *et al.*, 1994). On the basis of the evolution of the pathways and their anatomical distribution in the brainstem, it is possible to distinguish between two major systems: (a) the phylogenetically old pathways – the spinoreticular, paleospinothalamic, and propriospinal systems – which course medially through the brainstem (Figure 18), and (b) the newer pathways which maintain a lateral course in the brainstem and project ultimately to areas in the thalamus and thence to the cortex – the neospinothalamic, spinocervical, and dorsal-column postsynaptic pathways (Figure 19). The fact that most of these pathways, including the phylogenetically old ones, are still continuing to evolve (Noback and Schriver, 1969) suggests that each has distinctive functions.

The medial systems

The *spinoreticular system* (Figure 18) consists of short, multisynaptic chains of fibres that ascend in the ventrolateral spinal cord and, beginning at the medulla, course medially into the brainstem reticular formation and terminate mostly on reticular cells on the same (ipsilateral) side – although some penetrate to the opposite (contralateral) side (Kerr and Lippmann, 1974). Some of the fibres carry information exclusively about light touch or intense (noxious) tactile or thermal stimuli, but the majority are multimodal – that is, they carry information evoked by several kinds of stimuli, and respond with higher frequencies of firing as the stimulus intensity increases (see Dennis and Melzack, 1977). Generally, reticular cells have large receptive fields and exhibit a gross somatotopic organization (Soper and Melzack, 1982). Moreover, they receive inputs

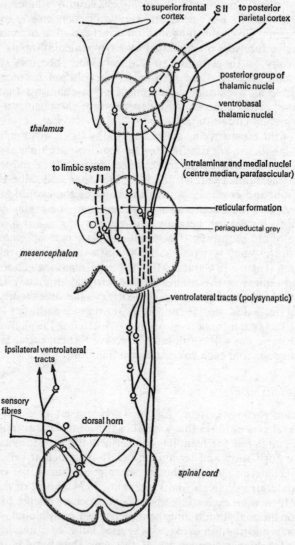

Figure 18. The slowly conducting somatosensory projection pathways. The breaks in the projection lines represent multi-synaptic connections. The propriospinal fibres are not shown, but consist of short fibres which are distributed throughout the cord. (adapted from Milner, 1970)

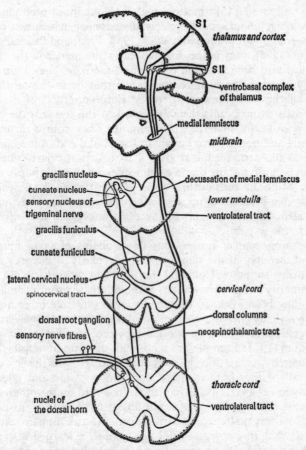

Figure 19. The rapidly conducting somatosensory projection pathways. The three main projection pathways are the dorsal column-medical lemniscal pathway, the dorsolateral tract (of Morin), and the neospinothalamic tract. The lower sections are shown on a larger scale than the upper sections.
(from Milner, 1970)

from other sensory modalities as well as from adjacent reticular cells and a variety of more distant brain structures.

The *paleospinothalamic tract* is a relatively small pathway which projects directly to the medial and intralaminar nuclei of the thalamus. This tract has many of the properties of the spinoreticular pathway – its fibres have large receptive fields and most of them carry multimodal information, with noxious input predominating.

The *dorsolateral spinomesencephalic pathway*, which was recently discovered by McMahon and Wall (1983, 1985) and Peschanski and Besson (1985), runs in the dorsolateral white matter in the rat, and has now also been found in the cat and monkey. The origin of this tract is lamina 1, which contains cells that lie in the termination zone of the unmyelinated afferents. Large numbers of these cells send their axons across the spinal cord to run towards the head in the opposite dorsolateral white column. They course through the medulla and pons and terminate in the caudal end of the midbrain, close to the periaqueductal grey. This is a particularly interesting region because it is the origin of many descending inhibitory control fibres. Midbrain cells in this region also project to the amygdala, a limbic area involved in negative affect and aversive behaviour. The area also projects to parts of the thalamus which are believed to play a role in pain.

The *propriospinal system* consists of chains of small fibres that ascend throughout the spinal cord, particularly in the grey matter, in contrast to the ventrolateral tracts we have just discussed, which lie primarily in the white matter. Although these propriospinal fibres have long been assumed to play an important role in pain (Noordenbos, 1959), they are elusive and difficult to study. Nevertheless, an ingenious study has shown that they are indeed involved in pain. Basbaum (1973) attempted to section all the long-fibre tracts in rats and thereby isolate the short-fibre system. He did this by cutting one half of the thoracic spinal cord on one side and later, at a slightly lower level, cutting half the spinal cord on the other side. In this way, only the chains of small fibres that carry signals through the spinal grey matter could carry information about pain. Basbaum showed that this operation did not abolish a learned response in which a painful electric shock made the rat turn its head to stop the shock. Even more remarkable was Basbaum's ability to train a rat to learn this response *after* the two hemisections of the cord. Of course, when the cord was totally cut through at a single level, the learned response was abolished. The evidence, then, suggests that a portion of the signals about pain are carried by short fibres that ascend diffusely through the cord, although their destination and other properties are unknown.

The lateral systems

In contrast to the medially projecting systems, the pathways that comprise the lateral group (Figure 19) are rapidly conducting and somatotopically highly organized. Although the three pathways – the spinocervical and neospinothalamic tracts and the dorsal column system – share many properties in common, there are also important differences among them.

The *spinocervical tract* ascends in the dorsolateral spinal cord. Many of the neurons in the tract respond to noxious mechanical and thermal stimuli. The majority of fibres from the lateral cervical nucleus cross the midline in the upper cervical cord and lower medulla and ascend in the medial lemniscus to an area in the lateral, posterior thalamus which is known as the ventrobasal complex (Figure 19). However, there is a small but definite projection to the rostral reticular formation (zona incerta), and to the posterior group and medial nuclei of the thalamus.

The *neospinothalamic tract* ascends to the thalamus from the ventral and ventrolateral regions of the spinal cord. Its cells respond to a wide range of stimuli (Price and Mayer, 1974; Yaksh, 1986); some respond exclusively to tactile or noxious stimuli, but the majority respond to both, with higher discharge rates to more intense stimulus levels. Although the neospinothalamic tract is more easily observed in monkeys than in cats, its existence in the cat, though less pronounced, is no longer in doubt, and the system clearly carries nociceptive information in both species (see Dennis and Melzack, 1977). In monkeys, the neospinothalamic tract is the most rapidly conducting somatic pathway. The majority of fibres of the neospinothalamic tract terminate in the ventrobasal thalamus. However, there are also substantial terminations in the rostral reticular formation and in the medial and intralaminar group of nuclei in the thalamus.

The *dorsal column postsynaptic system* was discovered as recently as 1968. Traditionally, the dorsal columns were believed to carry only fibres activated by innocuous touch and proprioception. However, Uddenberg (1968) discovered postsynaptic fibres in the dorsal columns which are activated by small to medium-sized receptive fields, and which produce a sustained, high-frequency discharge to noxious pinch. Later, Angaut-Petit (1975a) confirmed the existence of these neurons, and reported that they comprise about 10 per cent of dorsal column fibres and that most of them (77 per cent) respond differentially to both gentle and noxious levels of stimulation. About 7 per cent respond only to noxious stimuli, and the remainder only to light tactile stimuli. Cells with similar properties are also found in the rostral portions of the dorsal column nuclei (Angaut-Petit,

1975b). There is evidence, which we will review shortly, to suggest that such a system may exist in man and that it may play a role in pain. It is important to note that the dorsal column nuclei project not only to the ventrobasal thalamus but also to the posterior group of nuclei in the thalamus (Figure 18) and the midbrain reticular formation (see Dennis and Melzack, 1977).

Behavioural evidence

The behavioural evidence shows clearly that there are functional differences between the medial and lateral systems and even among the component pathways of each. Electrical stimulation of the ventrolateral spinal cord in people undergoing neurosurgery often, but not always, produces reports of sharp, burning pain. Electrical stimulation of the dorsal columns does not produce such reports, but mechanical stimulation often does (White and Sweet, 1969). Furthermore, Sourek (1969) found that insertion of a fine needle into the medial part of the dorsal columns produces pain sensations felt in the lower part of the body, while insertion of the needle into the more lateral portion produces pain sensations at higher levels. These sensations are felt on the same side as the needle insertion; when the midline is crossed, the pain shifts to the other side of the body. The data suggest that dorsal column postsynaptic fibres exist in man and that they play a role in pain perception and behaviour. At the midbrain level, electrical stimulation of the neospinothalamic tract in man produces pain described as bright and sharp. Surprisingly, stimulation of the medial lemniscus at high frequencies is described as hot and painful (Nashold *et al.*, 1969). In the rat, stimulation of the medial lemniscus produces clear signs of pain: cringing, writhing, running, jumping and some vocalizing, and the animals rapidly learn to press a lever to turn off the stimulation, indicating that it is highly aversive. In fact, there even appear to be two distinctly different aversive populations of fibres in the medial lemniscus of the rat (Dennis *et al.*, 1976).

Studies which produce lesions to reveal the functions of the ascending systems suggest that the pathways of the lateral systems are involved in pain. In man, attempts have been made to relieve phantom limb pain by sectioning the dorsal columns on the same side as the stump. Although cramping pain was relieved in some of the patients, the pain usually returned after several months (Browder and Gallagher, 1948). In monkeys, unilateral ablation of the dorsal columns briefly reduced reactivity to electric shocks of the legs on the same side (Vierck *et al.*, 1971). In cats, section of the dorsolateral cord (which included the spinocervical and spinomesencephalic tracts) temporarily impaired pain responses, and the effect lasted longer when a lesion was made of the whole dorsal half of the cord (Levitt and Levitt, 1968). These and other studies (see Dennis and Melzack, 1977) suggest that spinocervical and dorsal column lesions have at least temporary effects on some aspects of pain. The data of these studies, however, like those of all studies that involve lesions, must be treated with caution because the lesion often destroys adjacent structures as well as descending pathways. Nevertheless, the data, taken together, suggest that all seven pathways of the medial and lateral projection systems play a role in pain processes. The possible roles they play and the implications of multiple systems with similar (though not identical) properties will be discussed in Chapter 9.

Brain systems

Not long ago, when pain was still considered to be produced by a simple projection system, there was a hypothetical pain centre in the brain. Precisely where this pain centre was to be found was the source of considerable controversy. The favourite site of centres of all sensation was the cortex, but no such centre could be located. Wilder Penfield, the great neurosurgeon, electrically stimulated the exposed cortex thousands of times in hundreds of patients in the course of neurosurgical operations for epilepsy or tumours. On a few rare occasions, the patients reported feeling pain, but this happened so infrequently that few writers were willing to place the 'pain centre' in the cortex. Special attempts were made to place phantom limb pain in the somatosensory projection areas of the cortex, and these areas were excised in many patients. Nevertheless, the phantom limb pain usually returned, and the painless phantom itself was rarely altered, so that cortical ablations for phantom limb pain were soon given up.

If the 'pain centre' is not in the cortex, where is it? The next obvious site is the sensory thalamus which receives input from the major pain-signalling pathways that originate in the spinal cord. Head (1920) long ago proposed that the 'pain centre' resides in the thalamus and that the cortex exerts an inhibitory control over it. The thalamic syndrome, he suggested, could be due to vascular or other lesions that destroy cortico-thalamic fibres so that all inputs to the thalamus are unmodulated and cause excruciating pain. It was natural, then, that neurosurgeons would destroy thalamic nuclei in the attempt to abolish pain. The operation at first appeared successful but later turned out to be a failure (Spiegel and Wycis, 1966). The pain usually returned even after extensive lesions, and was often worse than before. Nevertheless, we now know that electrical stimulation of the somatosensory thalamus (Hosobuchi *et al.*, 1973; Turnbull *et al.*, 1980) or the fibres that fan out from it and project via the internal capsule to the cortex (Mazars *et al.*, 1976) can sometimes relieve chronic pain. These observations indicate that the sensory thalamus is involved in pain, but is not the pain centre.

It is now becoming increasingly evident that virtually all of the brain plays a role in pain. Even seemingly unrelated brain activities such as seeing, hearing and thinking are important. Seeing the source of injury, hearing the sounds that accompany a rifle shot or a falling beam, and thinking about the consequences of an injury all contribute to pain. Any satisfactory understanding of pain must include all of these processes which interact with inputs from the injured area or from deafferented neurons that produce pain signals when injury is absent.

Reticular formation

It is now well established that the reticular formation is involved in aversive drive and similar pain-related behaviour. Stimulation of nucleus gigantocellularis in the medulla (Casey, 1971a), and the central grey and adjacent areas in the midbrain (Spiegel *et al.*, 1954; Delgado, 1955) produces strong aversive drive and behaviour typical of responses to naturally occurring painful stimuli. In contrast, lesions of the central grey produce marked decreases in escape responses to noxious heat (Melzack *et al.*, 1958). Although these areas are clearly involved in pain, they may also play a role in other somatosensory processes. Casey (1971a) found that most cells in nucleus gigantocellularis responded to tapping or moderate pressure on the skin. The response pattern of the cells, moreover, was a function of the intensity of stimulation; the cells responded with a more intense and prolonged discharge to stimuli (pinch, pinprick) that elicited withdrawal of the tested limb. Similarly, Becker *et al.*, (1969) found that many cells in the midbrain central grey and tegmentum responded to electrical stimulation of large, low-threshold fibres. An increase in the stimulus level in order to fire the small, high-threshold fibres produced distinctively patterned responses showing high discharge rates, prolonged afterdischarges for several seconds, and the 'wind-up' effect (increasing neural response to repeated intense stimuli).

The role of the reticular formation in pain is especially clear in an elegant series of experiments by Casey (1971a and b; Casey *et al.*, 1974). He demonstrated a correlation between pain-related behaviour and single neuron activity in cells of the nucleus gigantocellularis of the medullary reticular formation. Cats with electrodes placed in this area were trained to cross a barrier to escape repeated single shocks to a cutaneous nerve. Weak shocks that did not elicit escape behaviour produced low-level discharge in the reticular neurons. However, the neural response increased when shock intensity was increased, and became maximal only when the shock elicited escape. Strong pinching was the only natural stimulus that excited some of these cells. Casey also found that direct electrical stimulation through the recording microelectrode was an effective escape-producing stimulus when delivered in or near the region of the responding cells. In a single set of experiments, then, Casey demonstrated a correlation between intense imputs that produce escape, a particular pattern of neural activity in reticular cells, and escape behaviour when the cells were directly stimulated.

Casey (1980) has recently proposed that reticular neurons are especially well suited to carry out integrated functions in the brain that are related to pain. A substantial number of reticular neurons have bifurcating axons that project caudally to the spinal cord and rostrally to the thalamus and hypothalamus. Stimulation of the reticular formation often elicits well-coordinated motor responses in animals deprived of forebrain function, and also produces marked changes in autonomic activity. In addition to being a major receiving station for pain signals and inputs from other sensory systems, it also exerts control over virtually all the sensory systems. Because noxious stimulation is so effective in influencing the discharge of these neurons, the reticular formation appears to be organized to play a major integrating role in pain experience and behaviour.

Limbic system

The reciprocal interconnection between the reticular formation and the limbic system is of particular importance in pain processes (Melzack and Casey, 1968). The midbrain central grey, which is traditionally part of the reticular formation, is also a major gateway to the limbic system (Figure 20). It is part of the 'limbic midbrain area' (Nauta, 1958) that projects to the medial thalamus and hypothalamus which in turn project to limbic forebrain structures. Many of these areas also interact with portions of the frontal cortex that are sometimes functionally designated as part of the limbic system. Thus the phylogenetically old medial ascending systems, which are separate from but in parallel with the newer neo-spinothalamic projection system, gain access to the complex circuitry of the limbic system.

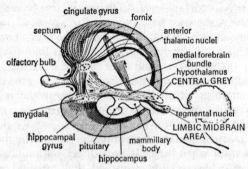

Figure 20. Schematic drawing of the limbic system, which is known to play an important role in emotional and motivational processes. The arrows indicate the direction of flow of nerve impulses through the system.
(adapted from MacLean, 1958, p. 1723)

It is now firmly established that the limbic system plays an important role in pain processes (Bouckoms, 1994). Electrical stimulation of the hippocampus, amygdala, or other limbic structures may evoke escape or other attempts to stop stimulation (Delgado *et al.*, 1956). After ablation of the amygdala and overlying cortex, cats show marked changes in affective behaviour, including decreased responsiveness to noxious stimuli (Schreiner and Kling, 1953). Surgical section of the cingulum bundle, which connects the frontal cortex to the hippocampus, also produces a loss of 'negative affect' associated with intractable pain in human subjects (Foltz and White, 1962). This evidence indicates that limbic structures, although they play a role in many other functions, provide a neural basis for the aversive drive and affect that comprise the motivational dimension of pain.

Intimately related to the brain areas involved in aversive drive, and sometimes overlapping with them, are hypothalamic and limbic structures that are involved in approach responses and other behaviour aimed at maintaining and prolonging stimulation ('self-stimulation'; Olds and Olds, 1963). Electrical stimulation of these structures often yields behaviour in which the animal presses one bar to receive stimulation and another to stop it. These effects, which may be due to overlap of 'aversive' and 'reward' structures, are sometimes a function simply of intensity of stimulation, so that low-level stimulation elicits approach and intense stimulation evokes avoidance. Complex interactions among these areas (Olds and Olds, 1962) may explain why aversive drive to noxious stimuli can be blocked by stimulation of reward areas in the lateral hypothalamus (Cox and Valenstein, 1965) or septum (Abbott and Melzack, 1978). In fact, in the lateral central grey, there is a strong correlation between current thresholds of brain stimulation to block pain and those for self-stimulation (Dennis *et al.*, 1980).

The role of limbic system structures is subtle and complex. Injury, in higher animals, occurs in a spatial and social context that often requires complex responses. Thus, the hippocampus appears to provide a 'cognitive map' in which spatial relations among objects in the environment are important in responses such as escape or hiding from dangerous predators or social rivals (O'Keefe and Nadel, 1978). The amygdala seems to provide an 'affective bias' as a result of matching incoming information against past experience, so that animals and people can respond adaptively to familiar or unfamiliar stimuli (Gloor, 1978). After ablation of the amygdala, monkeys unhesitatingly ingest hot, sharp, or otherwise injurious objects that normally, on the basis of past experience, elicit caution or avoidance.

Ventrobasal thalamus and its cortical projection

The medial pathways that project to the reticular formation and limbic system are not organized to carry precise somatotopic information about the location, nature, extent and duration of an injury. Yet an injury, initially at least, is usually precisely localized. A burn on a finger by a hot stove element from a pipe is immediately located and examined. A jab in the buttock by a sharp object similarly elicits a sudden movement of the hand to rub the precise point. If the reticular formation and limbic system are not organized to transmit precise information rapidly to the brain, it is reasonable to assume that the laterally projecting pathways are involved (Melzack and Casey, 1968; Dennis and Melzack, 1977). Indeed, recent studies suggest that the sensory-discriminative dimension of pain is subserved, at least in part, by the neospinothalamic projection to the ventrobasal thalamus and somatosensory cortex (Figure 19).

Neurons in the ventrobasal thalamus, which receive a large portion of their afferent input from the neospinothalamic projection system, show discrete somatotopic organization even after dorsal column section. Studies in human patients and in animals (see Wall, 1970) have shown that surgical section of the dorsal columns, long presumed to subserve virtually all of the discriminative capacity of the skin sensory system, produces little or no loss in fine tactile discrimination and localization. Furthermore, Semmes and Mishkin (1965) found marked deficits in tactile discriminations that are attributable to injury of the cortical projection of the neospinothalamic system. These data suggest that the neospinothalamic projection system has the capacity to process information about the spatial, temporal, and magnitude properties of the input.

Cortical functions

We have already seen that cognitive activities such as memories of past experience, attention and suggestion all have a profound effect on pain experience. In addition, there is evidence (reviewed in Chapter 2) that the sensory input is localized, identified in terms of its physical properties, evaluated in terms of past experience, and modified *before* it activates the discriminative or motivational systems.

The neural system that performs these complex functions of identification, evaluation, and selective modulation must conduct rapidly to the cortex so that somatosensory information has the opportunity to undergo further analysis, interact with other sensory inputs, and activate memory stores and pre-set response strategies. It must then be able to act selectively on the sensory and motivational systems in order to influence their response to the information being transmitted over more slowly conducting pathways. We have proposed (Melzack and Wall, 1965) that the dorsal column and spinocervical projection pathways act as the 'feed-forward' limb of this loop. The dorsal column pathway, in particular, has grown apace with the cerebral cortex (Bishop, 1959), carries precise information about the nature and location of the stimulus, adapts quickly to give precedence to phasic stimulus changes rather than prolonged tonic activity, and conducts rapidly to the cortex so that its impulses may begin activation of central control processes.

The frontal cortex may play a particularly significant role in mediating between cognitive activities and the motivational-affective features of pain (Melzack and Casey, 1968). It receives information via intracortical fibre systems from virtually all sensory and associational cortical areas and projects strongly to reticular and limbic structures. Patients who have undergone a frontal lobotomy (which severs the connections between the prefrontal lobes and the thalamus) rarely complain about severe clinical pain or ask for medication (Freeman and Watts, 1950). Typically, these patients report after the operation that they still have pain but it does not bother them. When they are questioned more closely, they frequently say that they still have the 'little' pain, but the 'big' pain, the suffering, the anguish are gone. It is certain that the sensory component of pain is still present because these patients may complain vociferously about pinprick and mild burn. Indeed, pain perception thresholds may be lowered (King *et al.*, 1950). The predominant effect of lobotomy appears to be on the motivational-affective dimension of the whole pain experience. The aversive quality of the pain and the drive to seek pain relief both appear to be diminished.

Similarly, patients who exhibit 'pain asymbolia' (Rubins and Friedman, 1948) after lesions of portions of the parietal lobe or the frontal cortex are able to appreciate the spatial and temporal properties of noxious stimuli (for example, they recognize pinpricks as sharp) but fail to withdraw or complain about them. The sensory input never evokes the strong aversive drive and negative affect characteristic of pain experience and response.

The data on the brain systems described so far suggest that there are specialized, interacting neural substrates for three major psychological dimensions of pain: sensory-discriminative, motivational-affective, and cognitive-evaluative (Melzack and Casey, 1968). An essential element in all of these interactions is descending inhibitory control mechanisms. Like every other aspect of pain, they are highly complex.

Descending systems

If the 1950s was the decade of discovery of multiple ascending pathways related to pain, then the 1970s was the decade that revealed the power of descending control systems. It was the exhilarating decade of the discovery of endorphins and enkephalins and, as a result, a better understanding of the mechanisms of analgesia than anyone would have dreamed possible at the beginning of the decade.

The story of the 1970s really begins in 1956, when Hagbarth (of Sweden) and Kerr (of Australia) worked together with Magoun (in the United States) to explore the recently discovered descending control functions of the reticular formation. Hagbarth and Kerr (1954) found that the responses evoked in the ventrolateral spinal cord could be virtually abolished by stimulation of a variety of brain structures including the reticular formation, cerebellum, and cerebral cortex. The implications were clear: the brain must exert an inhibitory control over transmission in the dorsal horns. In 1958, Melzack *et al.*, discovered, totally unexpectedly, that lesions of a small area of the reticular formation (the central tegmental tract adjacent to the lateral periaqueductal grey) produced hyperalgesia and hyperaesthesia in cats. That is, the cats over-responded to pinpricks and often cried and shook their paws as though in pain. The observers concluded that fibres in this area exert a tonic (or continuous) inhibitory control over pain signals; removal of the inhibition allows pain signals to flow unchecked to the brain, and even permits the summation of non-noxious signals to produce spontaneous pain.

These conclusions led David Reynolds, a young psychologist at the University of Windsor, Ontario, to test the hypothesis that the tonic inhibition from the central tegmental-lateral periaqueductal grey area could be enhanced by electrical stimulation, and might produce analgesia. In 1969, he reported that the stimulation did indeed produce a profound analgesia – sufficient to carry out surgery on awake rats without any chemical anaesthetic, and in 1970 he reported a replication of these results in higher species. Reynolds' observations met with scepticism and were generally ignored. In 1971, Mayer, Liebeskind and their colleagues, unaware of Reynolds' discovery, independently found the same phenomenon, which has come to be known as 'stimulation produced analgesia'. A series of brilliant experiments by Mayer, Liebeskind, Akil, Besson, Fields, Basbaum and their colleagues (see Liebeskind and Paul, 1977; Mayer and Watkins, 1981; Yaksh, 1986) led rapidly to reports that (1) electrical stimulation of the lateral periaqueductal grey and adjacent areas produces strong analgesia in awake animals; (2) the analgesia often outlasts stimulation by many seconds or minutes; (3) stimulation of the area inhibits lamina 5 cells in the dorsal horns, and acts selectively on noxious rather than tactile inputs; (4) the system seems to involve serotonin as a transmitting agent; and (5) the effects of stimulation are partially diminished by administration of naloxone, a morphine antagonist.

New discoveries followed in rapid succession. One set of studies showed that the injection of small amounts of morphine directly into the periaqueductal grey area produces analgesia (see Herz *et al.*, 1970; Mayer and Watkins, 1981), indicating that a major action of morphine is to activate descending inhibitory neurons in the brainstem. It was also found that the area that elicits analgesia has a broad somatotopic organization (Balagura and Ralph, 1973; Soper and Melzack, 1982). Moreover, there is evidence that stimulation of the area for several minutes before a painful stimulus is administered produces an enhanced analgesic effect, suggesting that some pharmacological substance is released into the area (Melzack and Melinkoff, 1974). It was also discovered that the brainstem inhibitory fibres descend through a distinct pathway in the dorsolateral spinal cord, that opiate analgesia and stimulation-produced analgesia are abolished or reduced by section of this pathway (Basbaum *et al.*, 1977), and that serotonin is the pathway's major transmitter (Basbaum and Fields, 1978). The picture that emerged is a relatively simple one despite the complexity of connections (Figure 21): the periaqueductal grey neurons, which are rich in enkephalin receptors and surrounding enkephalins, activate cells in the nucleus raphe magnus which, in turn, send fibres to the dorsal horns and inhibit dorsal horn cells by the release of serotonin (Fields and Basbaum, 1994; Yaksh and Malmberg, 1994).

During this period, the stage was set for a remarkable breakthrough in the whole field of analgesia and pain. Several biochemists and pharmacologists in the United States were convinced that the reason why morphine was a powerful analgesic was because there were specialized chemical receptors – opiate receptors – on nerve cells, whose structure was such that a morphine molecule fits into them like a key into a lock. After much research these opiate receptors were finally discovered (see Snyder, 1980). The next question was obvious: why would such opiate receptors evolve when the probability of a person or animal ingesting morphine is negligible? The answer, to Terenius (1978), Hughes and Kosterlitz (1977), and others (see Terenius, 1979; Snyder, 1980) was that the body manufactured its own opioid substances – chemicals similar in structure to morphine. And, indeed, when these investigators searched for such molecules, they found them, and called them endorphins (endogenous morphine-like substances) and enkephalins (opioid substances 'in the brain'). Soon, it was discovered that three large

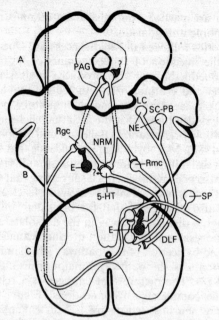

Figure 21. The endogenous pain control system as proposed by Basbaum and Fields (1978).

A: Midbrain level. The periaqueductal grey (PAG), an important locus for stimulation-produced analgesia, is rich in enkephalins (E) and opiate receptors, though the anatomical details of the enkephalinergic connections are not known. Microinjection of small amounts of opiates into PAG also produces analgesia.

B: Medullary level. Serotonin (5HT)-containing cells of the nucleus raphe magnus (NRM) and the adjacent nucleus reticularis magnocellularis (Rmc) receive excitatory input from PAG and, in turn, send efferent fibres to the spinal cord.

C: Spinal level. Efferent fibres from the NRM and Rmc travel in the dorsolateral funiculus (DLF) to terminate among pain-transmission cells concentrated in laminae 1 and 5 of the dorsal horn. The NRM and Rmc exert an inhibitory effect specifically on transmission neurons.

Catecholamine-containing neurons of the locus ceruleus (LC) in rat and subceruleus-parabrachialis (SC-PB) in cat may also contribute to pain-modulating systems in the DLF. (NE = norepinephrine.)

(from Basbaum and Fields, 1978)

protein molecules – 'prohormones' – give rise to the opioid peptides which fall into three families: endorphins, dynorphins and enkephalins. Their chemical structure has been determined, and many of them have been synthesized in the laboratory.

In the early enthusiasm following the discovery of these endogenous opiates, all forms of control of pain were promptly attributed to them. These phenomena included not only stimulation-produced analgesia but acupuncture, transcutaneous electrical nerve stimulation (TENS), the placebo effect, congenital analgesia and episodic analgesia. However, later research did not substantiate most of the claims (Wall and Woolf, 1980), although opiate involvement in TENS (Sjolund and Eriksson, 1979) has been confirmed. There is no doubt that the opiate systems exist and that they influence many biological activities, including the endocrine system, as well as pain. However, their functional role remains a deepening mystery in which it is not apparent when they come into action. Most surprisingly, chronic pain is completely uninfluenced by inactivating the endogenous opiate system by means of antagonists (Lindblom and Tegner, 1979).

Many sites have now been found in the forebrain and midbrain which induce behavioural analgesia when they are electrically stimulated. The best studied sites are the hypothalamus and the periaqueductal grey (PAG). Recently, Cohen and Melzack (1985, 1986) have found that stimulation of the habenula, a small structure which lies above the thalamus, produces striking analgesia. The circuitry by which these areas produce their effect remains uncertain. They may do so by ascending projections but it is clear that there are powerful descending projections which originate in the pons and medulla. These descend by way of the dorsolateral white matter to terminate in the spinal cord, particularly in the upper laminae of the dorsal horn. Here they inhibit the response of transmitting cells to injury.

The best known site of origin of the descending systems is in the rostral ventral medulla, which includes the serotonin-containing cells of the midline nucleus raphe magnus, and the nearby cells in the reticular formation. This area receives a major input from the PAG and its neighbouring midbrain reticular formation. The origin of another important descending system is in the dorsolateral pons where noradrenalin-containing cells project into the spinal cord. The descending systems appear to exert their action on the spinal cord by the release of serotonin and noradrenalin and possibly peptides. These substances cause the release of inhibitory compounds from spinal cells which include gamma-aminobutyric acid, enkephalin, dynorphin and, perhaps, dopamine.

The crucial question which remains is to understand when such systems actually become effective. One intriguing clue comes from studies (Fields and Heinricher, 1985) of the midline medulla cells under conditions where withdrawal behaviour was also observed. A type of cell was found which was continually active but became abruptly silent just before a withdrawal response occurred. They reasoned that these 'off' cells normally exert a continual inhibition of withdrawal reflexes. Only when they became silent were the spinal reflex circuits allowed to operate. This hypothesis of the existence of 'permission-to-respond cells' has wide-ranging implications. It suggests that the reason why electrical stimulation of the area is effective is that the 'off' cells are forced into continuous activity so that the cord circuits never receive their 'permission to operate'. In support of this hypothesis, Fields and Heinricher (1985) showed that analgesic doses of morphine or stimulation of the PAG also made the 'off cells' fire continuously.

One of the reasons for our relative lack of understanding of the functional role of the control systems may be that they have been studied during the wrong time-period. In previous chapters, we have stressed a three-phase process of reaction to injury: 1) the very rapid response of cells and organisms to injury; 2) the secondary reactions to the arrival of nerve impulses in C fibres; and 3) the greatly delayed responses associated with transport changes. It is often forgotten that narcotics are not analgesics in the sense that they are used clinically to prevent the first, rapid response to injury. A surgeon cannot operate on a patient who has received only morphine, even in large doses. The patient can still appreciate a pinprick and would certainly not permit a knife cut. Narcotics are excellent only for the delayed, late consequences of injury, not for the injury itself, unless massive doses of morphine are given. For this reason, Woolf and Wall (1986) examined the effect of a clinical dose of morphine on the flexion reflex in the spinal decerebrate rat, and found that it was not influenced. However, if they tried to exaggerate the flexion reflex with a conditioning volley in unmyelinated C fibres, this long-latency, long-lasting exaggeration was completely prevented by the narcotic.

Another example of this is seen in the formalin test, where a small amount of formalin is injected subcutaneously (Dubuisson and Dennis, 1977; Figure 22). This produces a sharp, stinging sensation which lasts for several minutes, followed by a prolonged, dull, unpleasant feeling which persists for more than an hour. It has been found, examining either behaviour or the responses of spinal cord cells, that the early response is little affected by morphine but the later phases are strongly depressed. It may be that the control

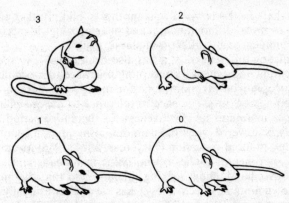

Figure 22. Typical responses used for rating pain intensity in rats. The animal's right forepaw has been injected with a dilute solution of formalin. Numerical values assigned to these responses are shown: 3, the rat licks the injected paw; 2, the paw is raised without touching the floor; 1, the paw is kept gingerly on the floor without full pressure; 0, the paw bears full normal weight as the rat ambulates in the cage. (from Dubuisson and Dennis, 1977)

systems, particularly those involving the endogenous opiates, react slowly and, once active, are prolonged in their action. Furthermore, the scientific search for the action of the control systems has concentrated too much on the initial, rapid-onset component of pain and has neglected the secondary later phases. The evidence on the effects of opiates on postsurgical pain suggests that they act on the prolonged pain associated with the incision rather than with sudden, rapidly rising pain that occurs when stitches are removed.

Recent studies with animals illuminate the distinction between the initial, fast-rising pain – exemplified by the tail-flick test for rats which induces rapid withdrawal of the tail from rapidly-rising heat pain – and the longer-lasting pain such as that seen in the second stage of the formalin test. For example, when the PAG is stimulated, much less electrical current is necessary to produce analgesia in the formalin test than in the tail-flick test (Dennis *et al.*, 1980a). This is astonishing, because the pain in the formalin test is more intense and prolonged. Furthermore, each test reveals a unique profile of effects when drugs are administered which are agonists or antagonists of major transmitters such as serotonin, noradrenalin, dopamine, and acetylcholine (Dennis and Melzack, 1980; Dennis *et al.*, 1980b). The formalin test is more sensitive to the effects of some drugs, while the tail-flick or hot-plate test is more sensitive to others.

It is not that one test is 'good' and another is 'bad'. Rather, each test appears to reveal different neural and pharmacological mechanisms and are influenced by different analgesic drugs.

By utilizing different tests, it has also been possible to shed light on the conflicting evidence concerning tolerance to morphine. Studies of people who take morphine for months or years to control cancer pain show little evidence of tolerance to the morphine. The same dose maintains its effectiveness for the entire period and, in fact, may be lowered when the pain diminishes due to spontaneous or therapy-induced remission (Twycross, 1974, 1978; Mount *et al.*, 1976). Experimental studies of morphine in humans and animals, on the other hand, show striking tolerance, so that the morphine dose, to maintain effectiveness, has to be continually raised (Goodman and Gilman, 1980). Abbott *et al.* (1982) investigated morphine tolerance in rats, using the formalin and tail-flick tests, and found rapid tolerance to morphine in the tail-flick test (confirming earlier studies) but little or no tolerance in the formalin test. Evidently, when morphine is given for moderate, continuous pain, there is virtually no tolerance, but when it is given for brief, just-perceptible pain, there is rapid tolerance. The results with the formalin test are clearly like those observed in people suffering chronic severe pain.

Summary

The physiological evidence shows that the receptors, fibres, and central nervous system pathways involved in pain are specialized to generate and transmit patterned information rather than modality-specific impulses. Injurious stimuli activate multiple fibre systems which converge and diverge a number of times so that the patterning can undergo change at every synaptic level. Nerve impulses in large and small fibres that converge on to the cells of the dorsal horns are subjected to modulation by the activity of the substantia gelatinosa. Similarly, the convergence of fibres on to cells in the reticular formation permits a high degree of summation and interaction of inputs from spatially distant body areas. Divergence also occurs; fibres fan out from the dorsal horns and the reticular formation, and project to different parts of the nervous system that have specialized functions. One of these functions is the ability to select and abstract particular kinds of information from the temporal patterns that are conveyed by the incoming fibres. Central cells, it is now also apparent, monitor the input for long periods of time. The afterdischarges, and other prolonged neural activity produced by intense stimuli, may persist long after cessation of stimulation, and may play a particularly important role in pain processes.

This convergence and divergence, summation and pattern discrimination all go on in a dynamically changing nervous system. Stimuli impinge on sensory fields at the skin that show continuous shifts in sensitivity. Furthermore, fibres that descend from the brain continually modulate the input, facilitating the flow of some input patterns and inhibiting others. The widespread influences of the substantia gelatinosa and the reticular formation, which receive inputs from virtually all of the body, can modify information transmission at almost every synaptic level of the somatosensory projection systems. These ascending and descending interactions present a picture of dynamic, modifiable processes in which inputs impinge on a continually active nervous system that is already the repository of the individual's past history, expectations and value systems. This concept has important implications: it means that the input patterns evoked by injury can be modulated by other sensory inputs or by descending influences, which may thereby determine the quality and intensity of the eventual experience.

The somaesthetic system is a unitary, integrated system comprised of specialized component parts. Several parallel systems analyse the input simultaneously to bring about the richness and complexity of pain experience and response. Some areas are specialized to select sensory-discriminative information while others play specialized roles in the motivational-affective dimension of pain. These parallel information-processing systems interact with each other, and must also interact with cortical activities which underlie past experience, attention, and other cognitive determinants of pain. These interacting processes produce the myriad patterns of activity that subserve the varieties of pain experience (Melzack, 1995).

Part Three
Theories of Pain

'The "real world" is a construct, and some of the peculiarities of scientific thought become more intelligible when this fact is recognized . . . Einstein himself in 1926 told Heisenberg it was nonsense to found a theory on observable facts alone: "In reality the very opposite happens. It is theory which decides what we can observe." '

D. O. Hebb, 1975

8   The Evolution of Pain Theories

So far, we have been concerned primarily with experimental and clinical observations related to pain. But facts alone fall short of providing a complete understanding of difficult problems. Books have been written which bring together all the known facts about pain, yet the puzzle persists. We grope towards understanding and, for that reason, invent theories that bring us closer to it.

Although the notion of a scientific theory sounds formidable, a theory is primarily an attempted solution to a puzzle or problem – like a guess made by a detective presented with an array of clues in a mystery. Several clues may lead to a theory or guess on the nature of the solution. The theory, in turn, may lead to a search for further clues that were previously not evident.

A theory alone, however, may not be enough to convince (or convict). New facts are tested against the theory to see whether or not they fit. If they support the theory, all the clues may fit together to make a coherent picture. In this chapter we will examine and evaluate the theories of pain that have evolved during the past century.

Specificity theory

The traditional theory of pain is known as 'specificity theory'. It is described in virtually every textbook on neurophysiology, neurology and neurosurgery, and is often taught as fact rather than theory. It is presented as though we already have the major answers to pain problems, and all that remain are a few minor questions that deal with therapy. It also proved to be a very powerful theory during the first half of this century, giving rise to excellent research and to some effective forms of treatment. It has several basic flaws, however, and new, more powerful theories have recently been proposed.

Specificity theory proposes that a specific pain system carries messages from pain receptors in the skin to a pain centre in the brain. To understand the theory, we must first consider its origins. The best classical description of the theory was provided by Descartes in 1664, who conceived of the pain system as a straight-through channel from the skin to the brain. He suggested that the system is like the bell-ringing mechanism in a church: a man pulls the rope at the bottom of the tower, and the bell rings in the belfry. So too, he proposed (Figure 23), a flame sets particles in the foot into activity and the motion is transmitted up the leg and back and into the head where, presumably, something like an alarm system is set off. The person then feels pain and responds to it. Despite its apparent simplicity, the theory involves several major assumptions, which we will examine shortly. First, however, we will see how Descartes' theory has evolved in the last three centuries.

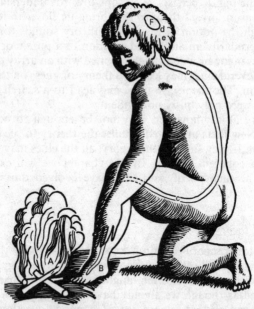

Figure 23. Descartes' (1664) concept of the pain pathway. He writes: 'If for example fire (A) comes near the foot (B), the minute particles of this fire, which as you know move with great velocity, have the power to set in motion the spot of the skin of the foot which they touch, and by this means pulling upon the delicate thread (cc) which is attached to the spot of the skin, they open up at the same instant the pore (d e) against which the delicate thread ends, just as by pulling at one end of a rope one makes to strike at the same instant a bell which hangs at the other end.'

The theory underwent little change until the nineteenth century, when physiology emerged as an experimental science. A major problem faced by sensory physiologists in the nineteenth century was this: how can we account for the different qualities of sensation? Our visual and auditory sensations are qualitatively different from each other, just as our skin sensations are obviously different from those of taste or smell. What is the basis of these different sensory qualities? As a result of studies by early anatomists and physiologists, it became apparent that the brain is aware of the outside world only by means of messages conveyed to it by the sensory nerves. The qualities of experience, therefore, are somehow associated with the properties of sensory nerves. It was Johannes Müller who first stated this proposition in scientific form, and his statement has become known as the 'doctrine of specific nerve energies'.

Müller's doctrine of specific nerve energies

Müller's monumental contribution (1842) to our understanding of sensory processes lies in his formal statement that the brain receives information about external objects only by way of the sensory nerves. Activity in nerves, then, represents coded or symbolic data concerning the stimulus object. Müller recognized only the five classical senses – seeing, hearing, taste, smell and touch – the sense of touch incorporating for him all the qualities of experience that we derive from stimulation of the body.

Müller was uncertain, at that time, whether the quality of sensation is due to some specific energy inherent in each of the sensory nerves themselves, or whether it is due to some special properties of the brain areas at which the nerves terminate. By the late nineteenth and early twentieth centuries, however, it was apparent that nerve impulses are essentially the same in all sensory nerves, and it was concluded that the quality of sensation is given by the termination of the nerves in the brain. The impact of all this was a search for a terminal centre in the brain for each of the sensory nerves.

Müller's concept, then, was that of a straight-through system from the sensory organ to the brain centre responsible for the sensation. Since the cortex is seemingly at the 'top' of the nervous system, a search was made for cortical centres. Visual and auditory projections to the cortex were found very early, and it was assumed that these cortical areas were the seat of seeing and hearing. The physiologists of the day were so convinced of the truth of this doctrine that DuBois-Reymond (see Boring, 1942) proposed that if the auditory nerve could be connected to the visual cortex, and the visual nerve to the auditory cortex, then we would see thunder and hear lightning!

It was at this time that Max von Frey, a physician, first began to contemplate these problems and between 1894 and 1895 he published a series of articles in which he proposed a theory of the cutaneous senses. This theory was expanded during the next fifty years, and is the basis of modern-day specificity theory.

Von Frey's theory

The way von Frey developed his theory (Boring, 1942) makes a fascinating story in the history of science. He had three kinds of information that he put together to form it. The first was Müller's doctrine of specific nerve energies. It was apparent to him, as it was to others, that Müller's notion of a single sense of touch or 'feeling' was inadequate. It was reasonable, then, for von Frey to expand Müller's concept to four major cutaneous modalities: touch, warmth, cold, and pain, each presumably with its own special projection system to a brain centre responsible for the appropriate sensation.

The second kind of information von Frey had was the spot-like distribution of warmth and cold sensitivity at the skin. He made two simple devices that are still used in neurological tests. He put a pin on a spring, and could gauge the pressure on the pin necessary to produce prick-pain, thus finding pain spots. He also put two-inch snippets of horse-tail hairs on pieces of wood and made 'von Frey hairs' to map out distributions of touch spots. Thus he believed that the skin comprises a mosaic of four types of sensory spots: touch, cold, warmth, and pain.

The third kind of information used by von Frey derived from the development, during the nineteenth century, of chemical techniques to study the fine structure of body tissues. Anatomists used particular chemicals to stain thin slices of tissue from all parts of the body, and then observed the tissues through a microscope. When they examined the skin in this way, they found a variety of specialized structures. To achieve immortality of sorts, some of the anatomists named the specialized structures after themselves. Thus, we still know these structures as Meissner corpuscles, Ruffini end-organs, Krause end-bulbs, Pacinian corpuscles and so forth. Two types of structure were so common that no one dared attach his name to them: the free nerve endings that branch out into the upper layers of the skin, and the nerve fibres that are wrapped around hair follicles.

The way von Frey utilized these three kinds of information is a remarkable example of scientific deduction. He reasoned as follows: since the free nerve endings are the most commonly found, and pain spots are found almost everywhere, the free nerve endings are pain receptors. Furthermore, since Meissner corpuscles are frequently found at the fingers and palm of the hand where touch spots are most abundant and most sensitive, they (in addition to the fibres surrounding hair follicles) are the touch receptors. The next association was an imaginative deduction: he noted that the conjunctivum of the eye and the tip of the penis are both sensitive to cold, but the conjunctivum is not sensitive to warmth and the penis is not sensitive to pressure; moreover, Krause end-bulbs are found in both locations; therefore, he concluded, Krause end-bulbs are cold receptors. Finally, he had one major sensation – warmth – left over, and one major receptor – Ruffini end-organs – so he proposed that Ruffini end-organs are warmth receptors.

Von Frey's theory dealt only with receptors. Others carried on, however, and sought specific fibres from the receptors to the spinal cord, then specific pathways in the spinal cord itself.

Extensions of von Frey's theory

Following von Frey's postulation of four modalities of cutaneous sensation, each having its own type of specific nerve ending, the separation of modality was extended to peripheral nerve fibres (see Chapter 5). Ingenious experiments (reviewed by Bishop, 1946; Rose and Mountcastle, 1959; Sinclair, 1982) were carried out to show that there is a one-to-one relationship between receptor type, fibre size, and quality of experience. The concept of modality separation in peripheral nerve fibres represents the most literal interpretation of Müller's doctrine of specific nerve energies. Since fibre-diameter groups are held to be modality specific, the theory imparts 'specific nerve energy' on the basis of fibre size, so that specificity theorists speak of A-delta-fibre pain and C-fibre pain, of touch fibres and cold fibres as though each fibre group had a straight-through transmission path to a specific brain centre.

Finally, a search was made for the 'pain pathway' in the spinal cord (Keele, 1957). Studies and operations on humans and animals suggested that the anterolateral quadrant of the spinal cord was critically important for pain sensation (see p. 64, on cordotomy). As a consequence, the spinothalamic tract which ascends in the anterolateral cord has come to be known as 'the pain pathway'.

The location of the 'pain centre' is still a source of debate among specificity theorists. Head (1920) proposed that it is located in the thalamus because cortical lesions or excisions rarely abolish pain. Indeed, they may make it worse. Thus, the thalamus is held by some to contain the pain centre, and the cortex is assumed to exert inhibitory control over it.

Analysis of specificity theory

Von Frey's designation of the free nerve endings as pain receptors is the basis of specificity theory. Its solution to the puzzle of pain is simple: specific pain receptors in body tissue project via pain fibres and a pain pathway to a pain centre in the brain. Despite its apparent simplicity, the theory has three facets, each representing a major assumption. The first of these, that receptors are specialized, is physiological in nature and has achieved the proportions of a genuine biological law. The remaining two assumptions, anatomical and psychological in nature, are not supported by the facts.

The physiological assumption

Von Frey's assumption that skin receptors are differentiated to respond to particular stimulus dimensions represents a major extension of Müller's concept of the 'specific irritability' of receptors. The assumption is that each of the four types of receptors has one form of energy to which it is especially sensitive. This concept of physiological specialization of skin receptors provides the power of von Frey's theory and appears to be the main reason for its survival through the decades. Sherrington (1900, p. 995) stated it in a manner that is acceptable to all students of sensory processes. He defined the specificity of a receptor purely in terms of the lowest limen (or threshold) for a particular stimulus to fire it, and made no assumptions concerning the eventual psychological experience. This concept of the 'adequate stimulus' (Sherrington, 1906) is so generally accepted that it is rightfully considered to be a biological principle or law.

The anatomical assumption

It is von Frey's anatomical assumption that is the most specific, the most obviously incorrect and the least relevant aspect of the theory. Von Frey assumed that a single morphologically specific receptor lay beneath each sensory spot on the skin and he assigned a definite receptor type to each of the four modalities. The crucial experiment of making a histological examination of the skin under carefully mapped temperature spots has been performed at least a dozen times (see Melzack and Wall, 1962), without a single investigator finding any support for von Frey's anatomical correlations.

The psychological assumption

It is the assumption that each psychological dimension of somaesthetic experience bears a one-to-one relation to a single stimulus dimension and to a given type of skin receptor that is the most questionable part of von Frey's theory (Melzack and Wall, 1962). Like all psychological theories, von Frey's theory has an implicit conceptual nervous sytem; and the model is that of a fixed, direct-line communication system from the skin to the brain – of distinct nerves and pathways of four different qualities (analogous to the differently coloured wires of an electrical circuit) running from four specific kinds of stimulus transducers in the skin to four specific receivers in the brain. It is essentially similar to Descartes' concept of pain (Figure 23) proposed three hundred years earlier. It depicts a fixed, straight-through conceptual nervous system. It is precisely this facet of the specificity concept, which imputes a direct, invariant relationship between a psychological sensory dimension and a physical stimulus dimension, that has led to attempts at repudiation of the doctrine of specificity in its entirety.

Consider the proposition that the skin contains 'pain receptors'. To say that a receptor responds only to intense, noxious stimulation of the skin is a physiological statement of fact; it says that the receptor is specialized to respond to a particular kind of stimulus. To call a receptor a 'pain receptor', however, is a psychological assumption: it implies a direct connection from the receptor to a brain centre where pain is felt, so that stimulation of the receptor must always elicit pain and only the sensation of pain. It further implies that the abstraction or selection of information concerning the stimulus occurs entirely at the receptor level and that this information is transmitted faithfully to the brain. The crux of the revolt against specificity, then, is against psychological specificity. This distinction between physiological specialization and psychological assumption also applies to peripheral fibres and central projection systems.

The facts of physiological specialization provide the power of specificity theory. Its psychological assumption is its weakness. This assumption will now be examined in the light of the psychological, clinical, and physiological evidence concerning pain (Melzack and Wall, 1962, 1965).

Psychological evidence. The psychological evidence on pain described in Chapter 2 fails to support the assumption of a one-to-one relationship between pain perception and intensity of the stimulus. Instead, the evidence suggests that the amount and quality of perceived pain are determined by many psychological variables in addition to the sensory input. For example, Pavlov's dogs that received electric shocks, burns, or cuts, followed consistently by the presentation of food, eventually responded to these stimuli as signals for food and failed to show 'even the tiniest and most subtle' (Pavlov, 1927, p. 30) signs of pain. If these dogs felt pain sensation, then it must have been nonpainful pain (Nafe, 1934) or the dogs were out to fool Pavlov and simply refused to reveal that they were feeling pain. Both possibilities, of course, are absurd. The inescapable conclusion from these observations is that intense noxious stimulation can be prevented from producing pain, or may be modified to provide the signal for eating behaviour.

The concept of four rigid modalities of cutaneous experience is wrong. We have already seen (Chapter 3) that the term 'pain' is a broad label for countless different perceptual experiences. Touches, tickles, itches and thermal sensations are also highly variable and rich in quality.

Clinical evidence. Phantom limb pain, causalgia, and the neuralgias provide a dramatic refutation of the concept of a fixed, direct-line nervous system. We have already noted in Chapter 4 that surgical lesions of the peripheral and central nervous system have been singularly unsuccessful in abolishing these pains permanently. Furthermore, gentle touch, vibration, and other non-noxious stimuli can trigger excruciating pain, and sometimes pain occurs spontaneously for long periods without any apparent stimulus. Moreover, new pains and 'trigger zones' may spread unpredictably to unrelated parts of the body where no pathology exists. These clinical facts defy explanation in terms of a rigid, straight-through specific pain system.

Physiological evidence. There is convincing physiological evidence (see Chapter 5) that specialization exists within the somaesthetic system, but none to show that stimulation of one type of receptor, fibre, or spinal pathway elicits sensations in only a single psychological modality. Specialized fibres exist that respond only to intense stimulation, but this does not mean that they are 'pain fibres' – that they must always produce pain, and only pain, when they are stimulated. The neuronography studies described on p. 87 have shown beyond doubt that there is no simple relationship between type of fibre and quality of sensation. Similarly, central cells that respond exclusively or maximally to noxious stimuli are not 'pain cells'. There is no evidence to suggest that they are more important for pain perception and response than all the remaining somaesthetic cells that signal characteristic firing patterns about multiple properties of the stimulus, including noxious intensity. The view that only the cells that respond exclusively to noxious stimuli subserve pain and that the outputs of all other cells are no more than background noise is purely a psychological assumption and has no physiological basis. Physiological specialization is a fact that can be retained without acceptance of the psychological assumption that pain is determined entirely by impulses in a straight-through transmission system from the skin to a pain centre in the brain.

Pattern theory

As a reaction against the psychological assumption in specificity theory, other theories have been proposed which can be grouped under the general heading of 'pattern theory'. Goldscheider (1894), initially one of the champions of von Frey's theory, was the first to propose that stimulus intensity and central summation are the critical determinants of pain.

Goldscheider was profoundly influenced by studies of pathological pain, especially those by Naunyn (1889) on *tabes dorsalis*, which occurs in patients suffering the late stages of syphilis. *Tabes* is characterized by degeneration in the dorsal spinal cord and dorsal roots, and one of its major symptoms is the temporal and spatial summation of somatic input in producing pain (Noordenbos, 1959). Successive, brief applications of a warm test-tube to the skin of a tabetic patient are at first felt only as warm, but then feel increasingly hot until the patient cries out in pain as though his skin is being burned. Such summation never occurs in the normal person, who simply reports successive applications of warmth. Similarly, a single pinprick, which produces a momentary, sharp pain in normal subjects, evokes a diffuse, prolonged, burning pain in tabetic patients.

Not only are the intensity and duration of pain out of proportion to the stimulus, but there is often a remarkable delay in the onset of pain. A pinprick may not be felt until many seconds later – usually a few seconds but sometimes as long as forty-five seconds (Noordenbos, 1959). Observations such as these had a powerful impact on Goldscheider, who was compelled to conclude that mechanisms of central summation, probably in the dorsal horns of the spinal cord, were essential for any understanding of pain mechanisms. The long delays and persistent pain observed in pathological pain states, Goldscheider assumed, are due to abnormally long time-periods of summation.

Several theories have emerged from Goldscheider's concept. All of them recognize the concept of patterning of the input, which is essential for any adequate theory of pain. But some ignore the facts of physiological specialization, while others utilize them in proposing mechanisms of central summation.

Peripheral pattern theory

The simplest form of pattern theory (Weddell, 1955; Sinclair, 1955) deals primarily with peripheral rather than central patterning. That is, pain is considered to be due to excessive peripheral stimulation that produces a pattern of nerve impulses which is interpreted centrally as pain. The theory proposes that all fibre endings (apart from those that innervate hair cells) are alike, so that the pattern for pain is produced by intense stimulation of nonspecific receptors. The physiological evidence, however, reveals a high degree of receptor-fibre specialization. The pattern theory proposed by Weddell and Sinclair fails as a satisfactory theory of pain because it ignores the facts of physiological specialization.

Central summation theory

The analysis of phantom limb pain, causalgia and the neuralgias in Chapter 4 indicates that part, at least, of their underlying mechanisms must be sought in the central nervous system. Livingston (1943) was the first to suggest specific central neural mechanisms to account for the remarkable summation phenomena in these pain syndromes. He proposed that pathological stimulation of sensory nerves (such as occurs after peripheral nerve damage) initiates activity in reverberatory circuits (closed, self-exciting loops of neurons) in the grey matter of the spinal cord. This abnormal activity can then be triggered by normally non-noxious inputs and generate volleys of nerve impulses that are interpreted centrally as pain.

Livingston's theory is especially powerful in explaining phantom limb pain. He proposed that the initial damage to the limb, or the trauma associated with its removal, initiates abnormal firing patterns in reverberatory circuits in the dorsal horns of the spinal cord, which send volleys of nerve impulses to the brain that give rise to pain. Moreover, the reverberatory activity may spread to adjacent neurons in the lateral and ventral horns and produce autonomic and muscular manifestations in the limb, such as sweating and jerking movements of the stump. These, in turn, produce further sensory input, creating a 'vicious circle' between central and peripheral processes that maintains the abnormal spinal activity (Figure 24). Even minor irritations of the skin or nerves near the site of the operation can then feed into these active pools of neurons and keep them in an abnormal, disturbed state over periods of years. Impulse patterns that would normally be interpreted as touch may now trigger these neuron pools into greater activity, thereby sending volleys of impulses to the brain to produce pain. In addition, emotional disturbance may evoke neural activity that feeds into the abnormal neuron pools. Once the abnormal cord activity has become self-sustaining, surgical removal of the peripheral sources of input may not stop it. Rather, clinical procedures that modulate the sensory input, such as local anaesthetic injections or physiotherapy, may again reinstate normal cord activity. There is no physiological evidence of functional reverberatory circuits, but Livingston's concept of sensory modulation to control pain has had a powerful impact on later ideas.

Sensory interaction theory

Related to theories of central summation is the theory that a specialized input-controlling system normally prevents summation from occurring, and that destruction of this system leads to pathological pain states. This theory proposes the existence of a rapidly conducting fibre system which inhibits synaptic transmission in a more slowly conducting system that carries the signals for pain. Historically (see Melzack and Wall, 1965), these two systems are identified as the epicritic and protopathic (Head, 1920), fast and slow (Bishop,

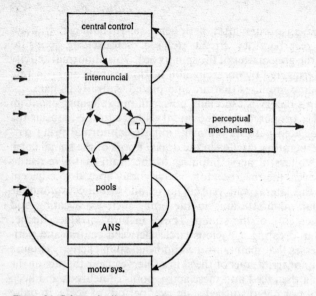

Figure 24. Schematic diagram of W. K. Livingston's (1943) theory of pathological pain states. The intense stimulation (S) resulting from nerve and tissue damage activates fibres that project to internuncial neuron pools in the spinal cord, creating abnormal reverberatory activity in closed self-exciting neuron loops. This prolonged, abnormal activity bombards the spinal cord transmission (T) cells which project to brain mechanisms that underlie pain perception. The abnormal internuncial activity also spreads to lateral and ventral horn cells in the spinal cord, activating the autonomic nervous system (ANS) and motor system, producing sweating, jactitations, and other manifestations. These, in turn, produce further abnormal input, thereby creating a 'vicious circle'. Brain activities such as fear and anxiety evoked by pain also feed into and maintain the abnormal internuncial pool activity.

1946), phylogenetically new and old (Bishop, 1959), and myelinated and unmyelinated (Noordenbos, 1959) fibre systems. Under pathological conditions, the fast system loses its dominance over the slow one, and the result is protopathic sensation (Head, 1920), slow pain (Bishop, 1946), diffuse burning pain (Bishop, 1959), or hyperalgesia (Noordenbos, 1959).

Noordenbos' theory represents an especially important contribution to sensory-interaction concepts. The small fibres are conceived as carrying the nerve impulse patterns that produce pain, while the large fibres inhibit transmission. A shift in the ratio of large-to-small fibres in favour of the small fibres would result in increased neural transmission, summation, and excessive pathological pain. Just as important as the input control by the large fibres, in Noordenbos' concept, is the idea of a multi-synaptic afferent system in the spinal cord. It stands in marked contrast to the idea of a straight-through system, and has the power to explain why spinothalamic cordotomy may fail to abolish pain. The diffuse, extensive connections within the ascending multi-synaptic afferent system, he proposes, can rarely (if ever) be totally abolished (unless the whole spinal cord is cut), so that there is always a 'leak' for impulses to ascend to the brain to produce pain.

Affect theory of pain

The theory that pain is a sensory modality is relatively recent. A much older theory, dating back to Aristotle, considers pain to be an emotion – the opposite of pleasure – rather than a sensation. Indeed, this idea of pain is part of an intriguing and usually neglected bit of history (Dallenbach, 1939). At the turn of the century, a bitter battle was fought on the question of pain specificity. Von Frey argued that there are specific pain receptors, while Goldscheider contended that pain is produced by excessive skin stimulation and central summation. But there was a third man in the battle – H. R. Marshall (1894), a philosopher and psychologist – who said, essentially, 'a plague on both your houses; pain is an emotional quality, or *quale*, that colours all sensory events'. He admitted the existence of a pricking-cutting sense, but thought that pain was distinctly different. For pain does not have just a sensory quality; it also has a strong negative affective quality that drives us into activity (Figure 25). We are compelled to do something about it, to take the most effective course of action to stop it, and, of course, this behaviour is in the realm of emotion and motivation.

The remarkable development of sensory physiology and psychophysics during the twentieth century has given momentum to the concept of pain as a sensation and has overshadowed the role of affective and motivational processes. The sensory approach to pain, however, valuable as it has been, fails to provide a complete picture of pain processes. The assumption that pain is a primary sensation has relegated motivational (and cognitive) processes to the role of 'reactions to pain' (Figure 25), and has made them only 'secondary considerations' in the whole pain process (Sweet, 1959). It is apparent, however, that sensory motivational, and cognitive processes occur in parallel, interacting systems at the same time. As we noted in Chapter 7, motivational-affective processes must be included in any satisfactory theory of pain.

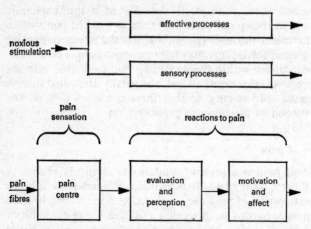

Figure 25. Top: diagram of Marshall's (1894) concept of pain as an affective quality or *quale*. Intense stimulation of the skin activates two parallel systems: one is the basis of the affective properties of the experience, the other underlies the sensory properties. *Bottom:* diagram of the concept, implicit in specificity theory, that motivation and affect are reactions to pain, but are not part of the primary pain sensation.
(from Melzack and Casey, 1968)

Evaluation of the theories

When we consider all the theories examined so far, we see that the 'specific-modality' and 'pattern' concepts of pain, although they appear to be mutually exclusive, both contain valuable concepts that supplement one another. Recognition of receptor specialization for the transduction of particular kinds and ranges of cutaneous stimulation does not preclude acceptance of the concept that the information generated by skin receptors is coded in the form of patterns of nerve impulses. The law of the adequate stimulus can be retained without also accepting a narrow, fixed relationship between receptor specialization and perceptual experience.

It is clear that von Frey made an important contribution that must be retained in any theoretical formulation. He proposed that the receptors of the skin are not all alike but are differentiated with respect to lowest threshold to particular energy categories. Indeed, recent evidence indicates a greater degree of receptor specialization than von Frey himself could ever have foreseen. Similarly, there can no longer be any doubt that temporal and spatial patterns of nerve impulses provide the basis of our sensory perceptions. The coding of information in the form of nerve impulse patterns is a fundamental concept in contemporary neurophysiology and psychology.

The concepts of central summation and input control have shown remarkable power in their ability to explain many of the clinical phenomena of pain. Goldscheider's emphasis on central summation mechanisms is supported by the clinical observations of extraordinary temporal and spatial summation in pathological pain syndromes.

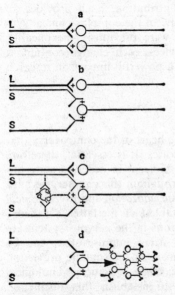

Figure 26. Schematic representation of conceptual models of pain mechanisms – a, von Frey's specificity theory. Large (L) and small (S) fibres are assumed to transmit touch and pain impulses respectively, in separate, specific, straight-through pathways to touch and pain centres in the brain – b, Goldscheider's summation theory, showing convergence of small fibres on to a dorsal horn cell. Touch is assumed to be carried by large fibres – c, Livingston's (1943) conceptual model of reverberatory circuits underlying pathological pain states. Prolonged activity in the self-exciting chain of neurons bombards the dorsal horn cell, which transmits abnormally patterned volleys of nerve impulses to the brain – d, Noordenbos' (1959) sensory interaction theory, in which large fibres inhibit (−) and small fibres excite (+) central transmission neurons. The output projects to spinal cord neurons which are conceived by Noordenbos to comprise a Multi-synaptic Afferent System. (from Melzack and Wall, 1970, p. 3)

Livingston's theory of spinal reverberatory activity that persists in the absence of noxious input provides a satisfactory explanation of prolonged pain. Noordenbos' concept that large fibres inhibit activity in small fibres is supported by the evidence that pathological pain is often associated with a loss of large myelinated fibres. These theories, nevertheless, fail to comprise a satisfactory general theory of pain. They lack unity, and no single theory has yet been proposed that integrates the diverse theoretical mechanisms.

However, when all the theories – from specificity theory onward – are examined together (Figure 26), is apparent that each successive theory makes an important contribution. Each provides an additional mechanism to explain some of the complex clinical syndromes or experimental data that were previously inexplicable. Despite the seemingly small differences, each change contains a major conceptual idea that has had a powerful impact on research and therapy.

On the concept of 'specificity'

The concept of 'specificity' lies at the heart of the controversy that surrounds the evolution of pain theories. It is essential, therefore, that we conclude by examining the concept in order to state unequivocally what we mean by it. Throughout this chapter, we have distinguished between *physiological specialization* and *psychological specificity*. The former is an indisputable fact; the latter is a theory for which there is no evidence. Neurons in the nervous system are *specialized* to conduct patterns of nerve impulses that can be recorded and displayed. But no neurons in the somatic projection system are indisputably linked to a single, specific psychological experience. Despite our attempts to establish this distinction (Melzack and Wall, 1962, 1965), many of our colleagues have failed to understand the distinction or continue to use the word 'specificity' in the sense of specialization but without saying so. If we can all agree that 'specificity' means physiological specialization, *without* implying that specialized neurons *must* give rise to the experience of pain and *only* to pain, or that pain can *never* occur unless they are activated, then we will have eliminated a major source of unnecessary controversy.

9 Gate-Control and Other Mechanisms

A new theory of pain, to be useful, must incorporate the known facts about the nervous system, provide a plausible explanation for clinical pains, and stimulate experiments to test the theory, including procedures that are potential new therapies. The gate-control theory, which we proposed in 1965, met these requirements. Subsequent experiments on the details of the theory support the general concept and elaborate upon it. Recent research has revealed new phenomena of plasticity in the nervous system which cannot be incorporated into the theory but which complement it and operate in addition to a gate-control.

Several facts, described in previous chapters, must be explained by any new theory: (1) the relationship between injury and pain is highly variable; (2) innocuous stimuli may produce pain; (3) the location of pain may be different from the location of damage; (4) pain may persist in the absence of injury or after healing; (5) the nature and location of pain changes with time; (6) pain is not a single sensation but has many dimensions; (7) there is no adequate treatment for certain types of pain, most of which fall into four categories: deep tissue damage (such as arthritis); peripheral nerve damage (such as amputation); root damage (such as arachnoiditis) and idiopathic pains, in which there is no sign of tissue damage and for which there is no agreed cause (such as most low back pains and headaches including migraine).

We shall first describe the gate-control theory, then the new developments, and finally we shall examine the adequacy of the theory and subsequent research in explaining the above list of facts about pain.

Mechanism 1: gate-control

The mechanism in which nerve impulses enter the spinal cord and proceed to the brain comprises five stages. In the following diagrams, the sign ⊣ indicates the end of an input at which one system influences the next. The symbol ○ indicates a group of cells involved in transmitting information or influencing its flow. The following are the five stages we used in developing the original model.

Stage 1

Small-diameter peripheral nerve fibres (S), which are the small myelinated A-delta fibres and the unmyelinated C fibres, are stimulated by injury. They deliver impulses, directly and indirectly, to transmission cells in the spinal cord (T) which transmit to local reflex circuits and to the brain:

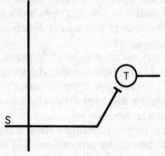

This stage incorporates all that is shown in Descartes' concept of pain (Fig. 23, p. 150).

Stage 2

No synaptic junctions in the central nervous system are as simple as that shown in Stage 1. All synaptic regions include cells which facilitate and inhibit the flow of impulses. It was necessary to propose that there are facilitatory cells in the region of the T cells because it was known that all cells in the dorsal horn of the spinal cord fire a prolonged burst of impulses after the arrival of a brief input volley (Wall, 1960). Furthermore, if this volley is repeated at regular intervals, the after-discharge becomes more and more prolonged (Mendell and Wall, 1965). The after-discharge and its 'wind-up' led us to incorporate an excitatory interneuron in the basic diagram:

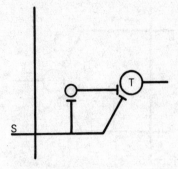

Stage 3

Early recordings from cells in the spinal cord (Wall, 1960) revealed cells which not only responded to the small, high-threshold fibres but were also excited by large, low-threshold myelinated afferent fibres (L). Later work showed that these cells with both L and S inputs were by far the most common of the centrally projecting cells which signal injury (Wall, 1967; McMahon and Wall, 1984; Yaksh, 1986). Since these cells respond to light pressure on the skin and increase their frequency of response as the pressure stimulus rises in intensity to a strong pinch, they have been called wide-dynamic range (WDR) cells (Mendell, 1966). There is also a minority of cells which are not excited by low-level stimuli and only respond when smaller afferent fibres are stimulated. These are called nociceptive specific (NS) cells. There is also a third group of cells which respond only to low intensity pressure stimuli. The specificity theorists concentrated on the NS cells as the only cells which could be involved in triggering pain. We, on the other hand, simply proposed that pain would be triggered if the firing rate of any group of cells exceeded a critical level determined by the properties of the brain. Much of the detailed work since 1965 has concentrated on the sensory roles of the WDR and NS groups of cells. When we discuss new developments in the theory, we will see that the most recent results support our original proposal in unexpected ways. In the diagram below, an excitatory large-fibre, low-threshold input is shown, meaning that the T cell is of the WDR type which responds over the full range of inputs. When the L input is missing or is inactivated, the T cell becomes an NS type:

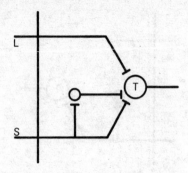

Stage 4

Generally, all synaptic regions contain both inhibitory and excitatory mechanisms which control transmission depending on the balance of their activity. The inhibitory cells are shown in the diagram (below) as a filled circle, while the facilitating cells are open circles. It was found that large-diameter afferents can excite as well as inhibit the T cells (Wall, 1964). This double effect is related to a spatial separation of inputs from large-diameter fibers in which those from the centre of the receptive field excite the cell, while those from a large surrounding area inhibit the cell (Hillman and Wall, 1969). In the dorsal horn of the spinal cord, close to the T cells, there is the densely packed layer of small cells, the substantia gelatinosa. None of the lamina 2 cells project over long distances, and are therefore candidates to be the inhibitory and excitatory interneurons. One type of inhibition was shown to be due to activity in the substantia gelatinosa (Wall, 1964); for this reason, we guessed that the inhibitory and excitatory interneurons are located in the substantia gelatinosa.

   When we proposed the theory, inhibition had been shown with certainty to occur at the terminals of afferent nerve fibres, which reduced their effect on the T cells (Wall, 1964). Postsynaptic inhibition, in which inhibitory cells act directly on the T cells, was assumed to occur but had not yet been demonstrated. Since presynaptic inhibition was the only one identified at the time, it was shown in the diagram of the gate theory while in the text we stated that postsynaptic inhibitions were also likely. Their discovery a few years later gave further strength to the theory:

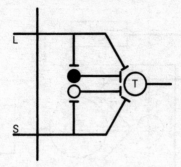

Stage 5

It has long been known that powerful influences descend from the brain and modulate spinal reflexes (Sherrington, 1906). In 1954, Hagbarth and Kerr showed that these descending effects also changed sensory messages travelling from the cord to the brain. Taub (1964) later showed that local stimulation in the midbrain and medulla inhibits the firing of T cells. Furthermore, there was evidence that a powerful, steady inhibition flowed continually from the brainstem on to T cells (Wall, 1967). It was therefore reasonable to include a descending influence on the inhibitory interneurons:

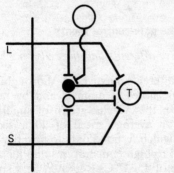

Finally, we assumed that ascending messages to the brain can influence the descending controls, thereby completing a loop from spinal cord to brain and back to the spinal cord. The first formulation of the gate-control theory in 1965 was shown thus:

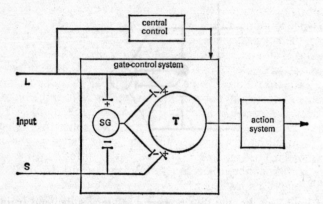

Figure 27. Schematic diagram of the gate-control theory of pain: L, the large-diameter fibres; S, the small-diameter fibres. The fibres project to the substantia gelatinosa (SG) and first central transmission (T) cells. The inhibitory effect exerted by SG on the afferent fibre terminals is increased by activity in L fibres and decreased by activity in S fibres. The central control trigger is represented by a line running from the large fibre system to the central control mechanisms; these mechanisms, in turn, project back to the gate-control system. The T cells project to the action system +, excitation; −, inhibition.
(from Melzack and Wall, 1965, p. 971)

Developments of the gate-control theory

Stage 1: Nociceptive afferents and the cells on which they end

The nociceptive afferents have been thoroughly investigated by dissection of single fibres in animals and by neuronographic recording in man. In the A-delta group of small myelinated fibres conducting with an average speed of 20 m/sec, there are large numbers of fibres which respond only to firm pinches. A fraction of these also respond to high temperatures and increase their firing in the noxious range of 45–47°C. Repeated heat stimuli sensitize the fibres so that they respond to smaller increases in heat. The un-myelinated C fibres in man, which conduct at less than 1 m/sec, respond to heavy pressure, to intense heat and to noxious chemicals, and are called polymodal nociceptors. Repeated stimulation leads to desensitization, unlike the A-delta fibres, which become more sensitive.

Those who wish to defend the old specificity theory have used the data from simultaneous recording from single peripheral neurons and reports of sensation when a person is given a shock to the skin. The defence amounts to the statement that the bigger the stimulus, the more the nociceptors fire and the greater the pain. This is hardly surprising. Wall and McMahon (1985) have used the same data to provide a strong defence of the presence of a gate control. Even in highly trained volunteer subjects there are at least three major mismatches between nociceptor firing and pain. First, the onset of firing does not coincide with the onset of pain. Second, the time course of firing relates very poorly to the time course of the pain. Third, identical pains evoked by different stimuli such as punctate pressure or heat are associated with strikingly different patterns of activity in afferent fibres. Specificity theorists carefully avoid discussing pathological pains, which, they admit, do not follow the rules of the normal nervous system. However, it seems totally unsatisfactory to explain 'normal' pain and leave the pains which matter, those of the suffering patients, for a later time and another explanation. Our conclusion from the experimental results as well as from patients' reports, is that pain is the result of an analysis by the central nervous system of the entire situation at the time, taking into account the firing of nociceptors as well as other data at its disposal. The beginning of that analysis starts as the afferent messages enter the spinal cord.

An obvious problem with the gate-control theory was that it grouped together the A-delta and C fibres. Specificity theorists have not done any better, since they simply assign 'fast pain' to the A-delta and 'slow pain' to the C fibres. They do not explain the significance of these two pains or why there should be two apparently redundant pain systems. At the end of this chapter we will review the new data which show that the myelinated and unmyelinated fibres have totally separate functions which are at least consistent with the gate theory but not with specificity theory.

Much more is now known about the precise terminations of the nociceptors. The C fibres end entirely on cells in the uppermost laminae. So do the A-delta fibres, but they also send a few deeply penetrating branches into deeper laminae. There is an amazingly accurate local map of these afferents so that each area in the periphery has its area represented by sensory terminals in the spinal cord. This precision mapping of locus of origin and of type of fibre allows an analysis of the firing of the cells on which the afferents end. As we shall see, there is not a hint of a simple, straight-through transmitting cell.

Stage 2: The presence of excitatory interneurons

There has been little progress in the further analysis of this stage. The basic facts of the after-discharge of dorsal horn cells have been repeatedly confirmed, but the interneurons which are responsible have not been found. This is not surprising since nerve cells have many functions which operate at different times so that it is difficult to trace serial links in which one cell always affects another in a fixed, reliable manner. Much more progress has been made in studies of inhibitory interneurons (Stage 4).

Stage 3: The convergence of excitation by low- and high-threshold afferent fibres

Three types of cells have been observed in the dorsal horn: 1) those which respond only to low-threshold afferents, 2) those which respond only to high-threshold afferents (nociceptive specific, NS), 3) those which respond to both low- and high-threshold afferents (wide-dynamic range, WDR). This has been repeatedly confirmed, but the number of cells in the three classes varies widely among different studies depending on the method of search and the excitable state of the nervous system. The significance of the results clearly depends on the attitude of the experimenter. If he or she accepts the idea of fixed, hard-wired lines, then the three classes of cells represent three kinds of anatomical contact of afferent fibres on to nerve cells. If, however, he or she accepts the idea that convergence onto cells is under excitatory and inhibitory control, then the three classes may represent three settings of the control mechanism. If the fixed-line approach were correct, similar numbers would be recorded over a wide range of experimental conditions. The facts show highly variable numbers, with the WDR cells becoming predominant in excitable spinal cords. The extreme examples are seen in recent studies. In one, the investigators were unable to detect any NS cells in conditions of light anaesthesia (Korzeniewska *et al.*, 1986). In another, it was shown that single cells moved from NS to WDR as anaesthesia increased (Collins and Ren, 1987). In a third, the modality of single cells moved from cutaneous to proprioceptive, depending on the presence of descending controls from the brain (Wall, 1967).

For the specificity theorist, it is obvious that pain is the consequence of the firing of NS cells. However, a study in man and monkeys involving stimulation of the spinal cord suggests that pain is related to the WDR cells rather than the NS cells (Mayer *et al.*, 1975). In a more direct study, both types of cell were recorded in monkeys trained to avoid noxious stimuli (Bushnell *et al.*, 1984); the NS cells were found to be much too insensitive to explain the discriminative behaviour of the animals, while the firing of the WDR cells matched the ability of the animal to discriminate. A third example relates to lamina 1 cells which are in the best anatomical position to receive synaptic contacts from the arriving nociceptive afferents, and which include the specific nociceptive cells believed by specificity theorists to be responsible for pain (Perl, 1985). It was discovered that the major projection pathway of such cells is through the contralateral dorsolateral white matter to the midbrain (McMahon and Wall, 1984, 1985). Unfortunately for specificity theory, section of the axons of these cells does not produce analgesia but, rather, a hyperalgesia, which suggests that they are part of a pain control circuit rather than the pain projection pathway.

The WDR cells may also play a role in referred pain. In the thoracic and lumbar spinal cord, cells which receive small afferents from the heart and abdominal organs also receive low-threshold afferents from the skin (Pomeranz *et al.*, 1968; Cervero, 1985). In other words, these WDR cells have their small-fibre input from one origin and their large-fibre input from another. This mechanism can explain referred pain, in which pain due to pathology in a deep structure seems to come from a cutaneous area which is often tender.

Stage 4: Inhibitory interneurons control transmission

Wall and Sweet (1967) tested this stage of the gate-control by stimulating nerves supplying a painful region with low-level electrical stimuli which are just sufficient to activate large low-threshold afferents. The patient feels tingling sensations in the area supplied by the nerve and, simultaneously, many pains are reduced to tolerable levels (Woolf, 1984). Stimulation of the appropriate nerve may be accomplished by transcutaneous electrical nerve stimulation (TENS), which has become a widely used treatment, or stimulation of electrodes implanted around a nerve, which is too complex for routine use. A simpler procedure is stimulation of the dorsal columns, a widely used technique in which an electrode is placed on the dura without surgery by means of an epidural catheter (Krainick and Thoden, 1994). These treatments support this phase of the gate-control theory, but go beyond it because the stimulation helps control not only pain but also abnormal muscle contractions associated with nerve or spinal cord damage.

The biological significance of both excitatory and inhibitory effects of large afferents on to T cells was revealed by Hillman & Wall (1969), who found that the excitatory large afferent fibres originate from the centre of a receptive field, while the fibres from the edge produce inhibition. This is a common type of organization, seen in visual, auditory and somatosensory pathways. It is a powerful way to achieve spatial discrimination of the size, shape and location of a stimulus. Even beyond the edge of a large receptive field of low-threshold afferents, intense stimuli have an inhibitory effect to counteract the excitatory effect of small fibres in the centre (Le Bars *et al.*, 1983). This phenomenon, which is called diffuse noxious inhibitory control (DNIC), is believed to involve an ascending limb to the brainstem which activates descending inhibitory systems that affect spinal cord cells. This interaction, in which an intense stimulus at one site inhibits an intense stimulus at a distant site, has been proposed to be the basis of pain-relieving procedures in folk medicine and 'counter-irritation' that use intense stimulation such as electric shocks and ice (Melzack, 1984b). Thus, there are two inhibitory interactions: the local inhibition of small-fibre excitation by large afferents as shown in the gate-control diagram and the distant inhibition by intense stimulation of small fibres as in DNIC.

It is now known that C-fibre function is more complex than that indicated in the gate-control diagram. Capsaicin has provided us with a tool to poison the majority of C fibres while leaving the A fibres intact. It immediately produces some analgesia to thermal stimulation but does not affect mechanical pain, which is not surprising since the A-delta fibres are intact. After some time, however, new excitatory connections are unmasked in the spinal cord (Fitzgerald, 1982) and the animal shows an increased reaction to nerve damage. We have, here, another example of the central nervous system increasing its excitability when an input fails, which we shall discuss later as one of the mechanisms of pain after nerve damage.

Soon after the publication of the gate-control theory with its emphasis on presynaptic mechanisms, it was discovered (as expected) that there is also postsynaptic inhibition. Surprisingly, it is still not known if and when these two types of inhibition occur independently in vertebrates, although it is certain in invertebrates. However, it is now generally agreed that the presynaptic inhibition involves the chemical gamma-aminobutyric acid (GABA) which is released from cells in the dorsal laminae and which depolarizes the afferent terminals, thereby decreasing their excitatory effect.

The inhibitory mechanisms which involve the endogenous opioids have been studied intensively. Opioids are released by cells in the substantia gelatinosa in the form of enkephalins or dynorphins. (*Opiates* usually refers to morphine and other opium derivatives, *opioids* to morphine-like substances such as endorphins, and *narcotics* is a loose term which refers to both groups of compounds.) The discovery of endogenous opioids, opioid receptors and descending inhibition, which depends on the release of endogenous opioids in the spinal cord, led to studies of narcotic action in the spinal cord. The highest concentration of these endogenous opioids is in the substantia gelatinosa. Micro-injection of morphine into the substantia gelatinosa produces inhibition which is abolished by the narcotic antagonist naloxone.

This was an exciting period in the development of the gate-control theory since it led to the chemical identification of one component and to the therapeutic use of narcotics applied directly to the cord to produce analgesia only in the segments bathed in them. We still do not know if this narcotic action is presynaptic, postsynaptic or both, and we do not know the natural circumstances that bring them into action. We must also keep in mind that many other endogenous inhibitory chemicals exist in the substantia gelatinosa and that the mechanisms of action of most of them remain unknown.

Stage 5: descending controls

Electrical stimulation of the periventricular hypothalamus, periaqueductal grey and medial lower brainstem produces analgesia in animals and humans (see Chapter 7). Fibres from these areas project through the dorsolateral funiculus of the spinal cord to the dorsal horns, where most fibres terminate in the substantia gelatinosa, and some penetrate more deeply into lamina 5.

The major physiological effect of these descending pathways is an inhibition of the deeper cells. However, there is also some excitation, particularly of cells in lamina 1, whose functional role is unknown. The inhibition of the deeper cells is selective; it reduces the excitatory effect of small-diameter afferents but does not affect excitation by the large low-threshold afferent fibres. Here we have the basis for a selective mechanism which produces analgesia to intense stimuli but does not affect signals evoked by mild stimuli. These controls go far beyond a simple gain control on cells which transmit information about one type of stimulus. As work proceeded on this phase of the gate-control, it became apparent that the type of stimulus to which the cell responded was under control to the extent that a cell sometimes signalled events from muscle and at other times events at the skin. The 'modality' control extends the simple gate-control into dimensions which were not originally considered.

These exciting discoveries raised the question: when do the controls operate? The answer is that they can be forced into action by local electrical stimulation or by locally applied chemicals. Gentle rubbing, TENS or dorsal column stimulation brings into action the local segmental control. Intense distant stimulation also produces descending inhibition which may involve ascending messages which in turn trigger the descending controls. These are all very crude phenomena which can hardly explain the presence of an elaborate, interconnected, many-factored control mechanism. Removal of the entire forebrain (decerebration), another crude manipulation, provides valuable clues. After decerebration, the remaining nervous system adopts an exaggerated sensory and motor posture in which the importance of muscle information is grossly exaggerated while that from skin is diminished. This shows the possibility of the brain's ability to provide a steady drive to the spinal cord which has the effect of exaggerating one class of message while almost abolishing another. Recent studies point to an even more subtle two-stage mechanism: 1) the brain gives 'permission' to local circuits in the spinal cord to respond if the situation merits the response, and 2) the local spinal cord circuits measure the input and trigger a reflex response if they are permitted to do so by the brain, and if the afferent input is sufficient. In any organizational flow chart there is a considerable difference between being permitted to respond and being ordered to respond.

Summary of gate-control developments

Each of the five stages which made up the gate-control mechanism have been supported by subsequent work. However, they are not sufficient to explain some of the basic facts about pain listed at the beginning of the chapter. Two completely different mechanisms were later discovered which have no relation to the gate-control but which add to it and do not contradict it. We shall now describe these two new factors and then return to examine how close we have come to understanding the basic facts about pain.

Mechanism 2: impulse-triggered prolonged pain mechanisms

In Chapter 3, we described the sensory consequences of a twisted ankle, with its early, sharp phase and a later deep, dull phase. The first phase is in a time epoch where the gate-control mechanism certainly plays a part, but we must now ask if it relates to the second phase.

There have been two traditional explanations for the second prolonged phase. First, local inflammatory changes produced by the injury affect the afferent nerve fibres in several ways: the original mechanical injury sensitizes the nociceptors so that their threshold falls; tissue breakdown products, such as the prostaglandins, sensitize nerve endings; substances leak from stimulated nociceptors which produce vasodilation, oedema and sensitization; stimulated nociceptors become sensitive to noradrenaline produced by the sympathetic nervous system. These changes provide a rationale for local therapy such as aspirin, ice packs, bandaging, and so forth. However, the changes are so widespread in terms of sensitivity and altered motor pattern that it is widely agreed that there must be some prolonged reaction in the central nervous system. This central change was believed to be due to 'reverberating circuits', but there is no evidence for this simple idea. Long-term changes beyond the first few seconds need an explanation other than the gate-control type which is dependent on classical synaptic transmission. We shall describe the observed facts beyond this classical period of the first few seconds. This work is described in a series of papers by Cook *et al.*, 1986a,b), Woolf (1983), Wall and Woolf (1984, 1986) and Woolf and Wall (1986).

The effect of a brief input volley on the flexion reflex

The flexion reflex (withdrawal of a limb from a noxious stimulus) is a stable response of the spinal cord. If a sudden, intense stimulus (which simulates an injury) is applied to the skin of the leg, there is an exaggeration of the flexion reflex which is explained by the gate-control mechanism. However, if the intense stimulation has occurred in deep tissue, the falling phase of the exaggeration is followed, after several minutes, by a second slow-onset phase which reaches a maximum after more than ten minutes and then persists for long periods. This fits the common experience that a skin injury such as a cut or a burn may hurt a great deal at the time, depending on the set of the gate, but later decreases, leaving a localized tender area in the limb. In contrast, a trivial deep injury such as a twisted ankle, persists and spreads, producing widespread tenderness and difficulty in using the limb. We shall now discuss this second phase of pain, which is the major source of misery for many chronic pain patients; they are not in continuous pain since they can find a comfortable position, but find that gentle, normal movement or touch triggers intolerable pain.

Studies of the input responsible for this second phase showed that it had to involve the unmyelinated afferent fibres, while the A-delta nociceptors produced only the immediate disturbance. There was found to be a range in the ability of different types of tissue to produce the prolonged spreading phase; joints (most effective) through periarticular tissue, viscera such as the bladder, muscle, deep fascia, to skin (least effective).

Prolonged sensitivity is triggered by nerve impulses but sustained by a central mechanism

That the prolonged second phase is sustained by a central mechanism is apparent in the observation that the prolonged effect could be initiated by a brief 20-second electrical stimulation of nerves in which no further afferent barrage occurs after the stimulus stops. In order to be certain that this was the case, the prolonged exaggeration was produced by briefly applying a chemical which stimulates C fibres to joints. When the prolonged sensitivity was fully established after 15 minutes, the joint was completely anaesthetized but the sensitivity continued. If the joint was first anaesthetized and then received the chemical stimulus, nothing happened. This latent period during which a central change is triggered has practical implications since it provides a rationale for early treatment of injuries. Sports medicine provides an example of this: small injuries are treated immediately with analgesics, ice packs and cold sprays which have been found to prevent the frequent consequences of small injuries – the crippling of athletes for days or weeks after the injury.

Mechanisms

Location
It is apparent that damage to deep tissue results in a rapid increase in sensitivity which then persists and spreads. No changes have been detected in the afferent fibres from the tender areas, either at their peripheral ends or in their terminals in the spinal cord. Since the

motor neuron reflexes are highly exaggerated, it is possible that the motor neurons have become hyperexcitable, but in fact they are completely unchanged. This leaves the interneurons as the likely location of the enhanced excitability. A brief input volley from unmyelinated afferents originating from muscle (but not from skin) is followed by a long-latency, prolonged spread of the receptive fields of these cells. A punctate injury is followed by the slow spread of receptive fields of cells which normally do not respond to the region of injury until they eventually incorporate it (McMahon and Wall, 1984). Most impressive are the results obtained with cells which respond only to noxious stimuli in the normal state. These cells also show a marked spread of their receptive fields and, in addition, become so sensitive that they now respond to innocuous stimuli as well as to noxious stimuli. This long-lasting conversion of NS to WDR cells is not only a refutation of specificity theory but, much more importantly, a likely mechanism for the tenderness – allodynia – which often follows small, deep injuries.

The prolonged sensitivity is not the consequence of injury-induced firing of the interneurons

Injury or stimulation of a peripheral nerve at sufficient intensity to involve unmyelinated afferents produces an initial burst of activity followed by a second phase of increased excitability which builds up as the firing dies down. It has been assumed that the second phase is a consequence of the initial firing, but experiments show that this is not the case. When a peripheral nerve is cut, there is an ensuing series of changes in the cut nerves and in the spinal cord. One of these changes is the disappearance of inhibitions in the spinal cord. A consequence of this is that stimulation of the cut nerve central to the cut produces a larger than normal level of central firing because the inhibitory components of the gate have failed. If the secondary excitability of the spinal cord were a consequence of the firing of the central cells, stimulation of a cut nerve should produce exaggerated central firing and an exaggerated second phase. The observation, in fact, is that the exaggerated central firing occurs but the second phase is completely abolished. We therefore need to postulate a double mechanism – a fast-acting mechanism which involves a gate-control and a long-latency, long-duration mechanism which is triggered by the arrival of impulses in C afferents and which does not depend on the rapid firing of interneurons or T cells.

Chemistry

The observations described above show that C afferents, particularly from deep tissue, have a double central action – rapid excitation followed by an independent, slow-onset, prolonged facilitation. The evidence so far suggests that the fast excitation is the consequence of the release of amino acids. However, C afferents also contain a variety of peptides which are excitatory, and it has been difficult to explain why the same fibres should emit two different classes of chemicals. However, now we know that C fibres produce two different effects in the spinal cord. In addition, it is well known that cutting a peripheral nerve depletes the C fibres of most of their peptide content so that we can now propose why such fibres retain their ability to produce the rapid excitation but lose their long-term effects. This points to a possible role for C fibres and their peptide content. It becomes even more intriguing to find that the peptide content of C fibres depends on the tissue from which the fibres originate. The peptide content of muscle C fibres, which produce prolonged facilitation, is very different from that of skin C fibres, which produce only a brief effect. Moreover, local application of peptides to the cord can convert the brief cutaneous C afferent effect to the prolonged muscle C afferent facilitation. This observation plays a key role in a new dimension of understanding of the function of narcotics. We noted earlier that narcotics act as analgesics partly by imitating a local peptide mechanism within the dorsal horn. A moderate dose of morphine, which has no effect on acute pain but which controls postoperative pain, has no effect on the flexion reflex or on the firing of interneurons but wipes out the long-latency, long-duration facilitation produced by C afferents. A picture is beginning to emerge of a second system of transmission control in the dorsal horn which is dependent on peptides.

Summary

The arrival of nerve impulses in the dorsal horn induces immediate excitations, reflexes and sensations by means of a gate-control mechanism. It also triggers long-latency, long-lasting changes in a different mechanism which sustains prolonged, widespread increases of excitability and sensitivity. The existence of this second mechanism may appear to be an unfortunate complication, but in fact it offers the exciting possibility of independent therapeutic control of acute pain and of its secondary consequences which relate to

peptides and the special properties of unmyelinated fibres that originate in deep tissue.

Mechanism 3: transport-controlled prolonged pain mechanisms

This mechanism, which we discussed in Chapter 5, operates in
parallel with the gate-control and the impulse-triggered control
mechanisms. Here, we shall briefly recapitulate the main facts.

(1) When a peripheral nerve is cut, a cascade of changes sweeps
centrally during the ensuing days and weeks which alters the
chemistry and physiology of the dorsal root ganglion cells, the
motor neurons and the central terminals of the sensory fibres.
(2) Changes in the afferents induce changes in the spinal cord
which include a reduction of inhibitions, a spread of receptive
fields and an increase of excitability.
(3) The delayed peripheral and central changes are not produced
by nerve impulses since they are not altered by prolonged
impulse blockade or by lesions, such as crush injury, which
imitate the changes of afferent barrage produced by nerve
section.
(4) The time course and other properties of the central changes
support the proposal that they are produced by changes in
chemicals transported within the axons of sensory fibres. Since
most of the changes can be produced by the specific C fibre
poison, capsaicin, it is believed that the unmyelinated afferents
play a particularly important role.
(5) The chemicals and their messages remain unknown although
nerve growth factor is a prominent candidate.

This brief summary of extensive work by many groups introduces
a new dimension to pain mechanisms. It relates to the special pains
associated with peripheral nerve and dorsal root injury. The first
hints of this axon transport mechanism came from the observation
that the central consequences of a crushed nerve are different from
those of a cut nerve. In a sense, the spinal cord seemed to 'diagnose'
the nature of the injury, even though peripheral axons are equally
interrupted in both lesions. It was recently discovered that when C
fibres are forced to grow into a new type of tissue, they take on the
characteristics of the new tissue and change their central actions
accordingly. This discovery tells us that C fibres are continually
sensitive to the type of tissue in which they end, and suggests that
they detect, by chemical means, not only the existence of grossly

pathological tissue but of subtle variations including the presence of normal tissue transplated to the 'wrong' place. This would give C fibres the role of 'chemical pathologist', reporting that all is well or that deviations from the normal are occurring. Peripheral abnormality detected by C fibres and signalled by a change of chemical transport could result in attempts by the central nervous system to compensate for the peripheral abnormality. This could obviously play an important role in pain mechanisms.

Implications of the three mechanisms in understanding pain

The three mechanisms we have just described make up the beginning of a theory to explain the basis of acute and chronic pain. They have stimulated experiments and speculation, and they must be checked against the seven aspects of clinical pain listed at the beginning of this chapter.

The relationship between injury and pain is highly variable

This obvious fact has long been a puzzle to specificity theorists. Any deviation from the expected one-to-one psychophysical relationship led to suspicions of a psychological abnormality. Generations of patients failed to impress their doctors with their pain. Those who did not feel pain in the presence of injury as well as those who complained of pain in the absence of injury were all condemned as psychologically suspect. The gate-control theory not only liberated thinking from this strait-jacket, but pointed to the dorsal horns as the place to look for the beginning of the basis of the variable relationship between injury and pain.

The three mechanisms, each with its own time epoch, operate within a range of variability that is determined by the demands of the environment and the needs of the brain. We must take into account, in understanding a response to injury, that the state of other tissue is important, and the state of the brain is equally important. Its job is to assess priorities of behaviour. In our motor performance, we are not puppets driven by strings; similarly, in our sensory world, we seek and select that information relevant to our needs, rather than being the passive recipients of whatever happens in our world.

This approach makes variability an expected, even welcome, phenomenon rather than a surprise to be denied. The effects of mood, culture, experience and expectation fall into place as part of a unified and integrated system and not as mysteries to be pushed aside or assigned to a totally separate mechanism of the mind. For example, the placebo effect – the actual relief of pain based on the expectation that pain will go away after treatment – is no longer magic or madness but a demonstration that the entire central nervous system, including the segmental reflex circuits, can adopt a 'no-pain' mode. The approach provides not only an explanation but, also, ample justification for the combination of psychological therapies along with direct intervention at the source of the pain and at transmission pathways.

Innocuous stimuli may produce pain (allodynia)

In several kinds of chronic pain, such as causalgia, tender areas become so sensitive that even a gentle touch evokes terrible pain. Specificity theory explains such a state by arguing that nociceptors have been converted into pathologically sensitive, low-threshold mechanoreceptors. While this sensitization undoubtedly occurs (termed primary hyperalgesia), the condition spreads so far from the area of injury that it is clear that the central nervous system has become hyperexcitable, so that normal impulses from normal tissue are handled by abnormal central circuits which grossly amplify the input. This is most obvious in referred pain where areas of skin distant from the disease become tender. Mechanism 2, in which unmyelinated afferents trigger prolonged, centrally sustained states, seems to be a probable origin of many such pains. The evidence that this mechanism involves particular peptides suggests that a selective drug action may some day be discovered which will counteract the mechanism and abolish the pain.

The location of pain may differ from the location of damage

We have already discussed the neural mechanisms that underlie many forms of referred pain (p. 54). Cells in lamina 5 of the dorsal horns receive a convergence of fibres from skin and viscera (Pomeranz et al., 1968), and the projection of the outputs of these cells to the brain would produce pain felt in both areas. Thus, cardiac patients, during an anginal attack, often feel pains in the upper chest and left shoulder and arm as well as a diffuse pain in the mid-chest region. However, the story is more complex. Within or near (or occasionally at a considerable distance from) the area of referred pain, it is often possible to find small 'trigger points' which are exquisitely sensitive and trigger severe pain when pressed on by a finger or punctured by a needle.

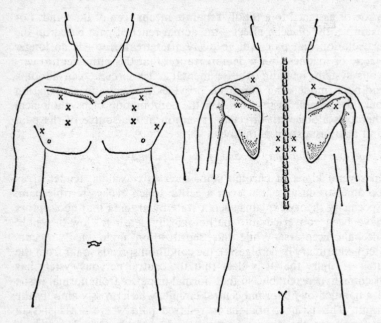

Figure 28. Kennard and Haugen's (1955, p. 297) chart of trigger spots (marked by Xs) in cardiac patients, showing the areas that are most frequently sensitive. Firm pressure on the trigger spots produces discrete, stabbing, 'hot' pain that sometimes persists for as long as several hours. Pressure at the same spots in non-cardiac patients often produces mild pain for several minutes.

Examination of cardiac patients by Kennard and Haugen (1955) revealed that most of them show a common pattern of trigger spots (Figure 28) in the shoulder and chest. Pressure on the trigger spots often produces intense pain that may last for hours. Astonishingly, similar examination of a group of subjects who did not have heart disease revealed an almost identical distribution of tender areas.

The patterns of referred pain are so consistent from person to person that physicians often diagnose the disease structure on the basis of the pain pattern. It is not surprising, therefore, that many trigger points are located in approximately the same place in most people (Travell and Rinzler, 1946, 1952). Pressure on these trigger points evokes pain in the referred area and injection of an anaesthetic in the trigger points removes the referred pain. There is a characteristic sequence to many of these referred pains. For example, in some

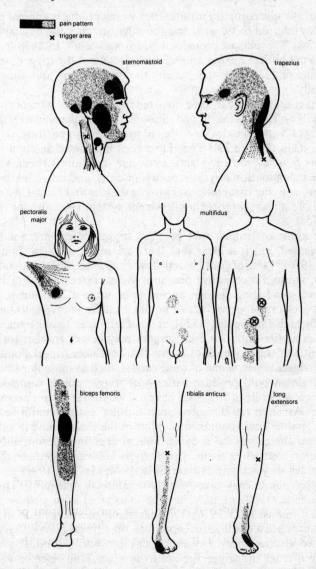

Figure 29. Typical myofascial pain patterns and their related trigger areas reported by Travell and Rinzler (1952, p. 425). When the referred pain pattern of a muscle is known, it can be used to locate the muscle that is the source of pain. The name of the muscle associated with each pain pattern is shown.

cases of chronic coronary insufficiency which produces anginal pain, the pain referred to the arm and shoulder becomes the outstanding symptom. The person protects the arm and tends to keep it in a rigid, fixed position. After anaesthetic injection of the trigger points, the pain relief allows the patient to use the arm and shoulder normally.

Trigger points appear to be involved in a variety of pain phenomena (Glyn, 1971; Travell and Simons, 1983), particularly those associated with muscles and the fibrous membrane (fascia) that covers them (Figure 29). They have been implicated in conditions such as muscle pain (myalgia), muscular (non-joint) rheumatism, muscle inflammation (myositis or myofascitis), and inflammation of the fibrous tissue that comprises muscle sheaths and fascial layers of the whole muscle-joint-tendon-ligament system (fibrositis or myofibrositis).

The kinds of trauma that produce trigger points are not fully documented, but it is clear that there are many of them (Simons, 1975, 1976). Loss of local blood flow (ischemia) due to a sudden sprain, unusual mechanical pressure, toxins, extreme cold or heat, and fever-producing diseases appear to be some of the causes. Persistent pressure on nerves at exit points, including nerve entrapment (Kopell and Thompson, 1976), is another. Scar tissue remaining from an earlier injury or even surgery may be yet another trauma that initiates the sequence of events that produces trigger points or larger trigger zones. Some of these causes, such as muscular stresses and strains, would produce patterns of trigger points common to most people, while others, such as scars, would vary from person to person. As Glyn (1971) notes, such 'insults' cause painful lesions which tend to heal spontaneously; but in the elderly, and in others in whom there may be a constitutional chemical abnormality in muscle or connective tissue, these trivial lesions perpetuate themselves until they become chronic (Sola, 1994; McCain, 1994).

Trigger points may involve only myofascial structures (Travell and Simons, 1983) or may become associated with pathological viscera (Simons, 1975, 1976). It is reasonable to assume that trigger points produce a continuous input into the central nervous system. Diseased viscera, then, may evoke an input which summates with the input from the trigger points to produce pain referred to the larger skin areas which surround the trigger points. Conversely, stimulation of the trigger points may evoke volleys of impulses that summate with low-level inputs from the diseased visceral structure, which would produce pain that is felt in both areas. These phenom-

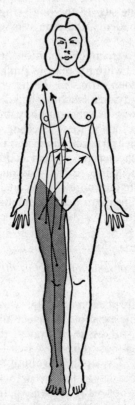

Figure 30. Patterns of referred sensation after cordotomy. The stippled area shows the region of analgesia produced by cordotomy in this woman. Heavy pressure applied to the analgesic skin produced 'an unpleasant form of tingling' that was felt at a non-analgesic part of the body. The sites of stimulation are indicated by dots, and the arrow from each dot indicates the point to which sensation was referred. (from Nathan, 1956, p. 88)

ena of referred pain, then, point to summation mechanisms which can be understood in terms of the gate-control and the slower, more prolonged mechanisms.

Referred pains may also occur after lesions of the central nervous system. Nathan (1956) studied patients who had undergone unilateral or bilateral cordotomy, mostly for the relief of cancer pain, and found that pinpricks applied to analgesic parts of the body, such as the leg, evoked pain that was felt at distant sites on the same or opposite side of the body (Figure 30). He also observed that, in some patients, the pain was referred to the site of an earlier injury.

Phenomena of mis-referral of sensation are also familiar to a small number of people who, for reasons unknown but presumably because of abberant connections in the nervous system, find that when they scratch a body area (such as the knee) they feel a curious itchy or tickling sensation in a distant body area, such as the upper shoulder. Observations such as these (Sterling, 1973) underscore the complexity of central neural connections and take us far away from simplistic concepts of the nervous system as little more than an old-fashioned telephone switchboard that has one plug-in connection for each telephone. Like our more complicated telecommunications networks, errors in connection occur, sometimes with trivial consequences and sometimes with painful, crippling, disastrous ones.

Pain may persist in the absence of injury or after healing of injured tissues

Attempts to explain this phenomenon are usually cautious because we lack adequate diagnostic tools to detect all forms of peripheral lesion, particularly in soft tissue. However, there is a long list of conditions in which the most diligent search has failed to find any peripheral abnormality. This applies to about 80 per cent of patients with low back pain. No lesion has been found that explains trigeminal neuralgia. It is not really known whether trigger points are the cause or the effect of the myofascial syndromes. In the search for the causes of headaches, it is generally agreed that the muscle tension and vascular changes are secondary rather than primary causes. This raises the possibility that these conditions may be primary disorders of the control systems. Any control system which normally operates by a push-pull mechanism to hold some activity at a steady level contains inherent dangers. If pushed by disease into a highly abnormal range, the control may itself be weakened and have insufficient power to restore the system into a normal working range. This occurs in heart failure and hypothermia. The disease may affect the control system itself, forcing the control into one extreme setting. This occurs in hyperthyroidism, some forms of hypertension, anorexia nervosa and epilepsy. The gate-control mechanism is not a likely mechanism to explain persistent pain, although it is possible to imagine some unknown disorder which permanently affected the inhibitory loops, thereby exaggerating the effect of normal inputs or leading to steady firing. However, the second control mechanism triggered by afferent impulses clearly involves local metabolic changes which could persist with positive feedback and an inability of inhibitory mechanisms to reverse the changes. The third mechanism, which depends on chemical transport, is certain to produce persistent change since, once established, there is no known restorative force. This type of control mechanism is highly likely to be involved where nerves, roots or central lesions are followed by persistent pain even when the original lesion seems completely healed. In every case of unexplained persistent pain, the proper scientific and therapeutic tactic is to search the periphery for some undiscovered source and, if this proves negative, to proceed centrally and to question the state of the control mechanisms.

Nathan (1962) reviewed several cases which indicate that somatosensory input may produce long-lasting effects similar to memories produced by visual and auditory stimulation. In one case, stimulation of the stump of an amputee who, five years before amputation, had sustained a severe laceration of the leg by an ice skate, later produced vivid imagery of the pain of the skating accident: 'It was not that he remembered having had this injury, he felt all the sensations again that he had felt at the time.' Similarly, phantom limb pain is sometimes felt in areas that had been painful prior to amputation. The pain of a sliver of wood under a fingernail or a tight cast on a foot has been reported as persisting in the phantom after amputation of the limb (Bailey and Moersch, 1941; White and Sweet, 1969).

The concept of a memory-like mechanism in pain is also supported by convincing experimental evidence. The most fascinating study (Hutchins and Reynolds, 1947; Reynolds and Hutchins, 1948) originated when dentists in the United States Air Force, during World War II, observed that aircrew often complained of toothache in a recently filled tooth when they flew in semi-pressurized airplanes. The first hypothesis – that air-pockets were trapped under the filling and exerted pressure on the tooth-pulp – was eliminated by carefully drilling and refilling the offending tooth, and finding that the painful episodes still persisted. It was then observed that the aircrew complained when they also had a sinus infection, so that changes in air pressure may have been exerting their effects by stimulation of receptors in the sinuses. In an ingenious set of experiments, volunteer aircrew underwent drilling and filling of diseased teeth, without local anaesthetics, on both sides of the mouth. It was then observed that pinpricks of the nasal mucosa, as long as seventy days later, produced pain in the treated teeth on the stimulated side. The effect was permanently abolished on one side by a single novocaine block of the trigeminal nerve, but persisted in the opposite, non-blocked side (Hutchins and Reynolds, 1947; Reynolds and Hutchins, 1948). These referred pains necessitate the assumption of a long-term central neural change. The data suggest that the treatment of the teeth evoked inputs that produced changes in firing patterns in the central nervous system. These changes, once initiated, were somehow capable of summating the continuous, low-level input from the treated teeth with inputs from more distant sources. The single block of a peripheral nerve, which could not have affected the teeth, permitted resumption of normal neural activity and the end of pain. That the *input* as such, rather than conscious awareness, was essential in initiating the abnormal central activity is evident in the observation that a subject who had four teeth extracted under nitrous oxide anaesthesia felt pain referred to the jaw when the nasal mucosa was pricked thirty-three days after treatment.

Similar observations were made by Cohen (1944) who studied patients who had anginal-effort syndrome, with pain referred only to the left side. He injected a small amount of hypertonic saline under the skin of the right side of the back which gave rise to a diffuse, deep-seated pain that soon disappeared. Two hours later, long after the pain had passed, exertion and anginal pain again caused its appearance.

The nature and location of pain change with time

Traditionally, explanations of all such changes were sought in peripheral mechanisms such as inflammation and scar formation. However, we have shown that, in addition to the peripheral sequence of changes, a cascade of changes also occurs centrally. Within minutes of injury, these are the impulse-triggered central changes which persist and grow. At a later stage, when a nerve has been injured, the effects of chemical transport become evident and secondary central changes develop during the following weeks or months. It is now suspected that abnormal tissue itself can signal its presence by chemical means to central structures even where there is no damage to major nerves. Each of these sequential central changes offers an explanation and a hope for a specific therapy.

Pain is not a single sensation but has many dimensions

One of the first effects of the gate theory was to destroy the idea that pain is a simple sensation subserved by a direct transmission line to a pain centre. The concept of pain as purely a sensory experience long overshadowed the affective and cognitive dimensions of the total pain experience. Typically, physiological and psychological textbooks dealt with 'pain' in one chapter and 'aversive drives' in another, as though both were entirely different processes. The gate theory, however, with its emphasis on parallel processing systems, provided the conceptual framework for integration of the sensory, affective and cognitive dimensions of pain.

The gate-control theory proposes that the action system responsible for pain experience and response is triggered when the integrated firing level of the dorsal horn T cells reaches or exceeds a critical level. Melzack and Casey (1968) have noted that the output of the T cells is transmitted towards the brain primarily by fibres in the ventrolateral spinal cord and is projected into two major brain systems: via neospinothalamic fibres into the ventrobasal thalamus and somatosensory cortex, and via medially coursing fibres into the reticular formation, the medial and intra-laminar thalamus and the

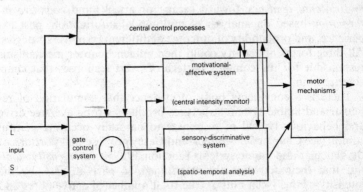

Figure 31. Conceptual model of the sensory, motivational and central control determinants of pain. The output of the T cells of the gate-control system projects to the sensory-discriminative system (via neospinothalamic fibres) and the motivational-affective system (via the paramedial ascending system). The central control trigger is represented by a line running from the large fibre system to central control processes; these, in turn, project back to the gate-control system, and to the sensory-discriminative and motivational-affective systems. All three systems interact with one another, and project to the motor system. (from Melzack and Casey, 1968)

limbic system. Stimulation at noxious intensities evokes activity in both projection systems, and discrete lesions in each may strikingly alter pain perception and response (Chapter 7).

Behavioural and physiological studies led Melzack and Casey (1968) to propose (Figure 31) that:

1 The selection and modulation of the sensory input through the neospinothalamic projection system provides, in part at least, the neurological basis of the sensory-discriminative dimension of pain.

2 Activation of reticular and limbic structures underlies the powerful motivational drive and unpleasant affect that trigger the organism into action.

3 Neocortical or higher central nervous system processes, such as evaluation of the input in terms of past experience, exert control over activity in both the discriminative and motivational systems.

It is assumed that these three categories of activity interact with one another to provide *perceptual information* regarding the location, magnitude, and spatiotemporal properties of the noxious stimulus, *motivational tendency* toward escape or attack, and *cognitive information* based on analysis of multimodal information, past experience, and probability of outcome of different response strategies. All three forms of activity could then influence motor mechanisms responsible for the complex pattern of overt responses that characterize pain.

There is a convincing body of evidence that stimulation of reticular and limbic system structures produces strong aversive drive and behaviour typical of responses to naturally occuring painful stimuli (see Chapter 7). Melzack and Casey propose that portions of the reticular and limbic systems function as a *central intensity monitor*: that their activities are determined, in part at least, by the intensity of the T-cell output (the total number of active fibres and their rate of firing) after it has undergone modulation by the gate-control system in the dorsal horns. The cells in the midbrain reticular formation are capable of summation of input from spatially separate body sites (Bell *et al.*, 1964); furthermore, the post-stimulus discharge activity of some of these cells lasts for many seconds (Casey, 1966), so that their activity may provide a measure of the intensity of the total T-cell output over relatively long periods of time.

Essentially, both kinds of summation transform discrete spatial and temporal information into intensity information. Melzack and Casey propose that the output of these cells, up to a critical intensity level, activates those brain areas subserving positive affect and approach tendency. Beyond that level, the output activates areas underlying negative affect and aversive drive.

The complex sequences of behaviour that characterize pain are determined by sensory, motivational, and cognitive processes that act on motor mechanisms. By 'motor mechanisms' (Figure 31), Melzack and Casey mean all of the brain areas that contribute to overt behavioural response patterns. These areas extend throughout the whole of the central nervous system, and their organization must be at least as complex as that of the input systems we have primarily dealt with so far. Even 'simple' reflexes, which are generally thought to be entirely spinal in their organization, are now known to be influenced by cognitive processes: if we pick up a hot cup of tea in an expensive cup we are not likely to simply drop the cup, but jerkily put it back on the table, and *then* nurse our hand.

There is no adequate treatment for certain types of pain

Our understanding of pain mechanisms may have improved, but until this knowledge is translated into adequate therapy, we must recognize the magnitude of our ignorance. In the remainder of this book, we shall describe how far we have come and, sadly for so many suffering people, how far we have yet to go.

Part Four
The Control of Pain

'Perhaps few persons who are not physicians can realize the influence which long-continued and unendurable pain may have upon both body and mind . . . Under such torments the temper changes, the most amiable grow irritable, the soldier becomes a coward, and the strongest man is scarcely less nervous than the most hysterical girl.'
S. Weir Mitchell, 1872

10 The Search for Drugs

The battle against pain has been fought with three major kinds of weapons: drugs, sensory-modulation techniques and psychological procedures. From early historical records of ancient Egypt, we know that the juice of the poppy pod – opium – has long been used. During the ensuing centuries, the ancient world discovered that pain produced by acupuncture needles, hot cups applied on the skin, and even stepping on electric eels to receive a jolt of electricity relieved aches and pains ranging from crippling back pains to severe headaches. This rich variety of drugs and sensory-modulation methods evolved in all cultures and countries against a backdrop of powerful psychological suggestion. The herbs, cuts and burns were administered with conviction by the healers of the time, who often combined religious chants and prayers with their medicines and instilled unquestioned expectation of relief of pain. The rhythmic, hypnotic chants, accompanied by the trappings of magic, enhanced the belief that the patient would improve – and he often did.

This effect – which we now call the placebo effect – is the common ingredient of all the healing arts. It is so powerful that modern-day pharmacologists have to demonstrate that their new drugs are better than the placebo – which is a real achievement. This chapter deals with recent progress in the continual search for new drugs; the sensory-modulation techniques and psychological methods are described later.

The search for new drugs to relieve pain has been pursued with great vigour and enormous expense. After all, the panacea we all dream of is a magic pill which abolishes all pain. In fact, we have many outstanding drugs, and a tremendous amount of pain is under control. Few of us can imagine the day, not so long ago, when people underwent surgery without an anaesthetic. Strong men immobilized the screaming patient on the operating table and the surgeon practised his craft – amputating a leg or a breast, or drilling a hole in the skull – with extraordinary speed. It is also difficult to imagine the time when teeth were drilled or extracted without an anaesthetic, or when women, during difficult labour, could only scream helplessly. The discovery of nitrous oxide, ether and chloroform to allow painless extractions and childbirths marked an incredible advance in the history of medicine. Until then, alcohol was imbibed as the only anaesthetic for surgery and many a patient was carried in a drunken stupor into the operating theatre.

We are now blessed with a wide variety of drugs: anaesthetics to produce general anaesthesia for surgery; local anaesthetics which block nerve conduction from an area; analgesics such as aspirin to take away headaches and toothaches; and narcotics to relieve severe pains such as those caused by surgery, cancer and heart attacks. Drugs exist in abundance; the tragedy, as we shall see later (in Chapter 13), is that they are often not used properly and there is far too much needless pain and suffering.

The majority of drug prescriptions come from only two families of compounds, the aspirin type and the opium type. This fact tends to be hidden by enthusiastic advertising for some new variant of one or the other family. The confusion is increased by the labelling of simple chemicals with trade-names and by selling mixtures of compounds with yet another trade-name. While these two families have survived, they are historically not the only anti-pain drugs. Plants were long the favourite source of medicine and these gave us the mandrake – a relative of the potato – which contains atropine and scopolamine which cloud consciousness. Henbane contains hyoscamine, another of these compounds. Hemp produces cannabis or hashish which has certain analgesic effects. Hemlock was used as a general soporific but was also thought to have a local action and was applied as a local poultice. Many plant oils, such as clove oil, have a strong local anaesthetic action. Of all plant derivatives, alcohol has surely been used and abused more than any substance for numbness and oblivion. But extracts of willow and of poppy have led to the most specific and useful drugs.

This chapter will deal with drugs that relieve pain without producing a loss of consciousness. The drugs that derive from cocaine and are used for regional anaesthesia shall be described in the next chapter, since they obviously provide a powerful method for the sensory modulation of pain and shall be discussed in that context. The drugs we shall describe here are (1) the mild analgesics, including aspirin and acetaminophen; (2) the more powerful analgesics – the opiates (or narcotics) – that derive from morphine; (3) the opioid compounds that are structurally like morphine but do not in fact derive from it; (4) psychotropic drugs; and (5) inhalant drugs such as nitrous oxide which can produce analgesia without the loss of consciousness.

Aspirin and other non-steroidal anti-inflammatory drugs (NSAIDS)

In 1763 a country clergyman from Chipping Norton in England, Edward Stone, wrote to the Royal Society in London to tell them that the extract of willow was good for rheumatism and bouts of fever. In 1827, Leroux isolated the active compound from the willow, Salix Alba, and named it salicin. Throughout the nineteenth century, many variations of this molecule were produced and used, and by 1899, Dreser produced acetylsalicylic acid. This was marketed by Bayer under the trade name of Aspirin. Many more variants have been produced in this century and the names of those commonly used include, in addition to the salicylates, the following: phenyl-butazone, indomethacin, mefanamic acid, ibuprofen, piroxicam and many others. This remarkable group has three therapeutic actions: (1) against pain; (2) against inflammation; and (3) against fever. They vary in their relative power to produce these three desirable effects, and also in the unfortunately large number of side-effects (Sunshine and Olson, 1994).

Rationale

The site of action of these drugs appears to be entirely on the injured tissue itself and there is no convincing evidence that thera-peutic doses have any effect directly on peripheral nerves or in the central nervous system. The most likely proposal to explain the action of aspirin-like compounds comes from research by Vane, first reported in 1971. In the 1930s, an active compound was dis-covered in semen and, since the fluid comes from the prostate gland, it was called prostaglandin. It was later discovered that there is a large family of these compounds and that they are synthesized from a fatty acid, arachidonic acid. When tissue is damaged, prosta-glandins are synthesized and released into tissues where they play a part in triggering the three classic signs of inflammation: (1) the blood vessels dilate, producing redness; (2) they leak fluid, producing swelling; and (3) nerve endings are sensitized so that they produce nerve impulses more easily and therefore increase pain. Aspirin blocks the synthesis of prostaglandins and therefore prevents the appearance of this crucial substance which announces that tissue is damaged. That is, it acts within damaged tissue itself and not on the nervous system.

Uses

The site of action in damaged tissue defines the uses of NSAIDs. Sudden injury sets off a chain of reactions related to pain. First, small molecules such as histamine and serotonin are released. Then, larger peptides such as bradykinen appear. Finally the prostaglandins are synthesized and released. Therefore, these drugs are effective against slow, prolonged tissue damage and its pain wherever it occurs. A broken leg, the socket of an extracted tooth, and an arthritic joint all have in common the same tissue reactions and, therefore, the same sensitivity to these drugs. Pain triggered by events which do not produce inflammatory reactions does not respond to the drugs.

Side-effects

Some people develop an extreme sensitivity to aspirin and show severe side-effects to normal therapeutic doses (Barnett *et al.*, 1982). The commonest of these is gastric irritation and bleeding, although this is reduced considerably by a special coating on aspirin tablets. Aspirin also affects the blood clotting mechanism and is used intentionally for this purpose. Two aspirin tablets (650mg) approximately double the mean bleeding time in normal adults. A positive effect is to prevent a second heart attack in cardiac patients; a negative one is to drink enough alcohol to produce a mild gastritis after which aspirin is taken for the hangover. Every hospital emergency room is familiar with this combination as the trigger for massive gastric haemorrhage. A frightening side-effect is the development of deafness after moderate to large doses. Since every household contains an array of aspirin-like compounds, accidental or intentional overdoses are common. These affect brain, liver, kidney and blood chemistry. Fortunately, intensive care units have become skilled at the reversal of these toxic effects if treatment is started rapidly.

Acetaminophen, the no. 2 mild analgesic

Because aspirin has potentially serious side-effects in people who suffer gastric disorders, another mild analgesic – acetaminophen –

has become increasingly popular. Acetaminophen (also known as paracetamol) is derived from phenacetin, another commonly used drug, and is the second most popular mild analgesic. It is sold under various trade names: Tylenol, Atasol, Empracet, Panadol, and others.

Unlike aspirin and other NSAIDs, acetaminophen and phenacetin have no significant anti-inflammatory actions. They are weak inhibitors of prostaglandin synthesis and are therefore less effective than NSAIDs for arthritis, skin injuries, and other causes of pain that involve major inflammation of peripheral tissues, including inflammation of blood vessels. Their site of analgesic action is unknown, but, pill for pill (in the usual packaging), acetaminophen and aspirin have equivalent analgesic potency. Although acetaminophen is easier on the stomach than aspirin, it has a different serious side-effect: at high doses, it can damage the liver.

Opiates, also known as narcotics

Opium, the extract of poppy, was known to the Sumerians in 4000 BC, but we know little about the uses to which it was put. The first medical document, the Ebers Papyrus of 1550 BC, recommends it for crying children. The Greeks dedicated it to the gods of night, death, sleep (Hypnos) and dreams (Morpheus) – hence the name 'morphine'. Hippocrates prescribed it as a hypnotic. However, in Roman times, it was used specifically against pain by Galen in the second century AD. The use of opium spread from Rome and so did its abuse. Avicenna, the greatest of the Arab physicians, died in 1037 from an overdose of opium and so did Clive of India in the eighteenth century.

As was apparent in the description of aspirin and local anaesthetics, the nineteenth century was rich in analysis and synthesis of simple organic molecules. In 1803, morphine itself was isolated by Sertürner from opium. Opium contains about ten per cent morphine and also smaller amounts of many other alkaloids, two of which are related to morphine. These are codeine and thebaine. From these three molecules, a very large number of synthetic compounds have been generated. At least twenty-five different compounds are listed in the pharmacopoeia and their most famous trade names include heroin, hydromorphone, oxymorphone, etorphine, oxycodone and dihydrocodone. The individual members of this group differ widely in their potency and duration, but they are fundamentally similar in their mode of analgesic action. All produce analgesia and, as the dose rises, varying degrees of drow-siness, change of mood and mental clouding.

Rationale

The site of the analgesic action of the opiates is undoubtedly in the central nervous system and has been discussed in Chapters 6 and 7. There are two clearly different sites of action with respect to pain. One of these is in the midbrain, where a system in the periaqueductal grey matter triggers a nearby system of descending controls which, in turn, inhibits the ability of the spinal cord to transmit messages about injury. The second area of action is in the spinal cord itself where high concentrations of enkephalins and opiate receptors exist in the substantia gelatinosa. The opiates are capable of producing local control of the transfer of messages about tissue damage from afferent fibres to the transmitting cells which send messages to the brain. There are undoubtedly many other brain areas which are directly or indirectly affected by opiates.

Uses

Narcotics may be given by mouth, by intramuscular injection or, for very rapid action, by intravenous injection. Oral administration is obviously the most convenient, even though absorption may be slow. Since narcotics are all very bitter tasting, they are taken with honey or a syrup to mask their awful taste.

Narcotics are most commonly used in emergencies with rapid onset of severe pain. They are injected for severe injuries, heart attacks and abdominal crises. They are also widely used to control post-operative pain and labour pain. Finally, they play a crucial role in the management of pain in terminal disease (which we shall discuss in Chapter 14).

The discovery that narcotics have a direct action on the spinal cord has led to a new method of administration (Yaksh, 1986). One tenth of the normal dose is injected into the fluid around the lum-bar cord. This produces a profound and long-lasting analgesia of the legs and pelvis without any of the psychedelic effects. It has also been found that morphine placed outside the cord in the epidural space produces analgesia in the nearest segments. Thus it is possible to obtain local analgesia without the an-aesthesia and paralysis produced by local anaesthetics (Findler *et al.*, 1982; Olshwang *et al.*, 1984; Moulin and Coyle, 1986). However, not all pains respond to epidural morphine, and the failures may tell us something of the mode of action. When pains originate from denervation, as in brachial plexus avulsion, the terrible pain is not in any way ameliorated, presumably because the narcotic receptors on the spinal terminals of the incoming sensory fibres are destroyed.

Addiction

More nonsense on narcotic addiction is written by both doctors and the press than on any other medical matter. The undoubted occurrence of addiction has led to a mass hysteria about its danger which has been very harmful for patients as well as for addicts. The reaction to intravenous narcotics by the great majority of normal experimental subjects who are not in pain is one of discomfort. One of the present authors has experienced this a number of times during pain tests and found the sudden onset of a flying drunken feeling with nausea and headache to be distinctly unpleasant and not at all fitting the popular expectation of a pleasant dream state. Patients in acute emergency pain frequently receive one or more injections and they experience a powerful relief of both their pain and anxiety and often drift off to sleep. A survey was made of the consequences of such injections given to the many thousands of Israeli casualties in the Yom Kippur War. Not a single case of narcotic addiction was found among these men in spite of the fact that most were in the age range most commonly at risk for social addiction.

But what of the patients who get narcotics over long periods of time? The usual hospital routine is to give a dose every four hours and this may continue for weeks or months in terminal cancer patients with multiple metastases. However, this intermittent medication may have disadvantages because the drug is gradually metabolized and the pain level varies over the four hours. To overcome this, a number of techniques of self-paced administration have been developed in which the patient is free to give himself regulated small doses at short intervals (Keeri-Szanto, 1979). When these methods were introduced, there was of course considerable fear that the patient would rapidly overdose himself since he could administer the very drug which is supposed to induce addiction with all its associated irresponsible behaviour. Therefore, narrow limits were built into the system, with continuous monitoring in order to follow patients' behaviour when given free access to injected narcotics. The result is very clear. Patients do not push their drug intake to the highest permitted dose. On the contrary, they bring their pain down to a bearable level at which they do not have mental clouding. Then they continue to give themselves the narcotic at the doses required to maintain this desired state. The overall result is that the patient gives himself less than the medical staff would administer.

Who then are the self-destructive and socially undesirable addicts? Let us look at the less emotional subject of alcoholism. Most of us are not alcoholics and do not have an internal struggle not to become addicted. Most of us have been drunk, usually on social occasions, while seeking release and euphoria. A few people feel miserable and inadequate all the time and have only felt pleased with themselves on certain rare occasions when drunk. Even fewer seek continuous escape, oblivion or dependency. Turning back to narcotics, one can see that their illegal use and abuse has marked similarities with alcohol. The Singapore Chinese merchant, just as clever and successful as his American counterpart, smokes opium before dinner or as a nightcap while the American drinks a martini or a brandy. Biographies reveal many distinguished Westerners as having been regular secret users of narcotics with no apparent effect on their health or effectiveness. A few people, who always show serious personality problems before using narcotics, feel a sense of fulfilment for a few seconds or minutes only after a sudden surge of narcotics. Some seek escape and oblivion. These people are generally sick, and are unhappy with or without narcotics or alcohol. Their existence is no reason for the doctor to withhold medicine from normal people in the fear that he will create monsters.

Tolerance

The most common rational reason given by physicians for withholding opiates from those in pain due to terminal illness is that patients develop such rapid tolerance to the drugs that narcotics should be saved until some extreme and final crisis. However, Twycross (1978) found that cancer patients require a gradually increasing dose only during the first few days of stabilization. After this initial period, the required dose levels out at a safe and acceptable level and from then on remains as stable as the patient's condition. If the patient's disease spreads, it may be necessary to increase the dose to some higher level which again stabilizes. If the patient's condition improves, spontaneously or due to therapy, the dose of morphine can be decreased without any objection from the patient. There is no evidence of tolerance in these patients who take steady doses of narcotics for months, even for years.

Most drugs have multiple effects and the onset of tolerance differs for each of the different effects. This is also a common problem with alcohol, in which the amount taken to produce a particular effect rises rapidly day by day. Unfortunately, the amount needed to produce euphoria rises much more rapidly than the amount needed to produce oblivion. This partly explains the number of pathetic alcoholics who can no longer achieve the desired happiness before they fall off their bar-stools. Similarly, the dose needed by the social narcotic addict to produce the sudden psychedelic effect is extremely large and approaches the lethal dose. This tolerance of the psychedelic effect actually works to the advantage of the cancer patient. During the first few days of regular narcotic administration, the patient may feel drowsy and have muddled thoughts. These unwanted effects pass but the desired analgesia continues.

This type of differential tolerance has been shown in studies with animals by Abbott *et al.* (1982). In rats, a test is used in which the tail is dipped in hot water and the time is measured until the animal flicks its tail out of the water. With rather high doses of morphine, the time which the animal leaves its tail in the water is prolonged. On repeated testing it is found that higher and higher doses of morphine are needed to produce this prolongation. However, in another test discussed in Chapter 7, a small amount of the irritant formalin is injected under the skin of a rat's paw and its prolonged behavioural reactions are recorded. Morphine in quite small doses decreases the animal's reaction to the irritant. In this test, unlike the tail-flick test, repeated testing and treatment with narcotics does not lead to tolerance. It therefore seems that the formalin test better imitates the chronic pain patient's failure to develop tolerance, whereas the tail-flick test better imitates those aspects of human response to narcotics which develop tolerance.

Tolerance is a widespread phenomenon which goes far beyond drugs. We have already noted (and will see again in later chapters) that chronic pain may recur even though the initial treatment is successful. This is particularly true after neurosurgical procedures. The body possesses a host of homeostatic mechanisms which maintain a stable level of many body functions. If some event occurs which disturbs the level of function, these mechanisms react to push the function back to the 'normal' level. For example, if the air temperature drops, skin vessels constrict to decrease heat loss and metabolism increases to raise heat production. If these measures fail to return the body temperature to normal, more vigorous and sophisticated reactions occur; shivering starts, a fire is lit, migration to Florida begins. Each of these reactions has a limited power which may be overwhelmed. If a man falls into the Arctic Sea, the heat loss exceeds the ability of the homeostatic mechanisms to protect the body, and temperature falls to a level where even the restorative mechanisms themselves fail.

We have continually stressed that pain, too, is under control by factors other than the input from injury. Some pains are best understood as a failure of control. When pain exists and a drug, a surgical lesion, physiotherapy or psychotherapy are initiated, the remaining control mechanisms will react in an attempt to re-establish the pain. This reaction may provide an explanation common to all eventual failures of therapy. A placebo which initially produces an excellent response fails on repeated administration. Many physiotherapies may do the same. An initially satisfactory dose of morphine may not be effective on the third application; but if the dose is raised, the effect may be strong enough to overwhelm the counter-reaction of the control mechanisms. The failure of surgery such as a cordotomy to control pain after some months of success may also be seen as due to a slow readjustment of control, in which there is enhanced use of previously minor pathways so that they can produce major effects.

Withdrawal

It is a common belief that the failure by those who take narcotics to maintain regular narcotic medication leads immediately to an intense and intolerable yearning, anxiety and terror. As with the fear of tolerance, this fear also turns out to be a gross exaggeration. We have already mentioned that a survey of several thousand military casualties given narcotics failed to identify a single case of addiction attributable to brief therapeutic exposure. Patients in severe chronic pain treated with narcotics may on occasion be successfully treated by a cordotomy, a nerve block or by physiotherapy. The common picture seen in such patients is that as soon as they obtain relief of their pain they request no further narcotics. Since they are indeed quite restless and jumpy, they are tapered off to normal within one or two days with rapidly decreasing doses of sedatives.

Side-effects

All drugs have multiple actions. Normally, nerve impulses release endogenous opiates at selected sites in the nervous system and in this way achieve a specificity of action. When a narcotic is injected or ingested to act on the whole body, all receptors come into action simultaneously producing not only the desired analgesia but also other results. Some of these are desirable, such as the decrease of anxiety. Outside the central nervous system there are mixed effects, good and bad. The narcotics tend to paralyse smooth muscle. The coronary arteries dilate so that morphine has two beneficial actions in a heart attack, in which the pain drops and blood flow to the heart increases. Similarly, the pain of renal colic is relieved by a direct action on smooth muscle as well as on pain. Constipation always occurs and nausea may be serious so that these side-effects have to be treated with other drugs.

Synthetic opioids

It is now known that narcotics such as morphine and codeine act by imitating the action of endogenously generated narcotics. Many of these have been found in the central nervous system and they fall into three families: the enkephalins, the dynorphins and the endorphins which have progressively larger molecules. All narcotics are believed to produce their biological effect by interacting with three major families of receptors known as the mu, kappa and delta receptors. Because the receptors are widespread throughout the body, narcotics have many actions other than the desired analgesia. These are nausea and vomiting, constipation, respiratory depression, sedation and difficulty in focusing the eyes. These side-effects are utilized to advantage in medicines against diarrhoea and cough.

In an attempt to isolate the desired analgesia from the unwanted side-effects, pharmaceutical companies have been active in producing variations of all analgesic drugs. They also wished to produce better uptake when the drugs were taken orally, better distribution to the brain or spinal cord and more prolonged or shorter action. They did this in three ways. The first was to modify the poppy plant molecules. The earliest and most famous result was heroin, but the list includes hydromorphone, leverphanol and hydrocodone. In the course of this search, they produced narcotic antagonists, such as naloxone, and some useful drugs which are mixed agonist–antagonists.

The second approach was to develop purely synthetic drugs which have narcotic actions and include meperidine, fentanyl, methadone, propoxyphene and pentazocine. The third and most recent approach has been to produce variants of the newly discovered endogenous narcotics. The dynorphins and endorphins are too large in molecular size for easy synthesis, and pharmacologists have therefore concentrated on the short chain peptides, the enkephalins. DADL (D-alamine-D-leucine enkephalin) is such a compound, with a longer life than the natural leucine enkephalin, which has been used to alternate with morphine applied on the spinal cord (Moulin *et al.*, 1985; Krames *et al.*, 1986).

Psychotropic drugs

People who suffer chronic pain frequently become depressed as a result of their problem. Depression is an understandable reaction in a healthy, vigorous person who develops severe arthritis, neuralgic pain or one of the many other kinds of debilitating chronic pain. The person is confronted with severe physical and social limitations because of the pain, in addition to any disability produced by injury. When careful medical examination fails to reveal a cause, which frequently happens, the situation becomes even more depressing. It is not surprising, then, that antidepressant drugs are often prescribed to patients with chronic pain, and that the drugs are frequently effective in relieving the pain as well as the depression.

It is now well known that antidepressant drugs, particularly the tricyclic antidepressants, produce analgesia quite separately from the reduction in depression (Monks and Merskey, 1984; Feinmann, 1985). There is convincing evidence, reviewed by Monks and Merskey (1984), that imipramine has a significant analgesic effect on chronic osteoarthritic and rheumatoid arthritis. Amitriptyline has been shown to be effective for migraine and chronic tension headaches. Other tricyclic drugs are effective for diabetic neuropathy, post-herpetic neuralgia and other pains. The analgesic properties of these drugs are believed to be due to their ability to raise the levels of amines such as serotonin in the central nervous system, thereby enhancing the activity of inhibitory mechanisms.

The major tranquillizers – the phenothiazines – are sometimes used alone or in combination with the antidepressants to treat a wide variety of pains (Monks and Merskey, 1984). In contrast, the minor tranquillizers, the benzodiazapines (valium, librium), are usually not effective and, indeed, may increase both depression and pain.

Combination analgesics

Because some drugs act at the periphery and counteract the release of prostaglandins, and others act on the central nervous system, it is reasonable to expect that a combination of both kinds of drugs would be more effective than each alone (Beaver, 1983). For this reason, aspirin is often combined with small doses of codeine and both together produce a much greater effect than either drug alone. There are several other combinations which are particularly effective, such as a mild narcotic plus a low dose of a tricyclic antidepressant. Many combinations derive from rational considerations of the cause of the particular pain for which they are prescribed, but sometimes the prescribing physician follows a 'hunch'. For example, painful diabetic neuropathy is sometimes reduced significantly by a combination of nortriptyline and fluphenazine (Gomez-Perez *et al.*, 1985), and desipramine enhances the effects of morphine for the control of post-operative pain (Levine *et al.*, 1986).

A particularly powerful combination is morphine plus dextro-amphetamine (a stimulant also known as 'speed'), especially in patients with cancer pain (Forrest *et al.*, 1977). This combination is rarely prescribed because both drugs have a bad reputation from their 'street' use. However, an increasing number of physicians are turning to this combination for patients with severe cancer pain and confirm its effectiveness. In the study that first reported the effect, the drugs were administered by injection. It is important to know whether the combination is as effective when taken orally. Another highly effective combination of drugs for cancer pain (when morphine alone, for example, has failed) is methadone, amitriptyline and a non-narcotic analgesic (Richlin *et al.*, 1987).

Inhalant analgesics

None of the drugs we have discussed so far produce analgesia that is sufficiently powerful to permit surgery to be carried out. Operations are usually done when the patient is given general anaesthesia that renders him unconscious or a local anaesthetic that blocks nerve impulses from an area as small as a wart or as large as the lower half of the body. In both cases, the patient reports feeling no pain, or any other sensation, even though major incisions cut through layers of tissue.

There is, however, a class of drugs that can produce unconsciousness when given in large quantities (and are therefore anaesthetics), but can also be administered in smaller quantities so that consciousness is not lost, yet the patient is analgesic to post-operative pain, labour pain, pain due to heart attack, and pains produced by injuries that bring patients into the emergency departments of hospitals (Sloan, 1986). These drugs include nitrous oxide. In recent years, a mixture of nitrous oxide and oxygen has been used increasingly for 'breakthrough pain' in cancer patients. Patients with some kinds of cancer, who are generally without pain, sometimes have severe, sudden pains that are difficult to control. In these situations, a mixture of nitrous oxide/oxygen is inhaled through a mask and pain is relieved in a few minutes (Fosburg and Crone, 1983). When the pain subsides, the mask is set aside, and the nitrous oxide is rapidly eliminated via the lungs.

Nitrous oxide/oxygen is being used increasingly in emergency wards, hospices for cancer patients, obstetrical wards, and dental surgeries. The mixture is remarkably safe, with few serious side-effects. Analgesia is rapidly induced and is dissipated just as rapidly by discontinuing inhalation of the mixture. It is to be hoped that nitrous oxide/oxygen, which is generally so safe, will be used for a variety of unpleasant or painful procedures that cause needless suffering. These include bone taps, sickle-cell anaemia crises, spinal punctures, injection into the lymphatic system and other such procedures. The pain is unnecessary and serves no useful purpose. The patient, in such a situation, could easily be given a nitrous oxide/oxygen mixture to inhale when necessary to eliminate pain. Careful monitoring of the patient is not needed, although the attending physician, dentist, nurse or other health professional maintains a check on the patient's condition. In general, the mixture is extremely useful for the management of temporary pain (as in minor surgery) as well as intermittent or spasmodic pain in cancer patients (Sloan, 1986).

Frontiers of the continuing search

Variants of aspirin

The remarkable effectiveness of aspirin has inevitably led to a search for safer forms of it. There is currently a great deal of interest in organic salicylates, such as lysine- and arginine-salicylic acid. These compounds are present in certain mineral waters from hot springs and may be the basis of the purported 'healing powers' of these waters, which are so popular with sufferers of arthritis, back pains and other aches and pains associated with inflammation of joints, muscles and other tissues.

Drugs that act on the sympathetic nervous system

Several drugs which act on the noradrenalin receptors in the sympathetic nervous system have been shown to produce analgesia. Two famous ones – propranalol and guanethidine – are discussed in the next chapter. Other drugs, which have so far been studied in animals only, appear to act as independent analgesics or as adjuncts to other conventional drugs. A particularly interesting drug is clonidine, which is commonly used to lower blood pressure and has also been found to be a very effective analgesic. All of these drugs have effects on major physiological functions such as blood pressure, heart rate, sweating, and so forth, so that thorough testing with animals is necessary before the drugs (or derivatives) can be prescribed for people.

Receptor-specific ligands

The receptors on cells in the nervous system to which morphine binds chemically and produces its effects come in different forms. For example, the μ (mu) receptors for morphine have two forms – μ_1 and μ_2; μ_1 is believed to mediate analgesia, whereas μ_2 receptors mediate morphine's side-effects of respiratory depression and constipation. Thus, various forms of morphine are being synthesized with the hope that one or more will act only on μ_1 receptors and therefore provide analgesia without the undesirable side-effects. Two other kinds of receptors – δ (delta) and κ (kappa) – bind with enkephalins and dynorphins respectively and there is an active search for drugs that will bind with them to produce analgesia.

Hormones

The naturally occurring steroids and their synthetic analogues can abruptly halt all aspects of the inflammatory processes, including the pain. However, inflammation has the useful property of fighting infection and repairing damage. Therefore, steroid therapy, whether general or local, has positive and negative effects. As we learn more about the various components of the inflammatory process, it may be possible to develop hormones or other similar compounds which would guide the process to leave the wanted aspects intact.

A number of cancers, particularly some from the prostate and breast, are dependent for their growth on the presence of hormones. This led to a number of therapies to slow cancer growth by starving them of the required hormones. The most radical approach was to destroy the entire pituitary gland since this indirectly controls the other hormones. Its destruction can be achieved surprisingly easily since the pituitary is in the base of the skull and is covered by thin bone which can be penetrated by a stout hypodermic needle directed through the nostril (Moricca, 1974). It was noticed that, in some cases, there is a rapid and profound relief of pain (Moricca, 1974; Katz and Levin, 1977; Corssen *et al.*, 1977; Lipton *et al.*, 1979). The mechanism of pain relief remains obscure because the pain may decrease without any apparent change in the tumour. It is suspected that the treatment may affect the hypothalamus which, apart from its control of the pituitary, has powerful interconnections with the limbic system and with descending control systems.

Drug delivery systems

Until recently, drugs were taken orally or given by injection. In special cases, they were given by means of a rectal suppository. Recently, however, there have been exciting developments in new ways to deliver drugs. One of these is to implant a small pouch, about the size of a circular powder compact, under the skin, with a flexible tube that slowly releases morphine or some other drug into the space around the spinal cord or even into one of the ventricles of the brain (Lobato *et al.*, 1985). The subcutaneous pouch has a reservoir and a microdrive mechanism run by a tiny battery, so that given amounts of the drug are injected continuously. The reservoir is filled as needed by a hypodermic needle containing the drug which is injected through a self-sealing membrane that covers the reservoir.

Another system, for patients who remain in bed, is to allow the patients to self-administer the drug by pressing a button on a small machine at the bedside (Keeri-Szanto, 1979; Tamsen *et al.*, 1982). This procedure at first aroused fears that patients would abuse the drugs, such as morphine, and take too much. Instead, they tend to take less than the nurse would have given. Yet another system, which is very simple, is the implantation of a pellet which has a special covering that allows a continual slow release of the drug.

All of these methods have advantages and drawbacks and, therefore, have given rise to vigorous debates between those for or against particular systems. However, they are clearly a blessing for patients who dislike the pain and discomfort of repeated injections. Most importantly, clever engineering minds are now hard at work in alleviating pain and suffering. The field needs all the help it can get and the introduction of engineers into drug delivery systems, as well as the electrical-stimulation systems (which shall be described in the next chapter), is most welcome.

It is clear that there is tremendous activity in the search for new drugs and the most efficient delivery systems. Our understanding of brain function, involving multiple ascending and descending systems, has led accordingly to a search for 'finer' tuning of drugs in relation to receptor and type of pain. There are now more brain transmitters than anyone would have dreamed of only a decade ago, when the discovery of endorphins and enkephalins led to a state of euphoria among scientists eager to find new drugs to relieve pain. There are not only a multitude of new neurotransmitters (people speak jokingly of the 'brain peptide of the month'), but we now understand that many substances serve as neuromodulators. For example, baclofen and the diazepans are part agonists of the inhibitory transmitter GABA. Recently it has been found that baclofen is often effective for patients with trigeminal neuralgia who cannot tolerate carbamazepine (Tegretol) at the usually effective doses (Fromm *et al.*, 1984).

These are exciting times, and there is no question that our new understanding is leading to our goal of abolishing pain. What stands in the way, as we shall see in Chapter 14, is ignorance about tolerance and addiction and the myths that surround them. We have the drugs, but all too often they are not prescribed appropriately or are given in such small doses as to be worthless. There is a great need for better education about drugs and their use.

11 Sensory Modulation of Pain

While drugs are able to keep most kinds of pain under control, there are several pain states which are not helped or which require such large doses that the patient becomes confused or drowsy and cannot function normally. Until recently, the most common medical procedure for the control of such severe, chronic pain was to destroy selected peripheral nerves or pathways in the central nervous system. These procedures were based on the concept of a specific pain system, so that it seemed logical to surgically interrupt the system to prevent 'pain impulses' from reaching the 'pain centre'. We now know that surgical procedures may be effective immediately after the operation, but pain tends to return, sometimes worse than before. A major change in concepts of abnormal physiological activity in the central nervous system as the basis of chronic pain (Livingston, 1943) led to the use of a series of local anaesthetic blocks of sensory pathways in the attempt to stop the abnormal activity and thereby allow normal patterning to resume. Blocks, which are not destructive, are commonly used with excellent results in a substantial number of patients.

The gate-control theory, after its publication in 1965, had a powerful impact on the treatment of pain. Its emphasis on a dynamic balance between excitatory and inhibitory influences, including feedback interactions between spinal and brain levels, has been the basis of new conceptual approaches to pain therapy and has suggested new forms of treatment. The gate theory, in recent years, has opened the way for a search for techniques to modulate the sensory input. It suggests that pain control may be achieved by the enhancement of normal physiological activities rather than their disruption by destructive, irreversible lesions. In particular, it has led to attempts to control pain by activation of inhibitory mechanisms.

Neurosurgical approaches to pain control

Destruction of peripheral nerves

Much ingenuity has gone into the destruction of peripheral nerves and central pathways. The sites for such lesions, which are akin to cutting the wires of a telephone system, are shown in Figure 32. Each site has its advantages and disadvantages. If the painful area is small and is supplied by a single nerve, a peripheral procedure is chosen and the operation is simple. Nerves can, of course, be exposed in open surgery, but with the development of techniques to inject substances onto nerves, less drastic operations become possible. After a temporary test of the effectiveness of the proposed lesion by injecting a local anaesthetic, it is possible to inject a toxic substance which will destroy the nerve fibres. Alcohol and phenol have been the most commonly used compounds. Another method is to burn a nerve by passing a high-frequency current through the tip of a needle, which produces intense heat. A prolonged block of nerves can also be achieved by cooling the nerve sufficiently to freeze it. If the painful area is large or close to the spine, it is necessary to move towards central structures. One possible operation is to section only the sensory roots (rhizotomy), leaving the ventral roots intact. This has the advantage of leaving movement intact, but involves major surgery. In rhizotomy, the ganglion which contains the cell bodies of the sensory nerve is separated from the spinal cord, so that the nerves degenerate and are permanently lost.

All surgical lesions of nerve roots and ganglia bring with them the disadvantage of total anaesthesia rather than selective removal of the pain. In addition, particularly with root sections, some of the patients develop unbearable new types of sensation of a peculiar nature which may be worse than the original pain and which are very resistant to treatment and to spontaneous cure. The mechanisms of these pains induced by nerve section have been discussed in Chapter 6. They lie partly in the region of the injured nerve which begins to generate abnormal nerve impulses and to produce unusual sensitivities. Furthermore, the cutting of peripheral nerves induces changes in the central nervous system, and the cutting of roots produces a major loss of nerve fibres which degenerate in the spinal cord following the lesion. The spinal cord cells which have lost their input begin to fire spontaneously and the nearest intact nerves increase their central influence. This means that an ongoing sensation is felt from the region which is totally anaesthetic while gentle stimulation of the edge of the anaesthetic area produces sharp pain.

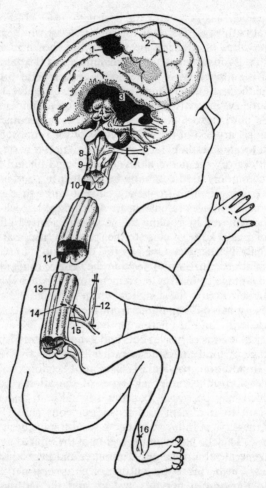

Figure 32. MacCarty and Drake's (1956, p. 208) schematic diagram illustrating various surgical procedures designed to alleviate pain: 1, gyrectomy; 2, prefrontal lobotomy; 3, thalamotomy; 4, mesencephalic tractotomy; 5, hypophysectomy; 6, fifth-nerve rhizotomy; 7, ninth-nerve neurectomy; 8, medullary tractotomy; 9, trigeminal tractotomy; 10, cervical cordotomy; 11, thoracic cordotomy; 12, sympathectomy; 13, myelotomy; 14, Lissauer tractotomy; 15, posterior rhizotomy; 16, neurectomy.

In seven cases of severe, chronic pain originating from peripheral nerve injury, Noordenbos and Wall (1981) have shown that meticulous surgery which excises the injured area in the peripheral nerve, including careful grafting of a section of new nerve, failed to remove the pain and in some cases made it worse. Here it is apparent that the peripheral nerve surgery was aimed at the wrong target because the seat of the trouble had already been transferred to the spinal cord.

Tic douloureux (trigeminal neuralgia), the terrible affliction of the face described in Chapter 4, requires surgery of the trigeminal nerve if drug therapy fails. Destruction of the sensory branch of the nerve produces a numbness of the face and the pain eventually recurs in many patients. Nevertheless, people who suffer these agonizing pains are often willing to take the risk. The most common method used by neurosurgeons is to insert a long needle through one of the foramina in the skull into the trigeminal ganglion, and a lesion of the ganglion is then made by injecting alcohol or glycerol or by passing an electrical current through the needle tip. In a more radical approach, the neurosurgeon exposes the ganglion by turning down a flap of skull under the temporal muscle. Then the temporal lobe and its dura are elevated to reveal the ganglion on the floor of the skull. Usually the nerve roots flowing toward the brain from the ganglion are cut. This exposure has allowed a number of new techniques and ideas to be tested, all of which work at least temporarily (Loeser, 1977). Some firmly massage the ganglion, while others decompress the ganglion by removing the dura which covers it. Most recently, the trigeminal nerve has been cushioned from the pulsation of the carotid artery which runs close by and is thought to produce mechanical damage. The temporary success of all these operations indicates the complex role of the sensory input.

Surgical or chemical destruction of spinal roots

We have seen that the site of neurosurgical attack moves toward the spinal cord as the site of origin of the pain becomes more diffuse. Unfortunately, this is a fairly common occurrence when cancer spreads to the thorax, abdomen or pelvis, or to the vertebral column and the adjacent roots and nerves. The large nerves peripheral to the ganglia contain a mixture of sensory and motor nerve fibres, so that cutting them results not only in an area of complete numbness but also in paralysis and wasting of muscles. The paralysis can be avoided by taking advantage of the divergence of the sensory nerves into dorsal roots as they approach the spinal cord, leaving the motor fibres to run in the ventral roots. Open surgery, which involves removal of the bony vertebral arches and opening of the dura mater, allows the surgeon to see the dorsal roots and to cut them. A recent variant of this procedure is to make electrolytic heat lesions of the dorsal root entry zone (DREZ) in the spinal cord, which destroy the cells in the dorsal part of the dorsal horn. This procedure produces good relief in about 60 per cent of patients with pain after brachial plexus avulsion and 50 per cent of paraplegic patients with pain (Nashold *et al.*, 1985). Because the operation is relatively new, its long-term effectiveness is not certain.

Because the body area served by one root overlaps with its neighbours, it is always necessary to cut at least three roots in order to achieve a complete anaesthesia of any part of the body. It can be seen that this involves major surgery which is clearly to be avoided, particularly in patients who may be desperately ill from the disease which is causing their pain. An alternative, much simpler method is to inject into the cerebrospinal fluid a solution of phenol and thick glycerine which can be made to soak the desired nerve roots by positioning the patient so that the viscous globule runs over one group of dorsal roots on one side. The most common roots to be approached in this way are the sacral roots supplying the pelvis, a frequent source of pain in cancer patients which can be treated by a simple lumbar puncture. This method is less accurate and less long-lasting than direct surgical section but is obviously far less disturbing to the patient.

There are unfortunate side-effects of these procedures in a high percentage of patients who survive for long periods of time. When a dorsal root is destroyed either by a knife or by chemicals, the nerve fibres central to the cut are isolated from their cell bodies which lie in the dorsal root ganglia. These isolated central parts of the nerve root degenerate and there is never any regeneration, unlike the regenerative process which can take place in peripheral nerves. This means that nerve cells in the spinal cord permanently lose the nerve fibres which normally activate them. Nerve cells which lose their normal drive demonstrate one of the many types of homeostatic mechanism, in this case called *denervation hypersensitivity*. It is as though the cell recognizes that it no longer receives its normal excitatory signals and therefore raises its own excitability to a stage where the cell begins to generate nerve impulses when no input signal is received. The consequence to the patient is that he first experiences the desired total anaesthesia in the region supplied by the cut roots, then develops a pins-and-needles feeling needles feeling which may gradually grow in intensity until he is in continuous pain. The surgeon has created on a small scale the same disorder which occurs with the common motorbike accident of brachial plexus avulsion in which, as we have described earlier (p. 10), the majority of patients with extensive root damage suffer severe pains.

Surgical or chemical destruction of the sympathetic system

All parts of the body are supplied by a special set of efferent nerves which originate in the chain of sympathetic ganglia which run on each side of the vertebral column from the top of the chest to the upper abdomen (Figure 6, p. 64). These nerves supply the blood vessels, glands and viscera and control their activity. The French surgeon, René Leriche (1879–1956), who wrote one of the first surgical textbooks on pain, believed that there are certain types of pain which are particularly influenced by the sympathetic system and proceeded to prove this by taking out the sympathetic ganglia related to the painful part, often producing dramatic pain relief. The success of this operation, particularly in causalgia, does not definitively demonstrate why it works.

The direct surgical approach to the sympathetic ganglia is always difficult and sometimes dangerous. As a result, anaesthesiologists have learned to insert long needles that reach the sympathetic ganglia. They then inject a test dose of local anaesthetic and, if the effect is satisfactory, the ganglia are injected with a destructive fluid such as alcohol or phenol.

Two mechanisms may explain why sympathectomy is effective. The first is that it decreases the noradrenalin which is released in the area of an injured nerve. This is consistent with the observation by Wall and Gutnick (1974) that damaged sensory fibres become highly sensitive to noradrenalin. It therefore appears that certain types of nerve damage allow the sympathetic system to trigger impulses in sensory nerve fibres by its release of noradrenalin, and sympathectomy would reverse this process.

The second way in which the sympathetic system is involved in pain is in its control of the diameter of blood vessels and its consequent effect on blood flow and blood pressure. If blood flow becomes inadequate for the needs of a muscle, pain occurs as in a cramp or in angina pectoris. Whatever the mechanism, it is now evident that virtually every type of pain is influenced by the sympathetic nervous system. Chemicals that block its activity (anti-noradrenergic drugs) decrease momentary pains as well as longer-lasting pains (Coderre *et al.*, 1984).

Cordotomy: the cutting of tracts in the spinal cord

Until recently, the most common neurosurgical procedure for the control of severe, chronic pain was 'cordotomy', in which the surgeon cuts axons in the ventrolateral spinal cord (See Figure 32). This part of the spinal cord was presumed to contain the specific 'pain pathway' to the thalamus, an assumption which was proved to be incorrect by the clinical results of cordotomy.

The major problem with the operation is that the effect fades as months go by. While fully justified in patients who are in the terminal stages of cancer from which they will die in weeks or months, the operation should not be done in patients who are likely to survive for longer times – partly because the pain returns, frequently accompanied by a variety of unpleasant sensations which are presumably generated by the deafferented spinal cord cells. In addition, the control pathways to bladder and rectum run in the ventral quadrants so that patients may have incontinence added to their other miseries.

The procedure to carry out a cordotomy was simplified by Mullan (1966). Under X-ray control, a needle is inserted between the cervical vertebrae until it lies in the cerebrospinal fluid on the ventral side of the cord. Its tip is located by injecting a fluid which can be seen by X-rays. When the position is considered satisfactory, a thin wire is pushed into the cord and the position is tested once again by using gentle electrical stimulation and asking the patient what he feels. Once verified as being in ventral white matter, a heat lesion is produced around the tip of the wire by means of an electric current. The immediate complications of this simple operation are less than those of open surgery, and the procedure is often effective for several types of severe cancer pain (Ischia *et al.*, 1984, 1985).

Cerebral operations for relief of pain

There are three major reasons why surgeons have operated on the brain in an attempt to produce analgesia. The first, and simplest, is that pains may originate from the upper chest, head and neck so that even bilateral cordotomies would fail to produce temporary analgesia in these areas. Second, it was thought possible that larger sections of the presumed pain pathways in the brain would produce a more profound and prolonged analgesia. Third, there has been a general belief that there is a 'pain centre' in the thalamus or cortex whose destruction should abolish pain.

Mesencephalic tractotomy

A very tempting target for those convinced that the spinothalamic tract is the 'pain pathway' is the confluence of spinothalamic fibres, just before arriving in the thalamus, on the lateral surface of the midbrain just below the inferior colliculus. White and Sweet (1969) report on thirty cases in whom this tract was cut at seven of the most distinguished centres of neurosurgery in the world. The appalling death rate of forty-one per cent shows the difficulty and danger of lesions in this region. While there was temporary pain relief reported in the survivors, forty-six per cent developed dysaethesias described as more severe than the original pain. These abysmal results led to the operation being abandoned but do not appear to have influenced in any way the thinking of those who moved on to the next target, the thalamus.

Thalamotomy

One of the founders of neurosurgery was Sir Victor Horsley, who developed a co-ordinate system and maps of the brain which allow wires to be lowered into the brain to end in the desired structure. This stereotaxic method has become a major technique for placing electrodes in deep-brain nuclei and tracts for recording or for lesion-making. Stereotaxic surgery allows an approach to any part of the midbrain and forebrain in man, with the needles inserted through a small hole drilled in the skull. The technique has become widely used by neurosurgeons to make lesions in the basal ganglia for movement disorders (such as Parkinson's disease), and obviously allowed lesions to be made in the thalamus for pain. However, although many of the lesions produced analgesia and pain relief for a brief period, tragically the pain returned in virtually all of the patients (Speigel and Wycis, 1966). Clearly, there is no evidence that the thalamus contains the pain centre.

Cortical lesions

Studies of the effects of cortical lesions on pain have led to the conclusion that the somatosensory cortex clearly does not contain the 'pain centre'. Large as well as small cortical lesions have no effect on pain (Casey, 1986). The long-held hope that phantom limb pain would be relieved by cortical excisions was given up long ago (White and Sweet, 1969).

Summary of surgical approaches

Acceptable long-term control of pain is rarely achieved by surgery. Not only does the pain eventually recur but additional unpleasant sensations appear as a result of denervation. Nevertheless, short-term control can, on occasion, be achieved, particularly with cordotomy, and is fully justified in patients with a short time to live, such as people in the terminal stages of cancer. However, neuro-surgical attempts to abolish other forms of chronic pain are often a disaster. One tragic case will suffice to show what can happen. A man developed phantom limb pain as a result of a brachial plexus avulsion. The arm was amputated – an unnecessary operation which was done in the incorrect belief that the paralysed arm had an abnormal effect on healthy, sensitive tissue. He then had a high cervical cordotomy. When this failed, it was repeated a second time in the belief that the first operation was not sufficiently extensive. He then had two operations on his frontal lobes which produced a definite, though temporary, psychological change but with no reduction of his pain. After destruction of the ventrobasal nucleus (Figure 19, p. 127) of the thalamus also failed, this unfortunate man committed suicide.

Our increasing knowledge of pain mechanisms now makes it clear that cutting the peripheral or central nervous system does not simply stop an input from reaching the brain. Surgical section of a peripheral nerve has multiple effects: it permanently disrupts normal patterns of input; it may result in abnormal inputs from irritating scars and neuromas; and it destroys channels that may be potentially useful to control pain by input modulation methods. Similar consequences occur after cordotomy, which is perhaps the most common operation to relieve pain. The reduction of input to the central nervous system, we now know, produces highly abnormal, bursting activity in the deafferented central cells – a condition that may persist long after the surgical section and which is conducive to prolonged pathological pain (Melzack and Loeser, 1978).

The complexity of brain activity also defies simple surgical solutions to pain problems. Pain signals project to widespread parts of the brain. If one area is surgically eliminated, there are others that still continue to receive the input. The nervous system, moreover, is able to form new connections and thereby provide new pathways for the sensory input. This plasticity is evident in physiological studies which show that after destruction of fibres to a central neural structure, the branches of neurons from adjacent areas now dominate the activity of the structure (Wall and Egger, 1971). The nervous system appears to have undergone some kind of reorganization so that the input, blocked from ascending through one pathway, is now projected through another.

Happily, the role of the neurosurgeon in the treatment of pain has been changing rapidly in recent years. Fewer rhizotomies and cordotomies are now being carried out, and neurosurgeons are turning increasingly to non-destructive approaches such as the use of devices to electrically stimulate nerves, spinal cord and discrete areas of the brain. A small number of neurosurgeons are carrying out pioneering work in these fields, and the results so far – which shall be described shortly – are highly exciting. They hold great promise for the patient in severe, intractable pain who is not helped by the traditional drug therapies (Gybels and Sweet, 1989).

Temporary local anaesthesia

For millennia, the leaves of *Erythroxylon coca* have been chewed by those who live in the Andes for their psychedelic effect. These leaves, which contain cocaine, were well known to produce a numbing of the mouth but this was generally ignored as an unwanted side-effect. The pure alkaloid was isolated by the middle of the nineteenth century, and in 1884 Karl Köller in Vienna was the first to use cocaine as a local anaesthetic, instilling it into the eye in order to carry out painless surgery. In 1884, Hall introduced local anaesthesia to dentistry, and in 1885 Halstead produced nerve blocks by injecting cocaine around nerves, which enabled him to carry out major surgery in the anaesthetized part of the body.

By 1905 the first synthetic local anaesthetic, procaine, was produced, which does not have the psychedelic effects of cocaine. Since 1948, procaine has largely been replaced by lidocaine which is more powerful and less toxic, and by a family of related compounds with slightly varying properties but all having '-caine' at the end of their names.

Procedure and uses

Local anaesthetics do not penetrate unbroken skin, and there is considerable doubt that they have any effect apart from the relief they produce by cooling the skin. However, local anaesthetics are able to penetrate mucous membrane tissue and are therefore incorporated in the innumerable nostrums for sore throats and haemorrhoids, and are even swallowed for hiccups.

By far the commonest use of local anaesthetics is by needle injection. Here the aim is to squirt the anaesthetic onto a nerve, or sometimes just to infiltrate a general area which one wishes to make numb. Most of us have experienced this technique when dentists inject close to one of the nerves supplying the teeth on which they plan to work. The injection is usually given in combination with adrenalin, which constricts the local blood vessels and slows down the absorption of the anaesthetic into the blood stream, thereby prolonging its local action.

Anaesthesiologists have become highly skilled in approaching most of the peripheral nerves in the body. They are now often aided in this procedure by using image-intensified X-rays so that they can follow the course of the needle tip with respect to bony structures. It is possible in this way to give a regional anaesthetic to a whole limb, but this involves extensive infiltration with quantities of local anaesthetic which approach the toxic limits. For the legs, chest, abdomen and pelvis a more economical approach can be used in which advantage is taken of the confluence of the sensory nerves as they pass into the spinal cord. As we have already mentioned, there is a space – the epidural space – between the inner side of the bony vertebral canal and the dura mater which covers the spinal cord. The nerve roots have to pass through this space and it is possible to place a fine catheter in it and to flood the region with local anaesthetic. Since these catheters can be manoeuvred to any segment of the spinal column, large areas of the body can be anaesthetized on both sides by this skilled but simple procedure of epidural block.

A more direct approach to achieve spinal anaesthesia for pain in the abdomen, pelvis or legs involves injection of the anaesthetic by way of a lumbar puncture needle. The needle is pushed through the skin in the midline of the lower back so that it slips between the vertebrae, passes through the epidural space, punctures the dura and enters the cerebrospinal fluid. In the adult, the spinal cord does not fill the entire spinal canal and the lowest part is filled with a bundle of nerve roots which supply the lower lumbar and sacral segments. This bundle, the cauda equina ('horse tail'), can be safely penetrated by a needle since the roots slide out of the way and it is possible to soak the entire region in local anaesthetic. As the amount of anaesthetic is increased, the level of anaesthesia on the body surface rises upwards. The limit is determined by the danger of paralysing the respiratory muscles in the chest. Here, then, we see that by taking advantage of the specialized anatomical flow of sensory fibres, it is possible to anaesthetize small or large areas of the body without interfering with other systems or with the patient's thinking processes.

Rationale

Local anaesthetics act by stabilizing the membranes of nerve and muscle cells which produce action potentials. After an injection, a high concentration of the anaesthetic is built up around the target nerve. The nerve membrane at rest maintains the separation of specific ions so that potassium ions accumulate on the inside and sodium ions on the outside. If the normal membrane is slightly disturbed by changing the voltage across it, this mechanism to separate ions is briefly altered, and sodium ions rush in while potassium ions flow out. This explosive flow of ions produces the nerve impulse and the impulse runs along the nerve membrane, followed in a few milliseconds by the restoration of the resting state. Local anaesthetics block the triggering mechanism by which these impulses are generated so that the nerve remains fixed in its resting state for as long as the local anaesthetic is present in a high enough concentration.

Side-effects

Great as this advance has been, there are certain limits to its usefulness. Local anaesthesia usually involves a complete block of all nerve fibres in the region. This results in a complete numbness of the area supplied by a nerve, but also in paralysis, since the motor fibres are also blocked. If the amount of anaesthetic rises generally in the body, other impulse-generating structures, such as the heart, begin to be affected by showing a decrease in excitability.

Since local anaesthetics produce such a satisfactory abolition of pain for an hour or more, there has been a search for methods of prolonging their action. Such drugs have been discovered but, unfortunately, they have toxic effects, including damage to the nerve which is blocked. The alternative approach has been to devise methods for continuous application of the short-acting drugs. This procedure succeeds over periods of days by using an indwelling catheter, and is utilized in some hospitals to suppress the worst of the pains after an operation or a wound. However, complications eventually set in and the treatment must end. One of the most interesting side-effects of these drugs is that in addition to blocking nerve impulses they also block the transport of substances along nerve fibres. This transport is necessary for the integrity of the nerve and for its target organs, and this secondary effect may therefore forbid the dream of a long-term local anaesthetic derived from this family of -caines.

Recently, morphine has been used in an unorthodox fashion for the relief of chronic pain. Normally, of course, it is injected into muscles such as the buttock or it is ingested orally. There is now evidence that morphine may bring about dramatic relief of some kinds of pain if a small amount is injected epidurally. Extremely severe pain due to spreading cancer in the pelvic region can sometimes be relieved to a significant extent by injection of a few milligrams of morphine in the lumbar epidural space (Cousins and Bridenbaugh, 1987). The results of this procedure, like all new techniques, seem extremely exciting. However, the method is new and requires more carefully controlled research before it can be recommended without reservation.

Despite the short-acting effect of an anaesthetic agent, anaesthetic blocks of the sensory input often produce pain relief that outlasts the duration of the blocks (Livingston, 1943; Kibler and Nathan, 1960). Successive blocks may relieve pain for increasingly long periods of time. Anaesthetic blocks of tender skin areas, peripheral nerves, or sympathetic ganglia would have the effect of diminishing the total sensory input that bombards the spinal transmission cells. They would, therefore, reduce the spinal cell output below the critical level necessary to evoke pain. These blocks, moreover, could bring about a cessation of self-sustaining, memory-like activity, so that temporary blocks would produce long periods of relief. Furthermore, the relief of pain would permit increased use of the body, allowing the patient to carry out normal motor activities. These, in turn, would produce patterned inputs (particularly from muscles) that would contain a high proportion of active large fibres that would further close the gate and delay the recurrence of pain. In addition, the motor 'commands' that descend from the brain to the spinal cord are accompanied by inhibitory descending control impulses which would also reduce the sensory input during movement.

The varieties of physical therapy

A multitude of techniques are practised by physiatrists (doctors of physical medicine and rehabilitation) and physiotherapists. The following (Zohn and Mennell, 1976) is a partial list:

1 Manual therapy: exercise; massage; manipulation; relaxation.
2 Mechanical therapy: traction; compression.
3 Heat: superficial heat: dry; wet.
4 Heat: deep heat: shortwave diathermy; microwave diathermy; ultrasound.
5 Cold: vapocoolant spray; ice packs; ice massage; hypothermia.
6 Electrotherapy: alternating current (Faradism); sinusoidal current; transcutaneous electrical nerve stimulation.
7 Electrotherapy: direct current (galvanism); interrupted galvanism.

These are the more widely used of many physical procedures, most of them requiring elegant and complicated-looking equipment. There is no doubt that they are effective for a wide variety of pains (Lehmann and de Lateur, 1994). The common feature among them is that they produce a sensory input – they generate nerve impulses that enter the spinal cord and brain and produce their pain-relieving effects for reasons that we shall examine later.

Massage and manipulation

Almost all societies practise variations of these two techniques in which mechanical pressure is used to relieve pain (Haldeman, 1994). While they are generally practised by highly skilled, trained professionals, there is not one of us who does not scratch an itch, stretch an aching back, or rub an area that hurts. These are our own, almost instinctive, manoeuvres which have developed into the various anti-pain procedures.

Massage

There are many massage techniques, each with its enthusiastic following. Some therapists move only skin with light repeated movements while others massage deep structures so vigorously that they produce pain. Massage may be given at the site of pain or at a considerable distance. A fascinating, recent discovery is that vaginal pressure produces a marked increase in pain threshold in rats (Steinman *et al.*, 1983) and women. Vaginal pressure in women raises the tolerance threshold to painful compression of a finger by 41 per cent and, when the pressure produces orgasm, by 75 per cent (Whipple and Komisaruk, 1985). Light mechanical vibrators driven by electricity and oscillating at the frequency of the mainline voltage are being used more frequently (Lundberg, 1984a, b; Sherer *et al.*, 1986). Deep massage involves heavy pressure and the stretching and pinching of ligaments, tendons and muscles. One of the main problems for an analysis of this and the following procedures is to know exactly what it is the therapist is doing and which of all the various pressures and movements are most effective.

Manipulation

Here the patient is subjected to a variety of stretchings, twistings and pullings. Some are gentle, some are quite violent. There are many practitioners, including osteopaths and chiropractors. However, physiotherapists, physiatrists and orthopaedists (bone specialists) also practise forms of manipulation. There are, in addition, faddist groups that practise special manipulations and massages. Each school operates on its own theoretical target. Some claim to be placing bones, especially the vertebrae, in their correct alignment but there is no X-ray evidence that the bones are out of place before the manipulation or that they are changed afterwards. Some say they are breaking up scar tissue which is trapping nerves while others state that they are putting muscles in their correct tensions. It is a pity that there is such a plethora of untested hypotheses since these manipulations on occasion produce quite dramatic relief. Yet the manipulators, the patients and the rest of us remain ignorant of exactly what was done to produce the disappearance of the pain or, for that matter, how to explain the many failures.

Heat therapy

General heating

Since neolithic times, people in all parts of the world have found ways of raising the body temperature and have used them for treatment of their pains. The North American Indians' hodown, the

Finnish sauna, the innumerable spas of Europe around hot springs (especially the thermae of Italy), the Roman baths with their hot and tepid rooms, the Russian and Turkish versions of the steam room, and the Japanese hot soaking tub all produce intense heat. The effect on pain is probably due to a general relaxation of tense muscles and a psychological feeling of well-being.

Local superficial heat

Great ingenuity has been used through the ages to apply and sustain local superficial heating. Since ancient times, poultices made of heated clay, stones, bread, dough, and towels have been shaped and placed on painful areas to heat them. In our modern age, we use electrically heated pads. We also produce vasodilation by rubbing herbs or drugs into the skin or by applying plasters made of mustard or cantharides (which is an extract of Spanish flies). Friar's Balsam and many liniments similarly produce a vasodilation of the blood vessels in the skin and, consequently, a feeling of warmth. Since the skin turns red as the blood vessels open up, these compounds are called rubifacients, or 'red makers'.

Local deep heat

Ultrasound

One of the uses of this modern technique is to raise the temperature in deep structures. The sounds that we hear consist of pressure waves in the air, and the highest tones we can hear are produced by wave frequencies of about fifteen to twenty thousand cycles per second. Pressure waves produced at high frequencies beyond our hearing range are called ultrasound just as ultraviolet is a type of light with a frequency beyond our ability to see. An ultrasound frequency of over one million cycles per second takes on a number of characteristics like light. It can be focused and beamed. It travels through water and soft tissues and, like an intense beam of light, it heats whatever absorbs it. The sound is produced by a rapidly vibrating crystal, like a crystal loudspeaker, which is placed on the skin. The sound enters the body and passes through the soft tissue with very little loss of energy. However, when the sound hits something solid like bone, it is absorbed and turned into heat. In this way, it is possible to gently warm the surface of bones and especially joints.

Diathermy

This is a method of heating a part of the body or a limb from the middle outward and it uses electromagnetic radiation rather than the pressure waves used in ultrasound. Radio waves are electromagnetic radiation at frequencies that pass through the body and most other structures, including walls in homes. The frequencies used in diathermy pass into the body but are absorbed in the deep tissues where the electromagnetic energy is transformed into heat. This property is used to the patient's advantage in diathermy where the middle of a limb can be gently warmed while leaving the skin virtually unaffected.

Mechanisms of action

Heat appears to be most effective for low-to-moderate levels of pain due to deep-tissue injuries such as bruises, torn muscles and ligaments, and arthritis. Whether it speeds up repair is not known, but it is doubtful. Despite the widespread use of heat to relieve pain, we do not know why it works. There are two hypotheses which both need to be tested. The first relates to the obvious vasodilation and the consequent increase of blood flow. It seems reasonable that, if there is damaged tissue or infection, the blood must bring cells and chemicals needed for the repair of injured or inflamed tissues and must sweep away the breakdown products of injury – such as histamine, bradykinin and prostaglandins – which we know contribute to pain. Even in the use of superficial heat for the relief of pain in deep structures, it is possible that deep blood vessels are dilated by 'somato-visceral' reflexes evoked by skin stimulation. This vascular hypothesis merits investigation because anti-inflammatory agents such as prostaglandin inhibitors are often effective analgesics, which suggests that the substances produced by inflammation and injury are built up at faster rates than they can be carried away by the blood flow.

The second hypothesis proposes that the heating of tissues generates nerve impulses which play a role in the afferent barrage and have an inhibitory effect by closing the gate in the spinal cord. This would explain how the application of heat at a distance from the source of the damage and pain can be effective. The nerve impulses stimulated by heating the skin travel into the spinal cord and, at convergent synapses, inhibit impulses that originate in damaged tissue much deeper than the heated skin. Therefore, it is possible that heat counteracts pain by stimulating nerve impulses which decrease the effectiveness in the spinal cord of the pain-producing nerve impulses.

The mechanisms that underlie the pain-relieving effects of most of the procedures of physical therapy remain a mystery. The most plausible hypothesis for all of them is that they produce sensory inputs that ultimately inhibit pain signals ('close the gate'). As we have seen, the gate theory proposes that this may occur (1) by activation of large fibres by gentle stimulation which has inhibitory effects at segmental levels; or (2) by activation of small fibres which project signals to brainstem areas which, in turn, send messages to the spinal cord that close the gate. Different procedures in physical medicine may be explained by either or both mechanisms. Considerable evidence about these mechanisms has been revealed as a result of the dramatic growth of research on transcutaneous electrical nerve stimulation.

Electrical stimulation of nerves, spinal cord and brain

The most obvious prediction of the gate-control theory was that stimulation of large, low-threshold fibres should inhibit cells which transmit injury signals. The large fibres in a peripheral nerve can be selectively stimulated by passing low-intensity electric currents through the nerve. The sensation produced by gentle electrical stimulation of normal peripheral nerves is a buzzing, tingling feeling which becomes painful only if the strength of stimulation is greatly increased to stimulate small fibres. Wall and Sweet (1967) therefore set about stimulating the large fibres in peripheral nerves, first in themselves and then in patients.

Transcutaneous electrical nerve stimulation

All nerves within about four centimetres below the surface of the skin can be stimulated by placing electrodes on the skin surface. These include the large nerves in the upper and lower arm, the nerves in the lower leg, and any superficial skin nerves. The electrodes, these days, are usually made of flexible conducting silicone and they make contact with the skin through a conducting paste. The electrodes are connected to a pocket-sized, battery-operated stimulator which puts out a continuous series of electrical pulses. The frequency and duration of the pulses vary among different stimulators, but in all of them the strength (amplitude) of the pulses can be varied by the patient, who raises the strength of stimulation until a comfortable tingling is felt in the area supplied by the nerve which is being stimulated.

This technique has now been used by hundreds of thousands of patients with machines made by numerous companies. There is usually a decrease of pain during the stimulation and this is satisfactory for the continuous control of the pain in a substantial percentage of the cases. The most clearcut responses have been obtained when there is skin tenderness associated with nerve damage or disease, or when there are tender muscle points. In patients with causalgia – the most dramatic example of pain associated with localized nerve damage – stimulation central to the area of damage produces a striking decrease in the skin's sensitivity, while stimulation peripheral to the damage increases the pain. In post-herpetic neuralgia, patients whose main complaint is an unbearable sensitivity of the skin report a satisfactory return of normal sensitivity when the main affected nerves are stimulated (Nathan and Wall, 1974). Since the procedure is so simple and free of side-effects, it has come to be used as an initial treatment for many chronic pain syndromes. It is also used in many centres for acute pains by applying the electrodes around the incision scar at the time of surgical operations; it often increases the patient's comfort and decreases the amount of narcotic needed to control post-operative pain. Similarly, the technique is used widely in Sweden during the first stages of childbirth when the mother frequently feels surges of low back pain during uterine contractions.

The mild increase of pain threshold, particularly in cases of skin tenderness, is sufficient to control pain in many patients during the stimulation. Of even more interest to some patients, particularly those with damage to nerves, the relief outlasts a brief period (15–30 minutes) of stimulation by many hours. This is a remarkable phenomenon in which a brief action produces a very prolonged relief.

There is no longer any doubt that transcutaneous electrical nerve stimulation (TENS) is an effective way to treat chronic pain. It is significantly more effective than a placebo machine when stimulation is administered within the painful area, over a related nerve, and even at a distance from the nerve (Thorsteinsson *et al.*, 1977). In a study of joint pain in patients with rheumatoid arthritis, stimulation near the painful joint at low intensity produced significant pain relief in 75 per cent of patients. When the stimulation intensity was increased, pain relief was obtained by 95 per cent (Mannheimer *et al.*, 1978). Intensity is clearly an important factor, and so is the frequency of the stimulation, although it may depend on the kind of pain. In a study of rheumatoid arthritis (Mannheimer and Carlsson, 1979), high-frequency (70Hz) stimulation was more effective than low-frequency (3Hz). In contrast, in a study of 123 patients who had pain due primarily to lesions of the nervous system, low-frequency stimulation was better (Eriksson *et al.*, 1979).

Perhaps the most exciting feature of TENS is that it produces relief in patients who received little or no relief by other methods, including neurosurgical procedures, anaesthetic blocks and so forth. In a group of 30 patients with post-herpetic neuralgia, Nathan and Wall (1974) observed that 11 were helped more by TENS than by any other treatment. In 9 patients, pain relief outlasted stimulation by 1 to 2 hours, and 2 patients were cured. Excellent effects are also reported for pain due to haemophiliac haemorrhages into joints (Roche *et al.*, 1985), anginal pain (Mannheimer *et al.*, 1986), and a variety of other types of pain (Woolf, 1984).

It is not yet possible to state the optimal frequencies or intensities of stimulation for each kind of pain problem, or the percentages of people helped. But it is clear that a high proportion is helped by appropriate stimulation, that TENS is more effective than any other form of treatment for many patients, and that the proportion may become higher when the correct form of stimulation is found for each pain syndrome, probably for each patient.

The original reason for introducing the technique still appears valid as a partial explanation of its success. Sensory nerve impulses have mixed effects in the central nervous system, producing both excitation and inhibition. A predominant effect is for the large-diameter afferents to raise the threshold of cells which respond to injury signals. As the continuous stimulation is applied, there is a gradual rise of the threshold of spinal cord cells in their ability to respond. Wall and Gutnick (1974) discovered an additional factor which may play a role in the stimulation of damaged nerves. Direct stimulation of a normal sensory nerve fibre at a distance from its receptive field generates nerve impulses which run in the normal direction towards the central nervous system, as well as nerve impulses which travel antidromically towards the periphery. As noted previously, the new sprouts which grow from the ends of damaged nerves take on several new properties. One of these is that nerve impulses that invade a sprout from the parent fibre tend to silence the sprout and raise its threshold to stimuli for a long time. Therefore, it may be that electrical stimulation of peripheral nerves, in addition to producing a central inhibition, also may decrease the abnormal excitability of the damaged parts of the peripheral nerve.

Dorsal column stimulation

Wall and Sweet (1967), realizing that it was essential to stimulate central to an area of nerve damage, implanted electrodes around major nerves and produced pain relief in several patients. They also stimulated large numbers of sensory roots as they enter the spinal cord. An anaesthesia needle was placed in the cerebrospinal fluid at the site where the roots run from the pelvis into the spinal cord. An electrode was then run through the needle to lie among the roots. For brief periods, these patients were given mild stimulation and they reported that their pain decreased while the stimulation was applied. These test results were sufficiently encouraging for Shealy *et al.* (1967) to develop a more radical procedure which would allow prolonged, permanent stimulation of the dorsal columns of the spinal cord. However, this procedure involved major surgery and was plagued by equipment breakdowns and by leakage of the cerebrospinal fluid through the hole in the dura through which the electrodes ran. Furthermore, a number of patients who initially responded very well for periods of weeks or months began to experience a return of their pain.

For these reasons, this radical form of dorsal column stimulation has been replaced by a much less intrusive technique – percutaneous dorsal column stimulation. In this method, electrodes are inserted through special epidural needles until they lie on top of the dura just above the dorsal columns. This is a highly skilled yet simple technique which requires no anaesthesia or major operation. Furthermore, the electrodes and the wires that lead to the surface of the body can be left in place for some weeks so that prolonged testing can be carried out. If the results are disappointing, the electrodes are simply pulled out. But, if the patient shows marked pain relief, the wires can be buried and attached to a radio stimulator during a relatively minor operation. A recent study (Urban and Nashold, 1978) has shown that of twenty patients who tried percutaneous epidural stimulation of the dorsal columns, seven reported excellent relief over a two-week trial period and were then given a permanently implanted receiver system. All but one of these patients experienced continuing pain relief throughout a long follow-up time of up to two years. What is impressive here is that the procedure is relatively simple, allows rapid identification of patients who will be helped, and produces excellent results in those for whom it is effective.

It is presumed that the major effect of this treatment is explained by the same factors we have described for peripheral nerve stimulation. The afferent sensory fibres in the dorsal columns all send branches into the spinal cord dorsal horn where they enter the cord. Each electrical pulse applied to dorsal columns sends impulses toward the brain, and other impulses which descend and enter the dorsal horn. It is assumed that the impulses entering the dorsal horn trigger an inhibition. Successful effects of dorsal column stimulation have been reported by Lindblom and Meyerson (1975) in patients with chest pain following the damage to nerves which may occur during chest surgery. In a beautiful series of careful tests, they showed that the effect is to readjust sensitivity to gentle stimuli which produce intolerable pain, while the normal actions of unaffected nerves are very little disturbed. As with successful gentle nerve stimulation, the successful effects of dorsal column stimulation appear to re-establish a normal balance of excitation and inhibition rather than to enforce a powerful blockade.

Brain stimulation

The discovery that electrical stimulation of the periaqueductal grey matter in animals produces a profound analgesia, which we described earlier, led to attempts to relieve chronic pain in human patients by similar stimulation. Some patients suffering chronic pain have now had electrodes implanted stereotaxically in the periaqueductal grey matter in the upper (rostral) portions of the brainstem and generally the results have been mixed. In one study of six patients (Hosobuchi *et al.*, 1977), five with cancer received complete relief of pain until they died three to eighteen months after implantation. The sixth patient, with facial anaesthesia dolorosa (severe pain in the face even though the skin is insensitive to stimulation), had only partial relief. Interestingly, although the chronic pain was relieved to some degree in all cases, pain due to pinprick or intense radiant heat was relatively unaffected except when the brain was stimulated at very high levels. The major limitation to the procedure is that the patients rapidly develop tolerance to continuous periaqueductal stimulation, so that it becomes ineffective.

Excellent relief of chronic pain is obtained by electrical stimulation of the posterior thalamus and adjacent internal capsule (Mazars *et al.*, 1974; Turnbull, 1984). Tsubokawa *et al.*, (1984) found that when tolerance occurred after prolonged stimulation, it could be greatly reduced by the drug L-dopa (which is usually used to treat patients with Parkinson's disease). As in peripheral nerve stimulation,

stimulation of the thalamus produces a tingling feeling in the affected body areas when it effectively relieves pain. This procedure is promising because pain is often suppressed for long periods of time after stimulation is stopped – as long as twenty-four hours in some patients (Young and Rinaldi, 1994). Interestingly, patients who receive partial relief report that intermittent attacks of sharp pain may disappear altogether, while the underlying constant ache tends to recur when stimulation is stopped. Resumption of stimulation again produces partial or complete relief. The mechanism of action of stimulation in the sensory thalamus is not clear. It is possible that descending inhibitory systems are activated indirectly by thalamic and cortical fibres that are known to project to the recticular formation. Another possible mechanism is that, because most of these patients have pain due to lesions of the nervous system, impulses evoked by stimulation disrupt abnormal firing in neuron pools in the brain that have been deprived of input and are therefore firing at excessive rates.

These procedures, so far, appear to be hopeful, and many of the problems have been overcome. The rapid development of tolerance to stimulation seems to be prevented or slowed down by reducing the duration of the periods of stimulation. Whether this strategy will work indefinitely, and for all patients, is not known. All surgeons have had failures and some have had no success at all. With careful selection of patients, however, the procedure has been highly successful. Since no destruction of brain tissue occurs, even those who fail to respond are not harmed.

Acupuncture and other forms of folk medicine

The study of folk medicine by anthropologists and medical historians has revealed an astonishing array of ingenious methods to relieve pain (Brockbank, 1954; Wand-Tetley, 1956). Every culture, it appears, has learned to fight pain with pain: in general, brief, moderate pain tends to abolish severe, prolonged pain. One of the oldest methods is cupping, in which a glass cup is heated up (by coals or flaming alcohol) and then inverted over the painful area and held against it. As the air in the cup cools and contracts, it creates a partial vacuum so that the skin is sucked up into the cup (Figure 33). The procedure produces bruising of the skin with concomitant pain and tenderness. Cupping was practised in ancient Greece and Rome as early as the 4th century BC, and was also practised in ancient India and China. Over the centuries, the method spread to virtually all parts of the world, and cups of various sizes, shapes and materials have evolved. Cupping has been used – and is still widely practised – for a large variety of ailments, including headaches, backaches and arthritic pains.

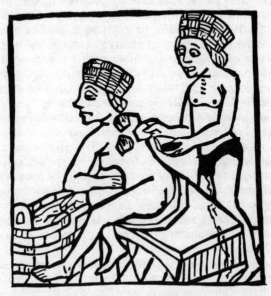

Figure 33. Cupping, shown in a German Calendar published in 1483. Note that the attendant holds a lighted lamp in his left hand. (reprinted in W. Brockbank (1954) from the Wellcome Historical Medical Library)

Scarification is another ancient practice in which the skin is cut by a sharp knife or by awesome devices with multiple blades. Scarification has been widely practised and sometimes is part of 'wet cupping', in which a hot cup is placed over the cut skin and sucks out blood. Wet cupping and scarification, like leech-induced bleeding, were often used to reduce the amount of fluid in the body, especially in cases of congestive heart failure. In addition, they were used to produce pain as well as local irritation and inflammation to combat disease and severe, chronic pain. Old medical texts describe the methods in great detail, and it is evident that they were used for common diseases as well as for the treatment of headache, backache, sciatica and other forms of chronic pain.

Cauterization is yet another ancient method. Generally, the end of an iron rod was heated until it was red-hot, and was then placed on the painful area, such as the foot in the case of gout, or on the buttock, back or leg in patients with low back pain. Often, however, the cautery was applied to specifically prescribed sites distant from the painful area. The procedure, of course, produced pain and subsequent blistering of the area that was touched by the cautery.

The same effect was achieved by two other procedures: rubbing blistering fluids into the skin, or applying a cone of moxa (made from the leaves of the mugwort plant) to a site on the body, setting the tip of the cone aflame, and allowing it to burn slowly until it approached or reached the skin ('moxibustion'). Again, the procedure produced pain and, while used for all kinds of diseases, was often prescribed specifically for painful conditions.

There are countless other methods that resemble the ones just described. It is evident that the one factor common to all of them is that they produce pain to abolish pain. The pain was usually brief and moderate, but its effect was to relieve or abolish a much more severe, chronic pain. These methods, of course, did not always work, but they obviously worked well enough to have survived throughout the world for thousands of years. Do these procedures work better than a placebo? There are no experimental studies, but the evidence from studies of acupuncture – a related procedure – suggests that they do.

The methods we have just described are generally known as 'counter-irritation', and some are still frequently used although there has not been (until recently) any theoretical or physiological explanation for their effectiveness. Suggestion and distraction of attention are the usual mechanisms invoked, but neither seems capable of explaining the power of the methods or the long duration of the relief they may afford. Because they involve painful or near-painful levels of stimulation to relieve pain, these methods have also been labelled as 'hyperstimulation analgesia' (Melzack, 1973).

Interest in folk medicine gained enormous impetus in recent years by the rediscovery of the ancient Chinese practice of acupuncture, which has been in continuous practice for at least 2,000 years. Basically, the procedure involves the insertion of fine needles (made of steel, gold or other metals) through specific points at the skin and then twirling them for some time at a slow rate. The needles may also be left in place for varying periods of time. The practice of acupuncture is part of a complex, fascinating theory of medicine in which all diseases and pains are believed to be due to disharmony between Yin (spirit) and Yang (blood) which flow in channels called 'meridians'. Acupuncture charts are extremely complex and consist, traditionally, of 361 points which lie on 14 meridians, most of which are named after internal organs, such as the large intestine, the heart, or the bladder (Kao, 1973). A great deal of mystery surrounds the practice of acupuncture in China, and the points chosen for treatment of a given malady are held to be influenced by the time of day, the weather and a multitude of other variables. The mystery, however, may hide one or more basic physiological principles.

Acupuncture was first described in the western world by the Dutch physician Willem ten Rhyne in 1683. After great initial enthusiasm, interest in acupuncture soon diminished. Since that time, acupuncture has been 'rediscovered' in the West about two or three times a century. In recent years, the major cause of the renewed interest in acupuncture was the description of its use in modern China to produce analgesia in order to carry out surgery. However, we now know that acupuncture is rarely effective for surgery (Bonica, 1974b), and the initial enthusiasm dropped rapidly. Nevertheless, visitors to China became more aware of its traditional use for various aches and pains, and often observed impressive results in cases of low back pain, myofascial pain, and some of the neuralgias.

Several kinds of evidence, obtained in western countries as well as in China, reveal the nature of acupuncture's action on pain. The first is the demonstration, in carefully controlled studies, that acupuncture has significantly greater effects on pain than placebo stimulation (Chapman *et al.*, 1976; Anderson *et al.*, 1974; Stewart *et al.*, 1977). Moreover, partial analgesia can be produced by acupuncture in animals such as monkeys and mice (Vierck *et al.*, 1974, Pomeranz *et al.*, 1977), and acupuncture stimulation inhibits or otherwise changes the transmission of pain-evoked nerve impulses at several levels of the central nervous system (Kerr *et al.*, 1978). However, an impressive number of studies show that acupuncture stimulation need not be applied at the precise points indicated on acupuncture charts. It is possible, for example, to achieve as much control over dental pain by stimulating an area between the fourth and fifth fingers, which is not designated on acupuncture charts as related to facial pain, as by stimulating the Hoku point between the thumb and index finger which *is* so designated (Taub *et al.*, 1977). The decreases in pain obtained by stimulation at either site are so large and occur in so many patients that it is unlikely that the pain relief is due to placebo effects. Rather, the results suggest that the site that can be effectively stimulated is not a discrete point but a large area, possibly the whole hand.

The same conclusion can be drawn from another study – a

double-blind experiment on the efficacy of acupuncture on osteo-arthritic pain – in which the control patients received 'placebo' acupuncture stimulation at sites just adjacent to the 'real' acupuncture points (Gaw *et al.*, 1975). Patients in both groups showed significant improvement in tenderness and subjective report of pain as evaluated by two independent observers, as well as in activity of the joint. Because there was no difference between the two groups, the improvement was attributed to a placebo effect. It is more likely, however, that it is stimulation within a large area and not merely at a point that has an effect. Similar conclusions can be drawn from an excellent study of acupuncture control over pain in patients with sickle-cell anaemia (Co *et al.*, 1979). It is the intense stimulation rather than the precise site that appears to be the crucial factor. This is exactly the conclusion drawn by several writers (Ghia *et al.*, 1976; Lewit, 1979) who showed that acupuncture stimulation of the painful area is as effective as stimulation at designated distant points. From all this it may be concluded that intense stimulation is the necessary factor, and the precise site of stimulation is less important than the intensity of the input. However, not every body area is effective. Stimulation of the outer ear (auriculotherapy) fails to produce greater relief of chronic pain than placebo stimulation (Melzack and Katz, 1984).

Hyperstimulation analgesia

The conclusion that intense stimulation can produce pain relief – 'hyperstimulation analgesia' – led to the investigation of other kinds of stimuli. The first study (Melzack, 1975b) examined the effects of brief, intense transcutaneous electrical nerve stimulation (TENS) on severe clinical pain. The data indicated that the procedure provides significant pain relief that frequently outlasts a twenty-minute period of stimulation by several hours – occasionally for days or weeks. Daily stimulation carried out at home by the patient sometimes provides gradually increasing relief over periods of weeks or months. That these effects are not due to placebo phenomena was demonstrated in a double-blind study (Jeans, 1979). Fox and Melzack (1976) then compared the relative effectiveness of TENS and acupuncture on low back pain and found that both forms of stimulation at the back and leg produce substantial decreases in pain intensity and both are equally effective.

Ice massage is yet another way to produce intense sensory input. At first, ice massage of an area makes it feel numb. If ice massage is maintained, however, it produces aching, burning pain and, therefore, may act like acupuncture or intense TENS. Melzack *et al.*, (1980a) treated patients suffering from acute dental pain with ice massage of the back of the hand (at the Hoku area, between the thumb and index finger) on the same side as the pain. The ice massage decreased the intensity of the dental pain by 50 per cent or more in the majority of patients. Furthermore, ice massage of the hand on the side opposite to the pain also produced significant pain relief (Melzack and Bentley, 1983). In another study, Melzack *et al.* (1980b) examined the relative effectiveness of ice massage and intense TENS for the relief of low back pain and showed that both methods produced significant pain relief in about 65 per cent of patients.

The fact that intense stimulation produces pain relief provides a link with a phenomenon we discussed earlier (p. 183): the relief of pain by stimulation of trigger points. Travell and Rinzler, in a classic paper published in 1952, summarized the work they carried out over a period of years demonstrating that 'dry needling' of trigger points – simply moving a needle in and out of the area without injecting any substance – produces striking relief of myofascial pain. At about the same time, Sola and Williams (1956) discovered that injection of normal saline is a highly effective way to relieve musculoskeletal pains such as shoulder and neck pains.

These observations led Frost *et al.*, (1980) to carry out a double-blind comparison of a local anaesthetic – mepivacaine – and saline injected into trigger points for myofascial pain. To their astonishment, the group that received saline tended to have significantly more relief of pain: 80 per cent of patients with saline reported pain relief, compared to 52 per cent with the anaesthetic. Furthermore, the average duration of relief was 3 hours for saline and 30 minutes for the anaesthetic. The saline was more effective, they proposed, because it irritated tissues, which is the essential ingredient of the treatment, while the anaesthetic actually blocked the irritating effect of the needle. Similarly, Lewit (1979) has observed that the effectiveness of trigger point injections bears little relationship to the agent injected, but is related to the intensity of pain produced at the trigger zone, and to the precision with which the site of maximal tenderness was located by the needle. While this sounds like torture, the brief shot of pain produced by the needle resulted in striking relief of pain.

The mechanisms that underlie hyperstimulation analgesia are not known. The most plausible hypothesis (Melzack, 1971, 1975b) is that the intense inputs activate brainstem structures that exert a descending inhibition on pain-signalling cells in the dorsal horns, and recent physiological studies (Le Bars *et al.*, 1983) support the existence of such a system. Intense electrical or thermal stimulation activates descending diffuse noxious inhibitory controls (DNIC) which could provide the basis for hyperstimulation analgesia. One of the major areas involved in these descending controls is the periaqueductal grey (PAG), which has been shown (Soper and Melzack, 1982) to have a rough somatotopic organization so that stimulation at a particular site in the PAG produces analgesia in large areas, such as a quadrant or entire half of the body. A mechanism such as this can explain how intense stimulation at a tender trigger point, which produces a deep, aching pain, can produce pain relief in the larger painful area associated with it (see Figure 29). Furthermore, since acupuncture points and trigger points have an astonishingly similar distribution (Melzack *et al.*, 1977), needling of acupuncture points (which also produces a deep ache) would produce an intense input that would activate the descending inhibitory controls. This would explain the fact that most acupuncture points for pain are found in or near the painful area (Melzack *et al.*, 1977). Of those at a distance, only a single point – the Hoku point for dental pain – has been shown to produce more effective pain relief than a placebo. Since the projections from the hand and jaw lie near each other in the brain, and presumably have interconnecting neurons, it is conceivable that stimulation of the hand could activate descending inhibitory controls over inputs from a large area that includes the jaw. However, stimulation of sites too distant from the painful area would not be expected to have any effect on pain; and, indeed, electrical stimulation of the outer ear (auriculotherapy) is no more effective than a placebo for the relief of pain (Melzack and Katz, 1984).

The physiology of the sensory modulation of pain

We have described four classes of sensory modulation therapy and can review the basis of each of these with a brief summary.

Therapy 1: Surgical section or anaesthetic blockade of sensory pathways

These therapies will obviously work when the source of the pain is an injury in the periphery. However, there are two serious problems.

First, peripheral section or anaesthetic block prevents the passage of all impulses and produces anaesthesia and paralysis as well as analgesia. Second, cutting pathways usually has a temporary effect because denervated central structures tend to become hyperexcitable and generate abnormal outputs in the absence of any input.

Therapy 2: Stimulation of low-threshold afferent fibres or the central pathways responsible for their inhibitory effects

As described in the gate-control theory, the arrival in the spinal cord of impulses in low-threshold afferent fibres produces some inhibitory effects. This can be achieved by rubbing, scratching, gentle massage, warmth, or by low-level TENS of the type described by Wall and Sweet (1967). We do not know if the electrical stimulation of midbrain structures also evokes this type of inhibition, since it is not known when the central descending control comes into action under normal circumstances. TENS, in this therapy, is aimed at stimulation of low-threshold afferents and the stimulation is applied to the region of the pain and not at a distance. The cause of the long-lasting effects is a mystery but may be related to the impulse-triggered, peptide-dependent, long-latency, long-duration effects described in Chapter 9.

Therapy 3: Stimulation of high-threshold afferents or their central pathways

The only known physiological basis for this is the descending diffuse noxious inhibitory controls (DNIC) described by Le Bars *et al.*, (1983). It is not known why the descending inhibition tends to persist for periods that outlast the duration of intense stimulation. The relatively widespread inhibition produced by this system (Soper and Melzack, 1982) provides a basis for the effectiveness of stimulation at a distance from the site of pain.

Therapy 4: The stimulation of trigger points

The basis of the effectiveness of this therapy is not known. At present, the mechanisms of therapy 3 provide a plausible explanation. Since the trigger point is highly sensitive, its stimulation produces an intense output that evokes descending inhibition over a widespread area. This hypothesis also provides a possible explanation of the pain-relieving effects of acupuncture.

12 Psychological Modulation of Pain

The evidence, reviewed in Chapter 2, shows unequivocally that psychological factors play an important role in pain perception and response. Suggestion, distraction, the meaning of the situation and the feeling of control are all capable of exerting a powerful influence on pain. On the basis of this evidence, psychologists and psychiatrists have developed a variety of new procedures to control pain. However, all of these procedures need to be evaluated in experiments to determine their relative effectiveness. For such research to provide meaningful data, it must meet the following essential criteria:

1 Carefully controlled studies, with patients suffering specific clinical problems, must demonstrate that the effect of the procedure is greater than the placebo effect that is part and parcel of every therapy – an effect known to be astonishingly powerful. Patients not only want to please the therapist, but suggestion, anticipation of relief, and diminished anxiety can all play a role in ameliorating any disease process.

2 The changes that the therapy produces must be of sufficient magnitude and duration to have clinical significance. If pain can only be reduced by ten per cent, or for periods that average 15 or 30 minutes per day, the therapy clearly has limited value, or perhaps none at all.

3 The procedure must be transferable from the laboratory or hospital milieu to the normal day-to-day environment. If a change that is demonstrated in the clinic cannot be reproduced in the home or office, the procedure has limited value.

4 Finally, it must be demonstrated that the psychological procedure, once acquired, will continue to be effective for many months or years. Even if a given procedure produces results that exceed the effect of a placebo, it must be able to produce those results for substantial periods of time. In short, follow-up studies

are essential to show that the procedure continues to be effective long beyond the training period itself.

We will now examine a variety of clinical procedures to see how well they meet the above criteria.

Relaxation

Relaxation is an essential component of most forms of therapy for pain. It decreases the activity of the sympathetic and motor nervous systems (Benson *et al.*, 1977; Jessup and Gallegos, 1994). Most of us are usually caught up in a state of tension and stress in a competitive world, so that we are constantly prepared for an emergency or 'fight-or-flight response'. This psychological stress produces muscle tension, as well as increased blood pressure, heart rate, respiratory rate, and adrenalin outflow. All of this activity feeds into the nervous system and produces feelings of tension and irritability, and may produce pain directly (such as tension head-aches and backaches) or indirectly by facilitating activity in neuron pools that project pain signals to the brain.

Benson and his colleagues have proposed that the 'relaxation response' is the basis of all meditative practices. Relaxation, they suggest, induces the subjective experience of well-being which is often referred to as an 'altered state of consciousness'. In contrast to Jacobson's method of 'progressive relaxation', in which people are taught to relax individual muscle groups in progression throughout a therapy session, Benson *et al.*, (1977, p. 442), have developed a simple technique based on a variety of historical religious practices. Their instructions for this non-cultic technique are the following:

1 Sit quietly in a comfortable position and close your eyes.
2 Deeply relax all your muscles, beginning at your feet and progressing up to your face. Keep them deeply relaxed.
3 Breathe through your nose. Become aware of your breathing. As you breathe out, say the word *one* silently to yourself. For example, breathe in . . . out, *one*; in . . . out, *one*; etc. Continue for twenty minutes. You may open your eyes to check the time, but do not use an alarm. When you finish, sit quietly for several minutes at first with closed eyes and later with opened eyes.
4 Do not worry about whether you are successful in achieving a deep level of relaxation. Maintain a passive attitude and permit relaxation to occur at its own pace. Expect other thoughts. When these distracting thoughts

occur, ignore them by thinking 'Oh well' and continue repeating 'one'. With practice, the response should come with little effort. Practise the technique once or twice daily, but not within two hours after any meal, since the digestive processes seem to interfere with the subjective changes.

This simple technique has now been shown (Benson *et al.*, 1977) to produce striking physiological changes characteristic of deep relaxation, such as decreased metabolism and lower blood pressure and respiration rate.

Are relaxation procedures effective for pain? Cox *et al.*, (1975) found that relaxation is more effective than a placebo for the relief of tension headache, and this conclusion is generally supported by other evidence (Turner and Chapman, 1982). Recently, Philips (1987) has shown that relaxation therapy produces significant decreases in a wide range of clinical pains, including low back pain. Relaxation procedures are easy to teach, and Philips makes a strong case for their inclusion as part of all therapeutic programmes for severe chronic pain.

Biofeedback

Few therapeutic procedures have created the enormous excitement and expectations of biofeedback. The discovery in the 1970s that it is possible to gain voluntary control over biological activities such as brain waves (EEG), blood pressure or heart rate was heralded by the news media as the panacea for a variety of illnesses. With the help of sensitive electronic equipment which monitors a person's EEG, heart rate, blood pressure, or muscle tension, it became possible to 'feed back' these biological signals to the person so that he knows, for example, that certain muscles are tense rather than relaxed. Then the person is taught to relax or use other stratagems to reduce muscle tension. The continuous feedback keeps the person apprised of how well he is doing in achieving control over these biological functions, some of which were previously thought to be 'autonomic' or beyond voluntary control. The expectations were enormous. People with high blood pressure could now learn to reduce it. People with abnormal heart activity could learn to control it.

Even pain, it was thought, could be controlled in this simple way – teach people to relax (for muscle-tension headache or backache) or to change their brainwaves to the 'alpha' pattern (steady 8–12 cycles per second) characteristic of relaxed meditational states, and the pain would vanish. Melzack and Perry (1975) carried out a study to test these claims. The patients they studied all suffered chronic pain due to a variety of injuries or diseases. Their main criterion in selecting patients was that they were in continuous pain of known physical origin as verified by the physicians who referred them to the study. Many of the patients had pain despite disc surgery, or the severing of pain pathways, and the pain was not substantially diminished by lying down or by drugs. In short, all the traditional pain-relieving procedures had failed.

A group of patients received alpha-biofeedback training to control their pain. Although the patients learned to produce significant increases in the amount of alpha rhythm in their brain waves, they did not experience greater reductions in pain than those which occurred in 'placebo' baseline sessions. In these sessions, given prior to the alpha training, the patients were allowed to relax in a comfortable reclining chair, were distracted from their pain by being given a thorough description of the training procedures they would receive later, and were given strong anxiety-relieving assurances that the biofeedback would diminish their pain. This placebo condition, then, was just as effective as the elegant, extremely expensive electronic biofeedback equipment and procedure.

This conclusion is now supported by an impressive amount of research. Several major reviews of the literature on biofeedback have recently appeared (Silver and Blanchard, 1978; Turk *et al.*, 1979; Jessup *et al.*, 1979; Turner and Chapman, 1982; Chapman, 1986), and all of them have concluded that relaxation training alone is as effective as biofeedback training for tension and migraine headaches, low back pain, and other chronic pain states.

Understandably, there has been an over-reaction to the excesses of the early claims. As we shall soon see, the biofeedback procedure *does* add something important to psychological therapy for pain. It is a useful vehicle for distraction of attention, relaxation, suggestion, and providing the patient with a sense of control over his pain, which may enhance other psychological approaches to the control of pain.

Hypnosis

Placebos are, without a doubt, the oldest form of pain therapy. Many of the herbs and medicines that have been used for thousands of years are now known to have no pharmacological value as analgesics, but their administration by doctors, medicine men or shamans has worked repeatedly. The results could only have been due to the powerful placebo effect. Hypnosis may be an equally ancient practice for the relief of pain. In primitive cultures, the rhythmic drumming and incantations that accompanied the medicines may well have had a hypnotic effect on the patient so that the strong suggestion that his pain would be relieved by the medicine would actually produce the desired effect. The use of repetitive incantations and music in the practice of medicine is as old as recorded history (Keele, 1957).

Modern hypnotic techniques, however, originated in the eighteenth century, and have been in continuous use as a way to control pain as well as to 'cure' a variety of disorders (Sheehan and Perry, 1976; Hilgard and Hilgard, 1986). In the mid 1800s there was enormous excitement and interest in the use of hypnosis to produce analgesia for major surgery – an interest which declined after the discovery of the inhalant anaesthetics, but was revived in this century through the remarkable growth of psychology and psychiatry. Yet, despite a vast amount of excellent research on the effects of hypnosis on experimentally induced pain, there is virtually no reliable evidence from controlled clinical studies to show that it is effective for any form of chronic pain (Hilgard and Hilgard, 1986; Spanos *et al.*, 1994). It remains to be shown that hypnotic suggestion is any better than a placebo pill or encouragement and moral support from the family physician or clergyman.

The number of people who are capable of undergoing major surgery with hypnotic analgesia is very small. It is sufficiently rare that the occasional operation performed under hypnosis without any drugs still merits newspaper headlines. This is not surprising because the proportion of people who are easily hypnotized – that is, are highly susceptible to hypnosis – is very small. Not more than fifteen per cent of the population falls into this category. The remainder can be hypnotized with varying degrees of difficulty, and a substantial proportion cannot be hypnotized at all. There is no reason to doubt the reports that hypnosis can be used effectively to control a wide variety of pain problems such as phantom limb pain, cancer pain, and low back pain. But these studies generally consist of a small number of individual cases, and do not make a statistically convincing argument. Nor do they meet the criteria listed on p. 224.

Melzack and Perry (1975, 1980) recently examined the effects of hypnotic training on patients suffering chronic pain such as low back pain, arthritic pain and cancer pain. The hypnotic training was administered by means of tape-recorded instructions which were played to the patients while they were seated comfortably in a reclining chair.

The hypnotic-training instructions took about twenty minutes and began with techniques that focused attention on relaxing various muscle groups. The taped message also included 'ego-strengthening' suggestions in which the patients were told:

As a result of this deep relaxation – this deep hypnosis – you are going to feel physically stronger and fitter and healthier in every way. You will feel more alert – more wide awake – more energetic. You will become less easily tired – much less easily fatigued – much less easily discouraged ... Every day you will become stronger and steadier – your mind calmer and clearer – more composed – more placid – more tranquil. You will find that it takes a lot for things to worry you – it takes a lot for things to upset you even slightly ...

These patients reported an average pain reduction of 22 per cent, which is not significantly greater than the 14 per cent reduction they obtained in the placebo-baseline sessions, which provided them with a sympathetic hearing of their pain problem, strong suggestion that their pain would be relieved and an opportunity to relax in a comfortable clinical setting. However, when the hypnotic training instructions were supplemented by biofeedback training (which by itself had no effect on pain), the combined treatments produced a statistically significant reduction in pain compared to baseline placebo sessions. The average pain reduction was 36 per cent, and 58 per cent of the patients reported pain decreases of 33 per cent or more (Figure 34). This is impressive when the population of patients is considered: they had all suffered severe chronic pain for years, had received a variety of treatments including orthopaedic and neurological surgery, and were referred to the study because their physicians had exhausted all the conventional medical approaches.

While these data make a strong case for using multiple therapies in combination, they indicate that hypnosis by itself does not have a sufficiently strong effect on clinical pain to be considered as a reliably useful therapy. Merskey (1983, p. 39), on the basis of the available clinical reports and personal experience, concludes that hypnotism is not 'worth using in anyone with pain of physical origin and very rarely in patients with pain which is psychological in origin'.

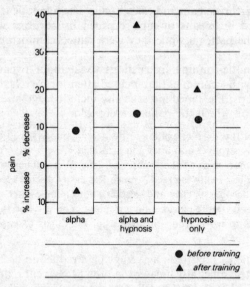

Figure 34. Average percentage decrease or increase in pain after placebo control sessions, and after treatments with alpha biofeedback training, hypnosis, or a combination of biofeedback and hypnosis. Only the combined treatment produced statistically more relief than the placebo control sessions.

Cognitive coping skills

Everyone, beginning at an early age, learns to cope with pain by using various strategies. The most common strategy is distraction of attention. For example, while sitting in a dental chair or waiting for an injection in the doctor's office, we often force ourselves to think about something else – such as a beautiful beach, a difficult chess problem, or some other absorbing thought. We may employ imagery by trying to conjure up the most vivid possible picture to distract our attention from the painful event. Alternatively, we may attend to the pain but give it a different quality by concentrating on the tingling, hot or pulsing qualities of the total pain experience rather than the unpleasant qualities (Turk and Meichenbaum, 1994).

In recent years, psychologists have devised a large number of ingenious methods that utilize different kinds of strategies or coping mechanisms. The following is a partial list of the strategies (Tan, 1982):

1 Imaginative inattention

The patient is trained to ignore the pain by evoking imagery which is incompatible with pain. For example, the patient is instructed to imagine himself at the beach, at a party, or in the country, depending on the image he can conjure up most vividly.

2 Imaginative transformation of pain

The patient is instructed to interpret the subjective experience in terms other than 'pain' (for example, transforming it into tingling or other purely sensory qualities) or to minimize the experience as trivial or unreal.

3 Imaginative transformation of context

The patient is trained to acknowledge the pain but to transform the setting or context. For example, a patient with a sprained arm may picture himself as a fighter pilot who has been shot in the arm while being chased by an enemy plane.

4 Attention-diversion to external events

The patient focuses attention on environmental objects and may count ceiling tiles or concentrate on the weave of a piece of clothing.

5 Attention-diversion to internal events

The patient focuses attention on self-generated thoughts such as mental arithmetic or composing a limerick.

6 Somatization

The patient is trained to focus attention on the painful area, but in a detached manner. For example, the patient may analyse the pain sensations as if preparing to write a magazine article about them.

These procedures are extremely clever. But are they effective for relieving pain? The evidence so far is encouraging but not conclusive. Of 27 studies carried out up to 1980, 15 indicated that these instructed coping strategies are superior to strategies generated spontaneously by subjects in control groups when laboratory pains are used (Tan, 1980). However, the fact that 12 of the studies failed to find significant differences indicates that the effect is not so robust that it always exceeds placebo effects. Nevertheless, it is evident that patients who are not instructed in particular strategies use their own strategies. In fact, even instructed patients may revert to strategies which they evolved themselves in the past and found useful. It is important, therefore, to have adequate control groups, and to examine the effects of the strategies on pain in real-life situations.

Two recent studies indicate that coping-strategy techniques are effective for clinical pain. The first (Horan *et al.*, 1976) investigated the effects of pleasant imagery, guided by a tape, on dental pain. The results showed that patients who utilized this strategy had significantly less discomfort than a control group which received no treatment instructions, and, more importantly, than a second control group instructed in 'neutral' imagery – that is, imagining numbers on a poster. The second study (Rybstein-Blinchik, 1979) examined patients who suffered severe pain due to amputation, rheumatoid arthritis, fractures, and other diseases or injuries. The results showed that patients who were trained in the coping strategy of imaginative transformation (or reinterpretation) of the pain had significantly less pain than patients who were taught two other strategies – diverting attention from the pain or concentrating on the pain (somatization). It is apparent, then, that particular procedures are effective for some patients, and for some kinds of pain. The approach is promising and may become more effective when patients' personalities are taken into account. For example, some people are less capable of generating imagery than others, and some people have a greater desire to cope personally with their pain than others, who may be more passive and prefer to have other people take full responsibility for its alleviation (Tan, 1980).

Operant-conditioning techniques

Operant-conditioning methods are based on observations that complex patterns of behaviour can be modified by the manipulation of rewards and punishments. Psychologists such as Wilbert E. Fordyce (1976) assume that pain consists of 'behaviours' that have been reinforced or rewarded, and the way to abolish 'pain behaviours' is to stop all such rewards. Fordyce, like other followers of the psychologist B. F. Skinner, is not concerned about the 'experience of pain', which he believes to be private information and not suitable for scientific study. Rather, he is interested in observable responses, stimuli, rewards and punishments.

What Fordyce says, in essence, is that people are often reinforced for having pain. When they complain of pain ('verbal pain behaviour'), they get attention and sympathy from family, friends and doctors; they don't do jobs they don't like; they can avoid people they dislike; they get medicines with impressive-sounding names; they may receive financial compensation without working; and they are often treated with a degree of respect they never had when they were well. In this way, the pain and other behaviour patterns associated with it (such as an abnormal gait) are reinforced. The task of the behaviour therapist, then, is to remove the reinforcements, to try to stop the patient from complaining of pain, and to induce the patient to resume normal behaviour patterns (Keefe and Lefebvre, 1994).

Fordyce (1976) has provided a thorough description of his procedures to re-train the patient who suffers chronic pain. The patient enters the hospital for a prolonged period (an average of eight weeks) and all the usual 'crutches' are removed. Pain behaviours such as complaints are ignored. All physical activity is rewarded with smiles and praise. And, during this period, medication is reduced to the barest minimum ('detoxification'). After the operant procedure, Fordyce reports, the patients are more active, complain less, take fewer drugs, work, and generally lead more normal lives. However, we are left with three vital questions that need to be answered.

First, does the patient actually feel less pain as a result of the training? That is, the patient is conditioned to diminish the frequency of certain 'pain behaviours'; but does that mean the patient feels less pain or simply learns to complain less or walk more in spite of the pain? Unfortunately, Fordyce dismisses the whole question by implying that the problem is basically philosophical and not one that an operant-conditioning psychologist need be concerned with. However, the problem is too important to be ignored; the failure to come to grips with it weakens the impact of the technique.

Second, how does the operant technique compare with other methods? Is it any better than a 'placebo' effect? It is hard to imagine a more powerful 'placebo' than the constant attention, encouragement, praise, and first-rate medical care that are an integral part of the complex operant procedure to diminish 'pain behaviours'. However, there have not been any controlled studies which compare Fordyce's operant technique to other therapeutic methods. The only attempt made to compare an operant-treatment group with a control group is so inadequate that no conclusions can be drawn. Roberts and Reinhardt (1980), in fact, used two so-called control groups: one consisted of patients who were rejected for treatment for reasons such as cardiac problems and severe mental disorders, and the other comprised patients who refused treatments. These are not control groups in any scientific sense. That is, they are not *matched* in any way to the experimental group to permit a comparison of the operant-conditioning treatment with a 'placebo' treatment or any other form of treatment.

Even in the absence of controlled data, the results are not impressive. In a study of a treatment programme essentially like Fordyce's, Anderson and his colleagues (1977) report that 74 per cent of the patients who completed the programme reported 'leading normal lives without drugs' when they were contacted 6 months to 7 years after discharge. However, the patients comprised a highly selected group, so that they were hardly 'typical' patients with chronic pain. Only 60 of 130 patients (46 per cent) referred to the programme were accepted for treatment. Only 37 (29 per cent) chose to enter, and 3 of these dropped out before the programme was completed. As Turk and Genest (1979, p. 305) point out, 'when Anderson *et al.*, report that 74 per cent of the patients treated were "leading normal lives", they are actually speaking of only 26 (19 per cent) of the original patients screened over a 7-year period'. It may be added that few conclusions can be drawn from a follow-up that ranges from 6 months to 7 years, without knowing how many patients were interviewed at each year after treatment.

The third question that concerns us is the cost of the 'operant-conditioning' programme. Even if the programme *did* work – and there is no evidence that it is better than a 'placebo' programme – it requires residence in a hospital for 4 to 8 weeks. The programme, then, is extremely expensive and requires a large amount of hospital space, time, and equipment. If this were the best of all possible worlds, this kind of treatment should be available to everyone. In fact, it is feasible for only a small number of patients, and well-to-do ones at that. Because of these limitations, it becomes important to determine the place of a technique such as this in societies that have limited funds for medical care.

These criticisms do not deny that patients in pain may use excessive amounts of drugs that actually harm rather than benefit them, that some patients may abuse a social system that pays financial compensation when people are disabled by pain, or that some people enjoy the sympathy, special attention and other 'rewards' of their pain. But Fordyce's programme is only one of many. Happily, there is evidence that simpler methods may produce effective results.

A recent study (Taylor *et al.*, 1980) has shown that patients with chronic abdominal or headache pain can be helped significantly by a relatively brief programme. The patients were first 'detoxified' – that is, all drugs were withdrawn on a schedule determined for each person. This procedure took 1 to 6 days, with an average of 3.7 days. The patients were then taught muscle-relaxation techniques and were given one or more brief supportive psychological therapy sessions. The average time spent in relaxation training was 1.5 hours and the time in supportive therapy was about 3 hours. The investigators found that this programme produced a significant reduction in pain in 71 per cent of the patients. At a 6-month follow-up, all (100 per cent) of the patients had less pain than before treatment, reported improvement in mood and increased activity, and were on significantly reduced medication. While these results are encouraging, they cannot be directly compared to those obtained in studies using 'operant-conditioning' methods, since these patients had primarily chronic abdominal pain while the others had preponderantly back and neck pain. Furthermore, the study did not have any control groups. Nevertheless, the evidence suggests that the reduction or elimination of drug intake can be accomplished in relatively short periods of time, and that additional simple procedures such as relaxation and brief supportive therapy may be effective for some patients with chronic, moderate levels of pain.

However, for severe pain, these procedures are not as impressive. Swanson *et al.* (1979) investigated 200 patients with severe chronic pain problems, primarily of the back and neck. The mean duration of the pain was 7 years, and 'the average patient was hospitalized 6 times, had had two surgical procedures, and had received treatment with some combination of physical therapy, traction, body casts, (anaesthetic) blocks, neuroablative procedures, electrostimulation, acupuncture, hypnosis, biofeedback, and psychotherapy'. The treatment, which required an average length of hospitalization of 20 days, consisted of behaviour modification (similar to Fordyce's 'operant-conditioning' technique), physical rehabilitation measures, medication management, education group discussion, biofeedback-relaxation techniques, family member participation, and supportive psychological treatment. At the time of dismissal from the hospital, 59 per cent of the patients had achieved moderate improvement or better. At a 3-month follow-up, 40 per cent were still doing well, and after 1 year, only 25 per cent continued to do well. Considering the severity of pain, this might be considered an achievement. But in the absence of any kind of control group, it is difficult to know whether 3 weeks of rest in the hospital with a daily programme of standard physiotherapy might not have done as well. Two conclusions can be drawn from studies such as this one: (1) complex, expensive programmes, in the long run, are disappointing in their effectiveness in relieving severe, chronic pain; and (2) no studies can lead to firm conclusions unless adequate, scientific, controlled procedures are used.

Psychological counselling

There is no evidence that the traditional psychological therapies, such as psychoanalysis, are effective for pain. Though chronic pain is sometimes diagnosed as a hysterical or conversion symptom (in which, for example, the tension of an unresolved sexual problem is presumed to be converted into manifest pain), the classical analytic therapies are rarely used (Merskey, 1983). We have seen (in Chapter 2) that patients are sometimes labelled as 'neurotic' when no obvious organic cause can be found for persistent pain. But we have also seen that the physiological basis of pain is often subtle and complex, with multiple interacting mechanisms that preclude simple causal labels (Pilowsky, 1994).

A particularly pernicious label is 'compensation neurotic', which is supposed to explain the frequent failure to help patients who have been injured in an accident and are awaiting legal action to receive compensation for their injury and pain. We now know, however, that these patients are not 'cured by a verdict' – that is, even when they are awarded financial compensation, the pain persists (Mendelson, 1982, 1986), which suggests a more complex basis to the pain. Compensation patients, contrary to traditional opinion, do not differ psychologically from people who do not receive compensation (Mendelson, 1984, 1994; Melzack *et al.*, 1985). Accidents which produce injury and pain should be considered as potentially psychologically traumatic, as well as conducive to the development of subtle physiological changes such as trigger points. Patients on compensation or awaiting litigation deserve the same concern and compassion as all other patients who suffer chronic pain.

The person who receives compensation is usually the victim of an accident who tries to cope with the resulting disability, pain, loss of income and disruption of day-to-day life. As a victim, he or she deserves the kind of psychological counselling that is now commonly advocated for victims of disasters such as floods or earthquakes (Everstine and Everstine, 1983). The sudden disruption in the person's normal working pattern, as well as in his customary role in the family and community, produces grief, sadness and bereavement over genuine losses. Accidents, whether large or small, underscore our sense of vulnerability. Even 'minor' losses, which occur after a mugging or a robbery in one's home, may produce long-lasting psychological effects. An accident that results in prolonged disability and pain has no less an impact on a person's psychological and physical well-being. Compensation is not a *cause* of pain, though it is often referred to that way. Malingerers and 'compensation neurotics' seem to be rare, and many unfortunate patients have been misdiagnosed, mistreated and allowed to suffer under the shroud of unfair labels, instead of receiving appropriate therapy.

Fortunately, there is increasing recognition of the diagnostic category labelled as 'post-traumatic stress syndrome' (Muse, 1985, 1986). About 10 per cent of patients referred to a general pain clinic exhibit the criteria of this syndrome, which usually begins with a sudden traumatic accident (Muse, 1985). However, all traumatic injuries do not necessarily give rise to this syndrome. Among burn patients, for example, about 40 per cent show the symptoms of post-traumatic stress syndrome, while 60 per cent do not (Perry *et al.*, 1987). Those who had the syndrome felt more personal guilt about the accident, even though they actually bore less responsibility for the burn.

Patients with post-traumatic stress syndrome appear to respond well to special treatment (Muse, 1986). They require multiple therapeutic techniques for a long period of time, including group supportive counselling and systematic desensitization procedures to cope with the terrible anxiety associated with the circumstances of the accident. Although this approach to patients with chronic pain related to a post-traumatic stress syndrome is relatively new, it appears promising (Muse, 1986) and merits further investigation.

Multiple convergent therapy

It is evident, from our review so far, that several psychological procedures are capable of diminishing pain. No one of them helps all people or abolishes pain completely. But each produces some degree of pain relief so that life for the suffering patient becomes more bearable. Even a few hours of relief a day, or a decrease in pain so that a bedridden person is able to carry out some of life's day-to-day activities, is a substantial help in allowing people in continuous pain to live with some degree of dignity. Because each procedure may help a little, it is natural to try two or more procedures in combination to see whether the effects of each are additive, Happily, the evidence suggests that they are (Gamsa, 1994).

It has long been known that placebo effects – which represent a powerful form of psychological therapy – enhance the power of any pain-relieving procedure. This has been substantiated beyond any doubt in the use of analgesic drugs (Beecher, 1959; Evans, 1985). A similar conclusion has been drawn from a study of the use of a combination of hypnotic training and biofeedback (Melzack and Perry, 1975)

Similar results have recently been obtained with a procedure known as 'stress-inoculation training' (Meichenbaum and Turk, 1976) in which patients are (1) given information that provides them with an understanding of pain and the stresses that accompany it; (2) trained in a variety of coping strategies (such as relaxation, distraction and imagery techniques) and allowed to choose the ones they prefer; and (3) rehearsed in the use of the strategies while they conceptualize the pain and stress at each phase of the total pain experience. An investigation (Hartman and Ainsworth, 1980) of the effectiveness of stress-inoculation training in patients with severe, persistent pain found that the training by itself did not reduce pain significantly, compared to pain-reductions that occurred during baseline control sessions in which the patients received only a form of relaxation training. However, when the stress-inoculation training was preceded by several sessions of alpha-biofeedback training, it produced significant reductions in pain compared to the baseline sessions. Once again, then, a *combination* of treatments was effective whereas a single procedure alone was not. The biofeedback sessions presumably facilitated the stress-inoculation training by providing the additional distraction, relaxation, suggestion and sense of control necessary to allow the patient to achieve a greater degree of pain relief.

Prepared childbirth training

The most famous of all psychological approaches to the control of pain is prepared childbirth training. We have seen earlier (Chapter 3) that labour pain is one of the most severe forms of pain, and several procedures have been developed to teach pregnant women how to cope with their pain when they are in labour. One of the methods, developed by Grantly Dick-Read (1944), is known as 'childbirth without fear'. More recently, Fernand Lamaze (1970) developed a programme for 'painless childbirth' which is widely known as 'Lamaze training'. Basically, these techniques include (1) providing detailed information on pregnancy and labour to the mother-to-be so that she knows what to expect and therefore experiences less anxiety; (2) relaxation training so that the woman can try to relax and calm herself when uterine contractions begin to increase in frequency, duration, and intensity; (3) coping strategies to distract attention from pain; and (4) breathing exercises which are useful to enhance relaxation and distract attention, as well as to aid in the process of giving birth.

Women in labour are subject to intense fears and anxieties related to their ability to bear the pain, to the possibility of medical complications, and to the baby's health. Prepared childbirth training, which is designed to reduce fear, anxiety and tension, should, therefore, also decrease pain. A recent study (Melzack *et al.*, 1981) demonstrates that it does, but the effects are not as great as people generally believe.

We observed earlier (Chapter 3) that some women report little pain during labour while others suffer severely. Several factors are significant predictors of labour pain. Women giving birth to their first baby (primiparas) generally have *less* pain if they (a) belong to higher socio-economic status groups, (b) do not have a history of menstrual difficulties, and (c) practised the procedures they learned in prepared childbirth training. Labour pain in multiparas (women who have given birth before) is influenced by the same factors, but it is especially important that the women feel that they have been adequately prepared for labour.

Figure 35 shows the average pain scores (Pain Rating Index) of primiparas who received prepared childbirth training (PCT) and those who did not. The results for individual PCT instructors are also shown. PCT, in all cases, consisted of a series of classes that included instruction in obstetrical physiology, breathing exercises, and relaxation techniques. Clearly, there is considerable variability among different instructors' groups in the scores obtained during labour. Discussions held with some of the women suggested that this is due partly to differences in the instructors' enthusiasm about PCT.

Figure 35 shows that PCT produces a significant decrease in total pain scores when compared to the scores of women who did not receive any training. Moreover, PCT does not merely diminish the affective dimension of pain, but also produces a significant decrease in the sensory dimension. A striking feature of Figure 35, however, is that the average scores of women who received PCT are still very high. The first instructor in the 'individual instructors' column, for example, was clearly the most effective of all; yet the mean total pain scores of her patients are at about the same level as the average totals recorded for out-patients with chronic back pain and cancer (see Figure 4, p. 43). Most significant is the fact that although this instructor strongly encouraged her patients to forgo epidural spinal blocks, five of the six women specifically requested an epidural block during the late stages of labour.

These observations should be interpreted in a positive sense (Melzack *et al.*, 1981; Melzack, 1984a). The fact that the current training procedures have statistically significant effects on pain is encouraging and indicates that psychological preparation is valuable. The additional fact that the average pain reduction is relatively small, means that there is need for further development of these obviously useful procedures.

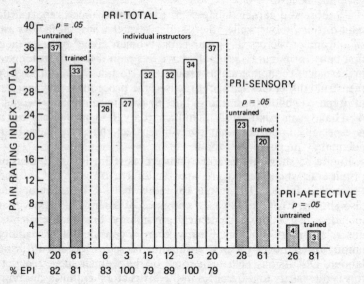

Figure 35. Left: mean P R I scores obtained by untrained and trained primiparas (Melzack *et al.*, 1981). Centre: the average P R I scores of trained women categorized by individual prepared-training instructors. Right: mean P R I scores for the sensory and affective descriptor sets of the McGill Pain Questionnaire (MPQ). The percentage of women who received an epidural block are indicated at the bottom.

Conclusion

There is no longer any doubt that it is possible to reduce many kinds of clinical pain by means of different psychological therapies. It is important to keep in mind, however, that these therapies rarely abolish pain entirely and are not equally effective for everyone. However, there are no perfect therapies of any kind. We have learned, as a result of literally hundreds of experiments, that there is a limit to the effectiveness of any given therapy; but, happily, the effects of two or more therapies given in combination are cumulative. Two therapies, each with slight effects that do not reach statistical significance, may produce significant reductions in pain when given together. For this reason, *multiple convergent therapy* is increasingly becoming the standard psychological approach to pain problems. Biofeedback, hypnosis and stress-inoculation training may each produce small effects. Two of the procedures together may have a large, significant effect. However, multiple convergent therapy does not refer only to psychological approaches. A psychological method may be used in combination with drugs or with sensory modulation procedures (Merskey, 1994).

The data indicate that multiple convergent therapy using several psychological procedures is effective because each kind of therapy may have its predominant effect on a different mechanism. Relaxation, for example, may reduce muscle tension and generally reduce activity in the sympathetic nervous system. Hypnosis, however, may have its predominant effect by activating control processes that modulate the input as it is transmitted through the brain. Procedures which involve the diversion of attention (so that even spinal reflexes may fail to occur) may, conceivably, activate the descending systems of the brainstem so that inputs are modulated at spinal levels. It is evident, then, that different psychological procedures may each have different predominant effects, so that several procedures together work better because more modulating systems are activated. It is also possible, of course, that each system may be increasingly affected as more procedures are used.

Whatever the precise mechanisms may be, the evidence reviewed in this chapter shows convincingly that psychological approaches can have powerful effects on pain. However, there are limitations to the procedures, and it is important to recognize them. By doing so, we set the stage for new approaches, or the use of old approaches in different combinations. The field is young and growing rapidly. It holds great promise as an approach by itself or together with the powerful yet simple methods of sensory modulation that we are also just beginning to understand.

13 Pain Clinics, Hospices and the Challenge of Needless Pain

While great strides have clearly been made in the control of pain, there are still many pain syndromes which are beyond our comprehension and our control. Back pains, especially of the lower back, are the most common kind of pain, and literally millions of sufferers are continually seeking help. Sometimes they obtain temporary relief, but most continue to suffer. Migraine and tension headaches similarly plague millions of people. New drugs and psychological techniques provide help for some, but the pains persist in the majority. Perhaps the most terrible of all pains are those suffered by some cancer patients in the terminal phases of the disease.

The inability to solve a patient's pain problem is deeply disturbing to both patients and therapists. At first, the patient respects the special knowledge of the various medical specialists, psychologists, physiotherapists, or other health professionals. But as the pain persists despite countless treatments, despite the claims often made in the media that sensational new pain cures have been found, and despite the best efforts by the therapists, the patient becomes understandably hostile. Respect is replaced by anger, hope by despair. This intolerable situation has recently led to two crucial developments in the control of pain – the pain clinic and the hospice.

The pain clinic as a response to the challenge of the chronic pain patient

Presently, few hospitals are organized to cope with the more complex kinds of pain. People suffering severe pain may be transferred from one doctor to another (from neurologist to neurosurgeon and finally psychiatrist) with little or no help. They may cycle through these specialists several times without experiencing any significant pain relief. What is needed is a concerted effort in which new modes of therapy can be attempted and evaluated. In short, what is needed are *pain clinics* in which specialists can work together to deal specifically with pain problems. In such clinics, an interchange of ideas can occur and the conditions are conducive to novel, imaginative approaches. Pain, in such a clinic, is not merely a symptom which each specialist perceives from his point of view. Rather, it is the pain syndrome that is itself examined, and the integration of many specialities to treat it is more easily achieved.

The idea of a pain clinic can be traced quite clearly to the experience and ideas of Dr John J. Bonica of the University of Washington Medical School, who is an anaesthetist and author of several seminal books on the treatment of pain. Bonica has always been interested in patients with particularly difficult pain problems. All too often, such patients would appear at his office with a 'thick file', having already been examined and treated by a succession of specialists. Bonica felt that this traditional approach was unsatisfactory and that a fresh approach was needed. He brought together a group of the traditional specialists who were particularly interested in the problems of pain. These included surgeons, neurologists, psychiatrists, psychologists, and so forth, who meet the patients both individually and as a group.

On visiting the pain clinic for the first time, the patient meets a single doctor who will from then on be responsible for all care and follow up. The doctor takes a history, carries out an examination and makes all the necessary tests. This doctor might come from any of the traditional specialties but has a particular interest in pain problems and is especially experienced with them. He has access to colleagues in all the relevant health-care fields, and thereby takes advantage of the crucial innovation of the pain clinic. The patient may be presented to a meeting of all the specialists, each of whom has received a detailed summary of the patient's condition. At these meetings, the combined experience of the specialists can be brought together and a step-by-step plan of treatment can be initiated.

The system brings with it three important advantages. The first is educational – the professionals can learn not only from a special group of patients but also from each other. In the best of these clinics, basic scientists are also present so that they too can experience the real nature of the problems rather than learn them second-hand. The second advantage to grouping together many pain patients and many concerned professionals is that it allows the development of new therapies. This has been particularly crucial for the beginning of psychological treatments directed at patients with chronic intractable pain. It has also encouraged the remarkable growth of the physical therapies involving sensory modulation. The third advantage of pain clinics is that they allow the accumulation of data – such as the relative effectiveness of different therapeutic procedures – that are often lost when the patient visits each specialist in his own clinic (Turk and Melzack, 1992).

The pain clinic allows the development of a battery of techniques to control pain. The pharmacological, sensory, and psychological methods of pain control do not exclude each other. A combination of several methods – such as electrical stimulation of nerves and appropriate drugs – may be necessary to provide satisfactory relief. The effective combination may differ for each type of pain, and possibly for each individual, depending on such factors as the patient's earlier medical history, pattern of spread of trigger zones, and the duration of the pain. But it is only in a clinic, where many cases are seen and complete data files are kept, that sufficient experience and knowledge can be acquired to allow the best judgement in each case. This is especially important when major decisions are made, such as the prescription of strong narcotic analgesics (methadone, oxycodone and others) to patients with severe non-malignant chronic pain. About sixty-five per cent of these patients receive excellent relief, with no evidence of tolerance or addiction (Portenoy and Foley, 1986).

The idea of pain clinics has spread during the past ten years. There is at least one in every major city of the western world. Obviously, each one differs depending on the personality and training of the professionals involved. The success of the idea of the pain clinic has inevitably led to the usual venal abuses of a good idea. Some specialists have simply re-labelled their old restricted services without enlarging the scope of their concepts or specialties in order to solve the patients' problems. A greater danger is already apparent in the appearance of the quack who possesses a single untested approach and re-labels his artifice with the modern, trendy title of 'pain clinic' and attracts the desperate patient who has received little relief from the more serious sources of help.

The hospice as a response to the challenge of the dying patient

There are few problems that are more challenging than the relief of pain in people with cancer – people whose lives are coming to an end. Many of us do not fear death but rather fear the pain that may precede it. Patients in the last stages of cancer have often come to terms with the knowledge that the end is near. Their worry is that they may not have the courage to bear the pain of their final weeks with the dignity they fought so hard to achieve in daily life. There is no merit to this suffering, no lesson to be learned.

The proportion of people who develop cancer is frighteningly high. Although it strikes primarily at older people, some forms of cancer occur in children and adolescents. Each year, in the United States about 700,000 new cases of cancer are diagnosed and about 400,000 people die from it (Bonica, 1980). Because tumours grow very slowly at first, cancer is rarely painful at its onset or during its early phases. In a large number of patients, however, cancer cells break away from the primary site and migrate to other tissues where they grow (metastasize) rapidly. Patients with metastatic cancer usually develop pain which increases in severity until it becomes relentless suffering. Furthermore, some patients develop pain directly or indirectly as a result of therapy. Bonica (1980) estimates that moderate to severe pain is experienced by about forty per cent of patients with intermediate stages of the disease, and by sixty to eighty per cent of patients with advanced cancer.

A major challenge that confronts physicians who treat terminally ill people is the judicious use of drugs. At present, this decision depends largely on the individual physician. One physician may seek any means, even major surgical operations, to avoid administering morphine, presumably out of fear of turning the terminal patient into an addict. Another may decide that a person's final weeks should be spent in tranquillity, and provide drugs such as morphine whenever they are requested by the patient. These are complex social issues and they may be handled best by a group of physicians and scientists who have gained familiarity with the ravages of prolonged severe pain on the human mind. As a result of this need in society, there has recently been a remarkable development – the hospice, whose sole aim is to provide care to terminally ill patients so that they can live the remainder of their days free of pain and other distressing symptoms. The concept of the hospice is best understood in historical perspective.

Up to the nineteenth century, the medical hospital was a place for care, for feeding and for isolation. Treatment played only a minor role. The patient lay in bed, awaiting the outcome of his disease, praying to his god for recovery or redemption, expecting few curative miracles from the surgeons and physicians. Quite obviously, a tremendous revolution has taken place in the actions of hospital doctors and in the expectations of the patients. Attention is now focused on active diagnosis and treatment. The enormous cost of occupation of hospital beds, largely because complex equipment and specialized services are extremely expensive, almost forbids the possibility of long stays in the modern hospital. Yet the need persists for a place for those beyond cure.

A revolution has taken place to meet the special needs of the terminally ill, and Cicely Saunders is the key figure in the revolution. In the course of her career Saunders gradually became concerned with incurable and terminally sick patients, and was deeply dissatisfied with what she saw. The patients, who were so deserving of loving personal attention in the last days of their life, were instead abandoned in isolated wards – in despair, depressed and facing death in utter loneliness. Her attitude was a totally different one and coloured all of her subsequent actions to help the dying patient: 'You matter because you are you. You matter to the last moment of your life, and we will do all we can to help you not only to die peacefully, but also to live until you die' (Saunders, 1976, p. 6).

Saunders worked first in existing hospices, and then with a team of powerful associates. Together, they collected money and built an extraordinary institution, St Christopher's Hospice in London. It opened in 1967 and has become a gathering point for those who wish to learn how to care for incurable people in the best possible way. It is important to add that she and many of her closest associates are deeply committed Christians. This is important because a commitment to religion, to the concept that death is a transition from this world to a more glorious one, greatly helps these people to work constantly with dying human beings and to cope with their own pain when their patients die.

There is another, almost political, aspect of the importance of religion for this group of people who set out to change the face of death. Their aim was to use every possible means to enhance the quality of their patients' lives until they died. In place of the lonely misery of dying in a large impersonal hospital, patients were encouraged to have contact with friends and relatives, and the medical emphasis was on relief of symptoms – especially pain – rather than cure, which was out of the question for these patients. Yet failure to try to cure has the inherent danger of being accused of 'killing the patient' by withholding treatment. Such an accusation is inconceivable against the group at St Christopher's, with their religious insistence on respect for life and their total rejection of mercy killing or euthanasia. Murder is an intentional act. However, excessive efforts to prolong the patient's life while adding to his misery, suffering, isolation and loss of dignity may equally be considered an assault on the patient. The key to the philosophy at St Christopher's is to allow the patient to die with the greatest possible dignity, not to prolong suffering and misery. There is a time in life when nature may be considered to have run its course. To try to prolong life in such a person now becomes unnatural and grotesque.

The patient's admission to St Christopher's is decided on by a hospice committee made up of nurses, doctors and other responsible people. Their job is to consider all aspects of the patient's case and to decide if it is time for admission to St Christopher's, or perhaps to another hospital with specialized facilities, or possibly to bring more aid to the patient's home. The majority of patients are in the terminal stages of cancer, but some may be admitted who suffer from diseases characterized by slowly progressing paralysis until they are beyond any self-care. The average period from admission to death is twelve days, which indicates the careful and successful selection of patients who have been treated comfortably at home until that time. The average figure, however, hides a very broad range, from a few who die very soon after admission to others who are not desperately ill but who have had some serious episode such as the onset of severe pain or paralysis.

On entering the hospice, the patient enters an atmosphere of intensive caring. From that point on, care and compassion are the constant features of living and dying. This is an important matter for friends and relatives as well as for the patient, because, now that continuous professional care is assured, they too can learn to approach. The staff become as skilled in helping the relatives in this matter as they do in teaching the patient to accept and expect communication and togetherness. With the exception of a few patients selected to be in single rooms for various personal reasons, the patients live in open wards with many beds rather than in the usual isolation cubicles. The effect is that patients become concerned with each other. A man within a few hours of death was asked how he felt and said, 'I'm feeling good but I'm worried about Jack in the bed over there.' A great deal of the fear of death is not so much a fear of the death itself but the idea of the indignity and agony of the period immediately before death. These patients witness other patients slipping calmly and quietly away and this itself is a tremendous relief to their own fears and fantasies.

None of this careful setting of the scene would have much meaning if the patient suffered symptoms which precluded a sense of dignity. People in agonizing pain, for example, scream out, weep, and want only to be alone in their misery. In those dying of cancer, there are many miserable symptoms, of which pain is the most common:

Table 4. Main symptoms felt by 607 patients admitted to St Christopher's Hospice with terminal cancer in 1976.

Pain	66%
Loss of appetite	62%
Cough	49%
Breathlessness	41%
Vomiting and nausea	41%
Insomnia	24%
Weakness	21%
Difficulty in swallowing	16%
Drowsiness	10%

The staff of St Christopher's have recently summarized their general approach and specifically their knowledge of symptom control (Saunders, 1978, 1984). In their treatment of pain, they have turned especially to the use of narcotic drugs. We have discussed these in detail in Chapter 10, but it is interesting to trace the history of the way this team approached the use of narcotics. The Brompton Hospital in London, which treated large numbers of terminal cancer patients in the nineteenth century, developed a mixture of drugs which has come to be known as the 'Brompton Cocktail'. More officially, it was called 'mist euphorians': the euphoria-producing mixture. It contained honey, gin, cocaine and heroin with some flavouring. It was given to suffering patients in the terminal stages of painful cancer and, not surprisingly, they were considerably relieved of their miseries.

The immensely useful Brompton Mixture survived into this century as an old-fashioned recipe used in the old-fashioned way. In recent years, due largely to the courage and determination of the St Christopher's team (including the outstanding pharmacologist Robert Twycross), the Brompton Mixture has achieved recognized medical status. It has now been shown beyond any doubt that the mixture is effective for the large majority of patients who have pain in the terminal stages of cancer. Just as importantly, it has been found that dependence (addiction) and tolerance are not problems in the treatment of pain in terminally ill patients. Once an effective dose has been found, it maintains its effectiveness for months. If the dose suddenly becomes insufficient to control pain, it is most likely due to a change in the patient's medical status (that is, spread or growth of the tumour) rather than to tolerance. In fact, it has been shown that the amount of morphine can be *reduced* without any ill effects when therapy (such as radiation therapy) produces a shrinkage of the tumour and a reduction of pain. The reduction of the amount of morphine is not accompanied by any evidence of withdrawal or other signs of addiction. Twycross has also demonstrated two other important facts: the narcotic is the essential ingredient of the mixture and – to everyone's surprise – morphine is as effective as heroin, possibly even more effective.

In a carefully controlled study, Twycross (1978) discovered that neither patients nor observers could tell the difference between equivalent doses of heroin or morphine. In fact, a careful analysis of the data showed that in males (but not females), morphine was more effective than the equivalent dose of heroin: the men on heroin had more pain and were more depressed. (Twycross attributes the increased depression to the presence of greater levels of pain.) The St Christopher's team, which had been active in the defence of heroin, have consequently dropped the drug from general use, retaining it only for one special circumstance. Heroin is more powerful milligram for milligram than morphine by a ratio of .5 to 1, and it is also much more soluble. Therefore, if a patient reaches a stage where he needs very large amounts of narcotic by injection, he receives a much smaller, more concentrated dose of heroin solution which hurts less after injection than the much larger volume needed to inject the equivalent dose of morphine. After all the controversy and the anecdotes surrounding heroin, careful experimentation now allows us to state calmly and concretely the merits and demerits of heroin.

As a result of a series of excellent studies, the Brompton Mixture was recognized by the 'British Pharmaceutical Codex' in 1973 as a legitimate elixir for the treatment of severe pain. The standard mixture contains a variable amount of morphine ('titrated' to meet the patient's needs), 10mg of cocaine, 2.5ml of ethyl alcohol (ninety-eight per cent), 5ml of flavouring syrup, and a variable amount of chloroform water, for a total of 20ml. As we shall soon see, morphine alone in water is as effective as the elaborate Brompton Mixture, and the much simpler morphine solution is now used increasingly because it is so easy for hospital pharmacies to prepare. These mixtures have the tendency to produce nausea, and are therefore given with drugs known as phenothiazines which enhance the analgesic properties of morphine *and* block the nausea. The mixture or solution is taken every four hours (or every three in some cases) and the dose of the narcotic is carefully adjusted ('titrated') over a period of days until a dose is found that not only takes the pain away but *keeps* it away; that is, each dose is taken *before* the pain returns. The pain, and the terror of its return, are gone. Yet the patient is lucid, able – indeed, often eager – to talk, to see relatives and friends, to clear up financial problems and even to reassure the soon-to-be bereaved.

While the idea of a hospice like St Christopher's is one of the great humanitarian advances of our century, it unfortunately represents an unachievable aim for all poor societies, and even many rich ones. Given the fact that a society has only a certain amount of money for health and welfare, there is a genuine debate, even in the most enlightened societies, whether a substantial portion of public funds should go towards care of the healthy or of the dying. Should a large sum of money given to health care be directed toward acquiring, let us say, a machine for a new and better kind of X-ray for a general hospital, or should it go into the development of a hospice? This problem has been confronted and debated by decent, well-intentioned people, and has often ended in stalemate. Few countries are as daring as Britain, or have a Cicely Saunders to champion and pioneer a great cause in the face of established medical practice.

Palliative care service

Several people in Canada and the United States have found an answer to the dilemma. The best known and most influential of them is Balfour Mount of Montreal's Royal Victoria Hospital, a teaching hospital of McGill University. Dr Mount, trained as a urological surgeon, became interested early in his career in the circumstances of dying in western society and found the same dismal conditions that appalled Cicely Saunders. In our western societies, a very large proportion (70 per cent in Canada) of people die in hospitals or related institutions. As a result the patient is removed from familiar surroundings and encounters isolation and depersonalization. Mount was disturbed by the number of dying patients who lie in some isolated ward, away from the people they love and with whom they would like to spend their last days or hours. As death approaches, interactions between staff and patients become strained. As a result, physicians visit less often and nursing care decreases. For example, it takes longer for a nurse to answer the bell rung by a dying patient than by a patient who will recover. In the absence of special training, all members of health care teams are subject to the fears and anxieties that are part of our death-denying, cure-oriented society.

Because few societies can afford a hospice like St Christopher's, Dr Mount took the next logical step: to integrate a specialized Palliative Care Unit (PCU) within a large general hospital. The concept is simple: a ward of ten or twelve beds is set aside in the hospital and is devoted solely to the care of terminally ill patients who have severe pain and special problems. Like St Christopher's, it is staffed by an astonishingly devoted group. To spend all one's working time caring for dying patients is a difficult task, and the team requires frequent opportunities for group discussions and to obtain help when they confront their own psychological problems. Once the unit functions well, however, its services are magnificent. Terminally ill patients receive constant care and attention, with pain and other problems continually monitored and ministered to. Volunteers of all ages become friends with the patients – talk to them, comb their hair, hold their hands, weep and laugh with them. The team helps bring the family together and assuage the feelings of guilt that trouble exhausted spouses, children or parents who must leave to get some sleep or food. The staff guide the bereavement process of all members of the dying person's family. Clergy of all denominations are also present to provide religious comfort when (and only when) it is requested.

At the same time, the unit is attractively decorated, and patients' friends and family are always welcome. In contrast to the rigid visiting hours in most large hospitals people can visit whenever they wish. Family members may stay overnight and, if the patient wishes it, may even share the bed in a private room. Children and pets are especially welcome. If a patient has a favourite dish, and the physician feels it can be digested without problem, then food may be brought in.

A marvellous feature of the PCU, which is described in detail by Ajemian and Mount (1980), is the fact that patients are able to go home when their condition stabilizes and for as long as is reasonable. The PCU, therefore, has been extended to form a Palliative Care Service beyond the confines of the hospital. The patients are given a bottle of the Brompton Mixture and instructions on how much to take and how often. A special homecare nurse visits often, or phones, and keeps close track of the patient. Any increase in pain or other change in the patient's condition results in a rapid return to the unit and the necessary attention to the problem. But while at home the patients are with people they love and in surroundings that are familiar and comforting. They are 'special' at home, and these days are precious.

The enormous success of the Palliative Care Unit and its auxiliary services is evident from the manifest gratitude of the patients and those close to them, and from the fact that similar units have been (or are being) developed throughout the world. A cost analysis of the PCU shows that society actually saves money by providing such a service. Unnecessary operations, X-rays, blood tests, and various treatments are not carried out. Feelings of guilt are understood and dealt with appropriately. The team effort means that services are provided efficiently. Time that the stabilized patient spends at home is time away from the hospital and therefore a saving of hospital funds. A well-run Palliative Care Service, then, is not only humanitarian but represents the most efficient way for a humane society to treat people who are terminally ill (Mount *et al.*, 1976). A further saving is now permitted by the finding that a solution of morphine in water is as effective as the Brompton Mixture (Melzack *et al.*, 1979). A small amount of alcohol is added as an anti-bacterial and anti-fungal agent. The morphine solution, because it is simple, is much cheaper and saves the time of the busy hospital pharmacist.

A special study was carried out to determine whether the PCU environment plays a role in the control of pain by the Brompton Mixture. Patients in two standard hospital environments – the wards and private rooms – served as 'controls'. Patients in the Palliative Care Unit comprised the 'experimental group'. The results showed clearly that the patients in the PCU had significantly less pain than those in the wards and in private rooms. None of the patients in the PCU had pain at distressing/horrible/excruciating levels, but 10 per cent of the private patients and 13 per cent of the ward patients had pain at these levels. Since the dosages of morphine and other ingredients were comparable for the three groups, the significantly greater effectiveness of the Brompton Mixture in the PCU can only be due to the psychological impact of the unit itself. The presence of a highly concerned staff, and the help of volunteers who provide comfort and good cheer, as well as all the other amenities of the unit must undoubtedly have had a strong psychological effect on the pain (Melzack *et al.*, 1976).

However, the Brompton Mixture (or morphine solution) is not the answer to every cancer patient's pain – unfortunately. About 10 per cent of the patients seen at the PCU in the above study had to be excluded immediately because the Brompton Mixture, even with high doses of morphine, did not control their pain: 1 had severe bladder spasms, 2 had sharp nerve-root pain that radiated into the legs, and 5 complained of severe pain, a major component of which was their despair and anguish at their impending death. These patients were treated with additional or other methods in the attempt to achieve physical and psychological comfort. The final results of the study showed that the Brompton Mixture was effective in controlling pain in 90 per cent of patients in the PCU and 75 to 80 per cent of patients in wards or private rooms. Clearly, the patients whose pain is uncontrolled represent a major challenge to clinical ingenuity. Other methods are necessary for those patients still in pain, and a variety of pain-control methods have been described (Cherny and Portenoy, 1994a, b; Breitbart *et al.*, 1994).

The nature of the clinical breakthrough

The development of pain clinics and hospices represents a breakthrough of the highest importance in the clinical control of pain. They are radical, new approaches to old problems. The gate-control theory of pain has provided, in large part, the conceptual background – the foundation – for new approaches to pain. The theory argues that pain does not have a single cause and is not even a single entity. There are multiple, interacting physiological and psychological mechanisms, and a rational approach to pain control requires multiple approaches that converge to produce a reduction in pain. Within this framework, the multi-disciplinary approach that is the hallmark of the pain clinic and the hospice takes on special significance. But still more, the pain clinic and the hospice represent an understanding that chronic pain and terminal pain each require a whole new set of challenges and skills. Acute pain, which is the basis of the traditional training of physicians, is wonderfully controlled by our modern-day drugs. Chronic pain, however, requires a new set of rules, and we are still novices in these new approaches to pain. Chronic pain and terminal pain are major challenges to the scientist and clinician. But the giant step has been the recognition that they are special problems. The challenges before us are clear: to conquer pain and suffering in all their forms.

The challenge of needless pain

New drugs, new techniques for sensory and psychological modulation, and pain clinics and hospices have brought pain relief to a greater proportion of suffering people than ever before. Yet there is still too much pain. Some of it is beyond the control of our present-day knowledge, and more research is urgently needed. However, a substantial part of it is due to misconceptions about addiction. The governments of many countries have enacted such stringent laws to prevent morphine and other analgesics from reaching street addicts that it is almost impossible for physicians to obtain the drugs for their patients. As a result, innocent patients are penalized by laws aimed at criminals.

We are appalled by the needless pain that plagues people in rich and poor nations alike. We now know that pain in cancer patients can be virtually abolished in 80 to 90 per cent of cases by the intelligent use of morphine. Many of those still in pain can be helped by using a variety of techniques such as inhalant anaesthetics, physical therapy, blocks and psychological procedures. The pain produced by the changing of dressings in burn patients, the pains of punctures of the spine or bone taps, labour pain, pain after major surgery – all of these can be blocked, or at least diminished, by the use of one or more of the many techniques that are now available. Yet many health professionals fail to provide adequate relief. Let us consider some of the major kinds of needless suffering.

Pain in children

Anyone who has watched a child suffer pain, whether due to minor diseases or major ones such as cancer, feels anguish and a sense of helplessness. We like to think that the health professionals who look after children do everything they can to prevent pain or to relieve it as much as possible. It comes as a shock, then, to find out that our ideas about pain in children are dominated by the myth that young children do not feel pain as intensely as adults, and therefore require fewer analgesics or none at all (McGrath and Unruh, 1987, 1994). In one study, more than 50 per cent of children who underwent major surgery – including limb amputation, excision of a cancerous neck mass, and heart surgery – were not given any analgesics, and the remainder received inadequate doses. Statistics such as these are found in virtually every study that examines the treatment of severe pain in children. Older children and adolescents are the butt of another myth – that they will become drug addicts if they are given narcotic drugs for severe pain – and do not fare much better.

We must learn to understand, assess and deal adequately with severe pain in people who are too young to describe their pain. Fortunately, major advances are being made (Barr, 1994; Houck *et al.*, 1994; McGrath and Unruh, 1987, 1994) which will inevitably lead to less suffering in young people.

Labour pain

We have already seen that labour pain is extremely severe in a substantial number of women. Epidural anaesthetic blocks are usually highly successful in reducing labour pain (Figure 36), yet many women choose to have their baby without an anaesthetic. Bonica (1994) has noted that prolonged, severe pain has a number of serious consequences which may increase the risk to the health of infants in difficult labours. It is interesting that the continuous low back pain reported by about a third of women in labour is more unbearable than the pains that accompany uterine contractions (Melzack and Schaffelberg, 1987). This fact suggests that the causes of labour pain are still not well understood. Studies on pain levels associated with different birth positions reveal that an upright position may be more comfortable during early labour and a supine position is preferred afterwards (Melzack *et al.*, 1991; Melzack, 1993).

Post-operative pain

Post-operative pain is not managed as well as it should be (Bonica, 1983; Melzack *et al.*, 1987; Cousins, 1994). Although the pain decreases rapidly in most patients during the three or four days following surgery, the high levels of pain during the first few days have led to studies of the causes. The most obvious cause is that inadequate doses of drugs are prescribed. Once again, the unfounded fear of addiction lies at the heart of the problem, so that physicians and nurses tend to prescribe and administer doses at the lower level of the range. Figure 36 shows the pain levels of patients before and after they were given drugs for post-operative pain. While pain scores are generally lower after drug administration, they are still high, particularly when compared to the decreases in pain achieved by other forms of therapy.

A recent study (Melzack *et al.*, 1987) has shown that surgical wards contain two populations: a young group that recovers quickly,

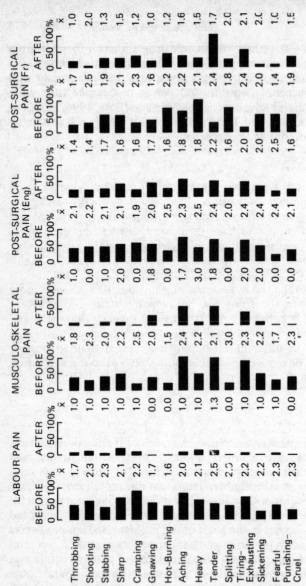

Figure 36. Profiles of the descriptors (and the relative intensities of each) chosen by patients with labour, musculo-skeletal and post-surgical pain. Bar graphs of the percentages of patients who chose each descriptor and the mean intensity (from 1 to 3) ascribed to each are presented. Data are shown before and after epidural block for labour pains, TENS for musculo-skeletal pain, and standard medication for post-surgical pain. The Short-form McGill Pain Questionnaire (SF-MPQ; see Figure 38)

and a group of older patients whose pain lingers on at high levels for many days beyond the expected 3 to 4 day recovery period. Despite the persistent, high level of pain in these older patients (presumably due to complications after surgery), they do not receive larger doses of drugs. Instead, they receive smaller doses at shorter intervals, but this strategy evidently fails to reduce pain adequately. These patients comprise about 30 per cent of the patients on a surgical ward at any time and therefore represent a substantial number of people who suffer needlessly high levels of pain.

Burn pain

It is not easy to imagine the severe pain of a burn, particularly when a large surface of the body has received third-degree burns that destroy all the layers of the skin. The pain suffered by these patients is extremely high (Choinière, 1988). In addition to the ongoing pain, there are daily sessions in which bandages and dead tissue are removed – a painful process called debridement. Although such pains are well controlled in some burn units, they are not controlled at all in others. Research is needed to determine the most effective drugs and doses and, equally important, the best time to carry out these procedures after the administration of the drug. Sometimes, a drug is given and debridement is started immediately, when in fact it may take an hour before the drug has its optimal analgesic effect.

Cancer pain

This still remains the most frightening kind of pain that can befall any of us. We have already described the hospice approach to pain control, which is the best of all possibilities. Unfortunately, there are not enough specialized services. People who face such pain should be aware of the help that is available. Morphine can be administered through various routes – orally, intravenously, by slow drip into a brain ventricle, or on to the spinal cord. If given orally, by far the preferred route, it should be 'titrated upward' in gradually increasing doses, until a dose is found which maintains continuous pain relief. The goal is to obtain a result like that shown in Figure 37, in which the patient is pain-free at all times. With some kinds of cancer, patients still have sharply-rising 'breakthrough' pains which are not kept under control by morphine. In these instances, nitrous oxide can rapidly be made available by using a small tank and mask; the patient breathes the nitrous oxide/oxygen mixture until the pains are gone. Even with this, about 5 to 10 per cent of people still have serious pain which underscores the need for more research.

The challenge to the patient

Pain is an individual, subjective experience and it is, therefore, the patient's responsibility to learn to communicate with health-care professionals, and to become knowledgeable about the kinds of therapy available for his or her problem. We have already noted (in Chapter 3) how difficult it is to describe pain. Nevertheless, the tools exist. The patient might describe the pain on a line from 0 (no pain) to 10 (worst possible pain), or simply with a number from 1 to 10. Since descriptive words often provide important clues to the cause and intensity of the pain, the patient could write down the appropriate words of the McGill Pain Questionnaire (Figure 3, p. 40) and present them to the physician, nurse or other professional care-giver. If the full MPQ seems too difficult to use, the patient may prefer the Short-form (SF-MPQ) shown in Figure 38. A copy

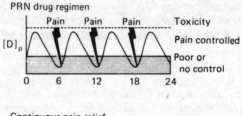

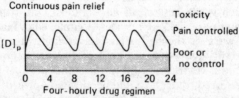

Figure 37. Diagram to illustrate PRN schedule in contrast to regular scheduling. (Twycross, 1984)

of it can easily be made and the patient can check the appropriate words and their intensities. This tells the care-giver how severe the pain is. Effective communication is an excellent beginning to making the correct diagnosis and finding the best treatment.

PATIENT'S NAME:_____ DATE: _____

	NONE	MILD	MODER- ATE	SEVERE
THROBBING	0) ____	1) ____	2) ____	3) ____
SHOOTING	0) ____	1) ____	2) ____	3) ____
STABBING	0) ____	1) ____	2) ____	3) ____
SHARP	0) ____	1) ____	2) ____	3) ____
CRAMPING	0) ____	1) ____	2) ____	3) ____
GNAWING	0) ____	1) ____	2) ____	3) ____
HOT-BURNING	0) ____	1) ____	2) ____	3) ____
ACHING	0) ____	1) ____	2) ____	3) ____
HEAVY	0) ____	1) ____	2) ____	3) ____
TENDER	0) ____	1) ____	2) ____	3) ____
SPLITTING	0) ____	1) ____	2) ____	3) ____
TIRING-EXHAUSTING	0) ____	1) ____	2) ____	3) ____
SICKENING	0) ____	1) ____	2) ____	3) ____
FEARFUL	0) ____	1) ____	2) ____	3) ____
PUNISHING-CRUEL	0) ____	1) ____	2) ____	3) ____

NO PAIN ├─────────────────────────────────┤ WORST POSSIBLE PAIN

PPI

0	NO PAIN	____
1	MILD	____
2	DISCOMFORTING	____
3	DISTRESSING	____
4	HORRIBLE	____
5	EXCRUCIATING	____

Figure 38. Short-form McGill Pain Questionnaire. (Melzack, 1987)

The challenge to the physician

Acute pain often requires immediate attention, and the physician's medical school training is oriented to the diagnosis and cure of such problems. Chronic pain, as we have seen, is highly complex, but the specialist should come only after the patient has seen a family physician who is expected to assume responsibility for the patient's health throughout his illness (and beyond). Interestingly, the philosophy of family medicine is fundamentally the same as that of a pain clinic: to treat the whole person, not just an organ, and to assess the patient in relation to his family and the society in which he lives (Turk and Melzack, 1992).

The family physician tends to treat chronic pain like acute pain, and when the procedures which are usually effective for acute pain fail to work, the physician, feeling inadequate to the task, sends the patient to an appropriate specialist. We have already noted how patients are often seen by a series of specialists without obtaining relief. It would be far better for the family physician to try to provide the therapy in a rational way before referring the patient to others (unless, of course, the cause of the problem is obvious and requires surgery, psychotherapy or other specialized treatment). The following is a plan for a rational approach to a patient with chronic, severe pain.

(1) Obtain a full medical history of all illnesses and injuries (including earlier injuries) which may provide clues about referred pain due to trigger spots, surgical scars, earlier operations on the viscera, and so on.

(2) Give the patient a thorough physical examination, and look for unusual signs such as hyper- or hypo-sensitivity of skin or other tissues, motor weakness, and any other signs that might provide an understanding of the problem.

(3) Treat the whole person, not just an organ or specific area, by considering psychological problems such as depression, anxiety and tension.

(4) Consider the effects of the pain on the interactions between the patient and his family.

(5) Do not make the patient feel guilty by saying 'the pain is in your head', with the implication that he or she is making up the pain for some questionable motive.

(6) Never allow the patient to lose hope; encourage future visits; brief chats may sometimes provide relief to a worried person who has pain with no discernible cause. Counsel patients who have been in accidents and feel stressed.

(7) Begin drug therapy with simple analgesics such as NSAIDs or acetaminophen, and prescribe antidepressants if they are needed. Use stronger medication, including narcotic drugs, if necessary. Do not under-prescribe; make sure that the patient receives proper, adequate doses.

(8) In cases of musculo-skeletal pain, always look for trigger points and try a series of local anaesthetic injections to see if the pain is diminished by such trigger point therapy.

(9) Use simple techniques of physical therapy and encourage the patient to experiment with them. These include massage, exercise, application of heat or cold, ice massage, transcutaneous electrical nerve stimulation.

(10) Keep track of the results of patient's visits to other physicians and health professionals. Chronic pain cases are like mystery stories – clues emerge at unexpected times, may sometimes suggest unorthodox therapies, and may lead to the solution of the mystery.

The reward for the physician for carrying out this difficult, time-consuming work is the pleasure of helping a patient in severe pain and preventing his or her life from being wrecked by it.

The challenge to society

The tragedy of persistent, severe pain inevitably affects the society of which the suffering patient and his family are a part. Chronic, disabling pain keeps people from work and the cost to society is not only the wages lost but also the medical expenses and the cost of supporting a wage-earner and all those who are dependent on him.

Pain research and therapy are dependent upon society for support. Governments provide the major share of the funds for research, particularly basic research in universities. It is this basic research, in fact, that has led to all the major breakthroughs in recent years, and these advances have led to the exciting new pain therapies which have helped so many people.

The recent growth of pain research and therapy has led to the development of an association called the International Association for the Study of Pain (IASP), which has more than 3,000 members worldwide, as well as many more members in local national chapters. The credo of IASP is that every human being has the right to freedom from pain to the extent that our knowledge permits this goal to be achieved. I A S P's aims are to learn more about basic pain mechanisms, to apply our knowledge to develop new therapies to relieve pain and suffering, and to transmit our knowledge to one another, so that these hard-gained benefits can apply equally to all mankind.

I A S P's members come from a diversity of backgrounds, representing virtually every field of the basic sciences and health professions. A common goal that motivates them is to educate one another in order to relieve pain and suffering. The I A S P's official journal, *Pain*, its international Congresses and its sponsorship of educational exchanges among countries, are all tools for achieving its mission.

The need to promote education is urgent. We have already described the inadequacy of pain treatment for so many people who suffer cancer pain, post-surgical pain, labour pain, chronic pains of myriad kinds. The most terrible aspect of so much of this suffering is that we actually have the means to relieve it and the costs are within the budget of even the poorest countries. The problem is not money but ignorance.

A concern of everyone who works in the field of pain is the ethics of research with humans and animals. For this reason, there are guidelines for ethical conduct in research. All research with humans requires 'informed consent' – a detailed description of the experiment is given to the patient or healthy subject by the experimenter, and written consent is given by the participant who volunteers to take part in the study. Animal research, of course, requires different guidelines (Zimmermann, 1984) and all major scientific journals require that the experiments adhere to the rules of ethical conduct to animals before they are considered for publication. 'Animal rights' movements remain dissatisfied with the rules of conduct and condemn all research with animals. There is no simple solution to this problem. This book has described many experiments with animals, and they have played a predominant role in all the important developments of pain research and therapy. Whether the experiments are justified or not depends on the priorities of each of us. At stake in this debate is the discovery of ways to relieve the terrible pain and suffering due to cancer, arthritis, strokes, and a multitude of other causes.

Since scientists generally believe that research on animals is morally justified, it is important that the information that is gained be used as widely as possible to relieve pain and suffering in humans. It is intolerable that the hard-earned gains of scientific research (for both animals and humans) should not be utilized throughout the world. The mechanisms for education thus become extremely important. The advances during the past two decades are impressive. The future, as we shall now see, looks even brighter.

14 The Future of Pain Control

The recent exciting advances in pain research and therapy indicate the direction of future developments. Our purpose here is not to make predictions of future breakthroughs (which, in science, rarely come true) but, rather, to discuss the problems and challenges that will inevitably be part of the story of pain research and therapy in the future.

The classification of pain syndromes

The foundation of any science is the proper classification of the phenomena it tries to understand. Merskey and his colleagues (1986), at the request of the International Association for the Study of Pain, have recently prepared the first 'Classification of Chronic Pain'. Its publication in the journal *Pain* is a milestone because, for the first time, it is possible to find an organized list of the known pain syndromes. This is only the beginning of the task because new syndromes are being discovered and some old ones need to be re-evaluated in the light of recent research.

The new syndromes are relatively rare and bizarre, but those who suffer these pains are grateful to know that they are not 'crazy', but have a syndrome in common with others. One recently discovered syndrome is 'painful legs and moving toes' (Spillane *et al.*, 1971), in which patients suffer terrible pains in the legs and feet, and show spontaneous, uncontrollable movements of the toes. It often happens that, when a new syndrome is discovered, the cause is found not long after. Thus, there is now evidence that this syndrome is due to nerve-root lesions that generate nerve impulses which spread in the spinal cord and are the basis of the pain as well as the continual motor outflow that evokes the incessant movements (Nathan, 1978). The discovery of this syndrome provided the clues for a related, mysterious pain which has now been classified as 'painful arms and moving fingers' (Verhagen *et al.*, 1985).

A terrible type of pain which was first described long ago but has only recently been established as a distinct syndrome is the 'burning mouth syndrome' (Grushka *et al.*, 1987a). It refers to a severe burning pain of the tip of the tongue which sometimes extends to the palate and lips. It is found predominantly in post-menopausal women, and has now been shown to be due to damage in the nervous system. The site of the damage has not yet been determined, but at least the earlier attribution of the pain to psychological causes has now been disproved (Grushka *et al.*, 1987b).

Another type of pain which appears to comprise a distinct syndrome is 'fibrositis' or 'diffuse myofascial pain syndrome'. Though described as long ago as 1904, it is still controversial (Smythe, 1979). It is characterized by multiple tender points at distinct, widespread sites on the body, as well as by disturbed sleep and morning fatigue and stiffness. It is found predominantly in middle-aged people who tend to have a perfectionistic, demanding life-style, and often begins after a precipitating stressful event, such as an accident. This syndrome may be related to the post-traumatic stress disorder which has recently been recognized in the psychiatric classification system known as DSM-III. Whether they are related or not, this syndrome indicates the difficulty of establishing the existence of a set of symptoms as a syndrome distinct from others. The vigorous debate about these syndromes is not academic – particularly to those who suffer from them. The future outcome of the debate will be the discovery of the causes of the syndrome, and valuable clues on ways to treat it.

In addition to new syndromes and contentious, barely established ones, considerable attention in the future will be devoted to a re-examination of the two most common ones which plague tens of millions of people: headache and low back pain. There is now considerable debate about the separation of tension and migraine headaches (Schoenen *et al.*, 1994). Some investigators argue that they are two distinct entities, while others hold that they lie on a continuum and vary only in intensity. Muscle tension seems not to be the cause of 'tension headache', and has been attributed, by Martin and Matthews (1978), to the same vascular causes as migraine. However, migraine headaches, which were once attributed to a sudden constriction followed by dilation of blood vessels in the head, are now a greater mystery than ever: the pulsating blood vessels seem not to be the cause of migraine, but are secondary to other unknown causes (Oleson, 1986). It is also clear, from the many different kinds of migraine headaches, that each may have different causes and represent distinctly different syndromes. Similarly, low back pain (see Chapter 4) is also a label for several distinct syndromes with different causes and symptoms that respond to different therapies (Grahame, 1980). Future investigators face the formidable task of finding new classification systems for the many kinds of headaches and backaches.

There are no panaceas

A major challenge in future research is to develop a proper perspective toward new therapeutic discoveries. The discovery of some new drug or technological advance in treatment is generally announced with great fanfare. Extravagant claims are made for one brand name of a drug over another, but basically we have a relatively small number of analgesic drugs. New compounds are always being discovered, but they need a great deal of clinical research before their place is firmly established in the pharmacopoeia of analgesics.

Scientists have long been aware that the 'coming out' of new therapeutic agents and techniques follows a characteristic sequence (Figure 39). In the first few years, the research data are exciting and the new discovery assumes Nobel-prize-winning proportions. Then there is a period of scepticism in which the drugs sometimes appear to be even less effective than the old ones. Finally, the research usually shows that a good – not great, but good – new analgesic drug or treatment has been found that can respectably take its place along with the others. In the course of all of this, it is evident that progress has been made, but not a major breakthrough. We must always keep this sequence in mind; there are no panaceas – not yet anyway. Even the endorphins and enkephalins, which were believed after their discovery to be the key to the whole puzzle of pain and the guideposts to the perfect analgesics, are now seen in perspective. They are, without a doubt, scientifically important steps to understanding pain and analgesia. A host of new opioid and other pain-related substances were discovered in an incredibly short time. But their roles in pain and analgesia are poorly understood and their practical implications for pain therapy are uncertain.

Just as there are no panaceas in the form of new drugs, neither are there panaceas in psychological techniques or any other foreseeable technological advance. Chronic pain is too complex, with too many interacting contributions, to expect to find some magical elixir or incantation that will abolish it all. A safe prediction is that the panacea for pain will not be found. Instead, the future of pain

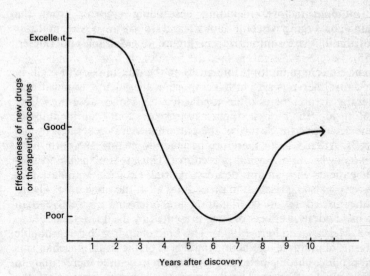

Figure 39. Diagram of the pattern of effectiveness after discovery of most new drugs or therapeutic procedures to control pain. Excellent results obtained in the first few years give way to poor results, followed by a period in which the drug or procedure is found to be another 'good' form of therapy for pain.

therapy appears to be in the rational use of multiple parallel therapies. Throughout this book we have seen that two therapies are better than one. The effectiveness of morphine is greatly enhanced by amphetamine (Forrest *et al.*, 1977) and cocaine (Mistra *et al.*, 1987). Ineffective doses of carbamazepine (tegretol) or phenytoin suddenly become effective with the addition of baclofen for treating trigeminal neuralgia (Fromm *et al.*, 1984). Similarly, hypnotic suggestion alone appears to have a weak analgesic effect, but may become highly effective when given with biofeedback (which by itself is ineffective) (Melzack and Perry, 1975). Indeed, every kind of therapy becomes significantly more effective when presented with the implicit suggestion of a placebo (Evans, 1985). The future of pain control, then, lies in the intelligent combination of the right kinds of treatments.

The gate-control theory has provided a conceptual framework for the multiple contributions to pain. In contrast to specificity theory which proposes that pain intensity is proportional to the severity of injury, the gate theory holds instead that pain intensity is determined by multiple factors, including descending controls from the brain, converging visceral inputs, and so forth. These multiple contributions are summarized in Figure 40 (Melzack and Loeser, 1978).

The concept of multiple influences on the transmission (T) cells in the central nervous system has important therapeutic implications. Therapy at present is often predicated on a one-cause-one-effect relationship. In contrast, Figure 40 indicates that multiple interactions determine the nature of the pattern which is generated by the T cells. Attempts can therefore be made to change the pattern by *simultaneous* use of several procedures. Thus, it is plausible to provide patients with an anti-depressant drug, electrical stimulation at trigger points *and* relaxation procedures all at the same time. Therapeutic procedures in combination are often more effective than the mere additive effects of each presented by itself (Melzack *et al.*, 1963; Melzack and Perry, 1975). This kind of approach is reasonable in terms of multiple interacting influences on the neural mechanisms that produce chronic pain, and it is certain to be used increasingly in the treatment of pain. The development of methods to assess the qualities of pain may play a future role in determining the kinds of therapy that are needed to selectively combat the different dimensions of the pain experience.

The future: a summary of the challenge of pain

The challenge remains so long as there are pains which we do not understand and which are inadequately treated. We can place the majority of these problem pains into three classes:

(1) *Pains where the cause is apparent but the treatment is inadequate:*
     Deep tissue disorders: osteoarthritis; rheumatoid arthritis; post-traumatic pains; inadequate blood supply (angina; claudication; Raynaud's disease).
     Peripheral nerve disorders: cancer infiltration; injury; amputation; neuropathies (diabetic; alcoholic; viral).
     Root and cord disorders: arachnoiditis; post-herpetic neuralgia; brachial plexus avulsions; spinal injuries.

(2) *Pains where the cause is not known but the treatment is adequate:* trigeminal neuralgia; 'tension' headaches.

(3) *Pains where the cause is not known and the treatment is inadequate:* most back pains; fibromyalgia; idiopathic cystitis; idiopathic pelvic and abdominal pains; migraine.

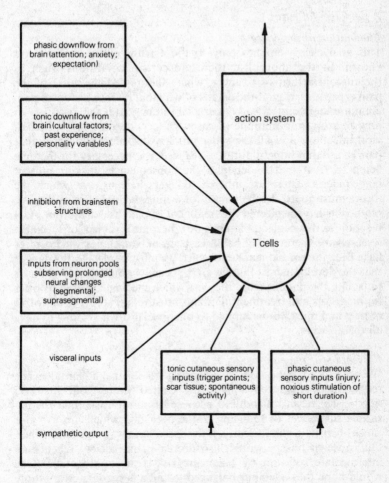

Figure 40. Diagram of the concept of multiple influences on the transmission (T) cells in the central nervous system. The concept suggests that attempts can be made to change the pattern of output of the T cells by simultaneous use of several therapeutic procedures.

These pains are indicative of our ignorance about pain mechanisms and therapy. To achieve adequate understanding and treatment in the future, we need to define our goals and the path which should best be followed to achieve each of them.

A fundamental cure

Elimination of the cause

This goal clearly applies only to those pains where the cause is known. In the above list, there are certain conditions, such as rheumatoid arthritis or cancer, where the immediate cause of the pain is obvious, even if the details of why that disease produces pain are not understood. Clearly, a crucial future goal is the discovery of how to stop auto-immune diseases, cancer, degenerative diseases, viral infections and all the other primary disorders which produce pain. Until that hopeful future is realized, it is necessary for the time being to treat and understand the consequences of our present inadequacies. There are inherent dangers here against which the future must guard. In the search for a fundamental cure of disease, physicians have neglected the treatment of pain as a symptom. As a reaction to this neglect, pain has now become a subject of specialist research and therapy. The helpful aspects of pain clinics and hospices have been the consequence. However, we must be alert to the danger that the development of a new pain specialty could swing so far as to isolate the patient from the best which medicine is able to offer for diagnosis and treatment. Patients must retain access to *all* forms of help and must not be limited to one specialist who claims to have all the answers.

Prevention of the cause

We need to learn the skills of balancing risk against advantage. The reduction of the speed limit in the United States from 70 to 55 m.p.h., which was introduced because of an oil crisis, had the desirable side-effect of reducing traffic accidents which are a major cause of chronic pain. Clearly, if the speed limit was reduced further, this cause of misery would also decrease; but society reaches an intermediate solution by balancing risk against advantage. One would hope that a similar balanced formula is considered by those who indulge in warfare and violent sports.

In many human activities the advantage is obvious but the risk is more difficult to analyse. Almost every occupation has risks which may produce painful disorders, and these need much closer attention. Machines have eliminated some kinds of muscular pains but have produced other kinds. Innocent sports, from jogging to football, frequently produce long-lasting pain. Squash, with its sudden changes of direction, has a particularly bad record. Even the arts produce victims. A recent survey of professional musicians showed a majority struggling to play or sing in conflict with pain associated with their necessary posture. The highest rate of occupational pain is found in ballet dancers and nurses.

Perhaps the saddest of all pains are those produced by doctors in the course of treatment. In the largest New York cancer hospital, about 20 per cent of the pains are produced by the treatment. These iatrogenic pains are not accidents but the result of a calculated benefit/risk equation. The search for pain relief entails a struggle to devise effective therapy in which the risk in minimal.

Prevention of progressive pain
Many pains disappear spontaneously. There is, therefore, a logical, conservative tradition that intentional inactivity by both patient and physician is the best tactic. This approach is supported by the fact that many treatments are expensive and painful, and not without risk. However, we have shown that many disorders are progressive, with the nervous system reacting in stages to accommodate to the pain-producing mechanism. It will therefore be necessary in the future to investigate the advantages of early, vigorous treatment. Contrary to tradition, it may be that in the long run early mobilization is superior to inactivity.

The intensely painful phase of acute herpes zoster usually ends after three or four weeks in the majority of people, but turns to a miserable, chronic condition in a minority. There are indications that early sympathetic block not only relieves the acute pain but decreases the long-term consequences (Colding, 1969). Similarly, the majority of cases of nerve injury do not have pain, but it might be better to attempt to treat all cases in order to prevent the terrible consequences in the minority who develop chronic, disabling pain. These pre-emptive treatments will require full co-operation between basic scientists and clinicians, and will require prolonged, multi-centre clinical trials.

Complete analgesia
It is conceivable that extremely powerful, long-lasting, local or general analgesic medicines or procedures will be developed. The idea of using genetic engineering to some day produce pain-free people is also appealing. But there are two reservations about such ambitions. Pain retains a biological function in arresting injury, in learning to avoid future injury and, much more subtly, as an inherent part of the processes involved in recovery from damage. Therefore, the fight to abolish the unacceptable aspects of pain has to be

matched with a preservation of the body's recuperative powers. The second aspect of this goal is that it contains an implicit concept which we believe to be wrong. That concept proposes that the nervous system contains a separate specific pain system, independently incorporated in the brain like an alarm system installed in a building. In contrast, we have tried to describe an integrated nervous system in which pain is not produced by injury alone but is profoundly influenced by a variety of psychological and social factors.

Discovery of the causes of pain

Science has only recently begun a serious investigation of the mechanism of pain (or any other sensation for that matter). It is, therefore, not surprising that the contribution of science to new treatments has so far been minimal. Most treatments remain pragmatic, often derived from ancient practice, as with aspirin or opium, or from ancient common sense and humanity, as in nursing care, distraction, massage, heat, cold, structural support, rest and encouragement. Science has often trailed behind established practice providing a *post hoc* rationale for what was already being done. As science moves into a new phase, there is the hope that it will generate new therapy based on new understanding. The recognition of a gate-control, with its inhibitory components, produced transcutaneous electrical nerve stimulation; the gate's local inhibitory circuits provided a rationale for the infusion of intrathecal and epidural morphine; its descending control produced a reason for brain stimulation. However, the pace of new understanding has been accelerating. It is now apparent that the gate-control mechanism may explain the very rapid shifts of excitability but we must now face at least two slower processes triggered by tissue damage. One evidently operates with a long latency and long duration related to impulses in unmyelinated fibres and to peptides. Here may be the source of tailor-made therapies directed at the secondary tenderness and pain which follows tissue damage. The other new mechanism involves the transport of chemicals within the axons of nerve fibres. The identification of those chemicals and their transport mechanisms offers a fundamental opportunity to propose genuinely new therapies which are not derived from any existing treatment and which manipulate the newly recognized plasticity of the adult nervous system.

Science can also play a role in identifying the secondary processes which impinge on the primary process of detection of tissue damage and triggering of pain. Psychological factors such as attention, distraction, fear and memories of past experience are the products of brain mechanisms which are not yet understood but will be revealed by future research.

The discovery of adequate treatments in the future

Medicines
Directed at the periphery. We now know there are four classes of events in damaged tissue related to pain, and each offers new possible treatments. The first class is the direct action of pressure, heat and chemicals on nerve endings. The second is the action of tissue breakdown on nerve endings. At present, only aspirin (and related NSAIDs) and steroids attack this effect, but they do not seek out the many specific types of chemical which are now being recognized as pain producers. The third is the role played by chemicals released by damaged nerve fibres, which leak out and produce a neurogenic component of inflammation. These chemicals (probably peptides) are targets for therapy. Lastly, the sympathetic system plays a role in producing pain when tissue is damaged by releasing a variety of chemicals which may be separately manipulated.

Directed at nerve fibres. Now that we recognize that nerve fibres play a role in pain not only by transmitting impulses but also by chemical transport, there is the possibility of manipulating these chemicals. The chemical transport mechanisms comprise a message system by which abnormal tissue signals its presence to the central nervous system. They must certainly play a role in the spinal cord and brain as the cascade of changes slowly shifts from the original area of damage to distant parts of the nervous system.

Directed at nerve cells. The present central analgesics have only a limited range of targets and these targets are very widespread. Fortunately, it now appears that there are many control systems whose pharmacology will be better understood in the future and could lead to new analgesics. Furthermore, there is much to be done in finding ways to direct drugs selectively to the structures where their action is required, without flooding the whole body where they may produce unwanted side-effects.

Surgery
The traditional art of surgery has specialized in excision, relieving pressure due to oedema or vascular accidents or restoring mechanical stability to weakened or broken bones. However,

surgeons have moved to replacement surgery, with particular success in joint replacement. While this will clearly flourish, there is a new future in the replacement of injured or destroyed tissues and structures. As the principles of cell growth, recognition and differentiation become understood, the possibility of tissue culture followed by transplantation in damaged areas of the nervous system offers a new future for replacement surgery. Surgeons have also just begun to explore stimulation procedures using a variety of central electrical and chemical techniques in which targeted inhibitory systems can be brought into action. These procedures hold enormous promise for furture attacks on some kinds of pain.

Physiotherapy

This area has been treated with insufficient respect by the medical profession and inadequate scientific rigour by its own proponents. Now that it is becoming understood that sensory-modulation techniques and active movement can bring inhibitory systems into action, the rationale for the various therapies will become better understood. Furthermore, as the effective component of each kind of therapy is analysed, treatment will be targeted at specific disorders that are precisely diagnosed.

Psychological treatments

We have shown that psychological processes play an integral part in pain mechanisms beginning at the earliest stages. This liberates the role of psychological therapy from a secondary position (to be used only when all else fails) to playing a part in all forms of therapy. This move has placed psychological therapy, even the placebo effect, in a position of respectability, so that rational approaches to pain management in the future will take advantage of powerful psychological controls which we are just beginning to understand.

A final statement

A basic tradition of medicine has been to seek a single diagnosis and a single therapy. However, there are pathological situations in all disease states in which the underlying mechanisms are so powerfully locked into an abnormal state that no one therapy can move the situation back towards normal. In treating pain, as in treating heart failure or kidney failure, it is fully justified to use a combination of therapies which push and pull the system toward normality. We are learning to accept that pain is not produced by the simple activation of a single specific, isolated signalling system but is subject to a series of controls acting in the context of a whole integrated nervous system. It therefore becomes necessary to combine all the available resources to allow the nervous system to move toward a normal, pain-free mode of operation.

Glossary

Definitions with an asterisk (*) are reproduced from Merskey (1986):

ablation The removal by surgery of any part of the body. In neurosurgery, refers to removal of part of the brain.

afferent fibre Nerve fibre which conducts nerve impulses from a sense organ to the central nervous system, or from lower to higher levels in sensory projection systems in the spinal cord and brain.

allodynia* Pain due to a stimulus which does not normally provoke pain.

anaesthesia Total loss of sensation in all or part of the body.

anaesthesia dolorosa* Pain in an area or region which is anaesthetic.

anaesthetic As an adjective, refers to an area that has lost all sensitivity. As a noun, refers to drugs that induce the total loss of sensitivity either in a localized area or in the whole body after loss of consciousness.

analgesia Loss of sensitivity to pain without loss of other sensory qualities or of consciousness.

analgesic As an adjective, refers to an area that is insensitive to pain. As a noun, refers to any pain-relieving drug.

antidromic Propagation of a nerve impulse along an axon in a direction that is the reverse of the normal direction of transmission.

arthrogram A procedure to obtain an X-ray of a joint after injection of a special dye that facilitates visualization of the structures of the joint.

asymbolia Loss of the ability to appreciate some aspect of the sensory world. *Pain asymbolia*: inability to appreciate pain – that is, feel it in the normal way or grasp its implications.

axon The part of a nerve cell (neuron) which is the essential conducting portion. Often called simply the 'nerve fibre'.

brachial plexus The nerves to and from the arm at the level of the shoulder before they connect with the spinal cord.

brainstem The part of the brain that lies between the spinal cord and the cerebral cortex. Generally refers to those parts of the brain called the medulla oblongata, pons, and midbrain. Sometimes it is used to include the thalamus.

causalgia* A syndrome of sustained burning pain, allodynia, and hyperpathia after a traumatic nerve lesion, often combined with vasomotor and sudomotor dysfunction and later trophic changes.

central nervous system In mammals, refers to the spinal cord and brain.

central pain* Pain associated with a lesion of the central nervous system.

clonic From the word 'clonus' referring to rapid alternate contraction and relaxation of a muscle.

commissural fibres A tract of neurons that connects two areas on opposite sides of the brain or spinal cord.

contralateral On the opposite side.

conversion hysteria Transformation of an emotional disturbance into a physical manifestation such as paralysis, anaesthesia of part of the body, or pain.

cortex The outer layer of an organ. Thus, *cerebral cortex*: the layers of nerve cells at the outer part of the brain.

cutaneous Relating to the skin.

decompression The relief of pressure within an organ by means of an operation to release excessive fluid. Thus, *subtemporal decompression*: the release of cerebrospinal fluid or blood through a burr-hole near the temporal (or lower side) part of the skull.

dendrite The part of a nerve cell (neuron) which conducts nerve impulses toward the cell body.

dermatome The area of skin innervated by a single sensory root of the spinal cord.

dysaesthesia* An unpleasant abnormal sensation, whether spontaneous or evoked.

ecchymosis Bruise; bleeding under the skin, usually after injury.

efferent fibre Neuron which conducts nerve impulses away from the central nervous system (to muscles or glands), or from higher to lower areas in the nervous system (such as a neuron that transmits from the brain to the spinal cord).

electroencephalogram (EEG) A recording of electrical activity of the brain, usually through electrodes placed on the scalp.

encephalon The brain. Thus, *encephalopathy*: any disease of the brain.

ephapse An artificial synapse (junction) between two conducting fibres that may occur after injury.

evisceration Removal of viscera (abdominal and thoracic organs).

ganglion An aggregate of nerve cell bodies. Thus, *sympathetic ganglion*: nerve cell bodies associated with the sympathetic nervous system.

herniation (of a disc) Protrusion of the intervertebral disc so that it presses against nerve roots and usually produces pain in addition to other symptoms.

hyperaesthetic Excessively sensitive, so that even non-noxious stimuli (such as a light touch) evoke pain.

hyperalgesia* An increased response to a stimulus which is normally painful.

hyperpathia* A painful syndrome, characterized by increased reaction to a stimulus, especially a repetitive stimulus, as well as an increased threshold.

hypoaesthesia Decreased sensitivity to all somatic stimulation.

hypoalgesia* Diminished pain in response to a normally painful stimulus.

iatrogenic Pain or other medical problems produced inadvertently as a result of medical treatment.

introspection The analysis, by a person, of the sensory, emotional and other qualities of conscious experience.

ipsilateral On the same side.

jactitations Jerking, paroxysmal movements.

lumbar The part of the back and sides of the body between the lowest pair of ribs and the top of the pelvis.

median nerve One of the three major nerves that supply the hand. The other two are the radial and ulnar nerves. The sensory area innervated by the median nerve is complex but may be described roughly as the middle portion of the hand, particularly the middle and index fingers and the adjacent portions of the thumb and ring fingers.

metastases Secondary tumours that have spread from the initial primary site.

myelin A fatty substance surrounding nerve fibres, thereby forming an insulating sheath. *Myelinated*: covered by a myelin sheath.

neuralgia* Pain in the distribution of a nerve or nerves.

neuraxis The central nervous system from lowest to highest levels.

neuritis* Inflammation of a nerve or nerves.

neuroma A nodule at the end of a cut nerve when regeneration fails.

neuron The structural unit of the nervous system, consisting of a nerve cell and its conducting dendrites and axon.

neuropathy A disturbance of function or pathological change in a nerve.

nociceptor* A receptor preferentially sensitive to a noxious stimulus or to a stimulus which would become noxious if prolonged.

noxious A noxious stimulus is one which produces or is potentially capable of producing tissue damage.

orthodromic Propagation of a nerve impulse in the normal direction; in axons, away from the cell body.

pain threshold* The least experience of pain which a subject can recognize.

pain tolerance level* The greatest level of pain which a subject is prepared to tolerate.

paraesthesia* An abnormal sensation, whether spontaneous or evoked.

peripheral nerves Bundles of nerve fibres that connect sensory or motor organs to the central nervous system.

pinna The external part of the ear.

placebo Latin word that means 'I will please'. Usually a pill or injectable solution of sugar or salt given in place of an analgesic agent.

polysurgical addiction Refers to patients who appear to have a compelling need for surgical operations.

post-tetanic potentiation From 'tetanus', which refers to the continued contraction of a muscle, which can be produced by a rapid succession of electrically excited nerve impulses. Post-tetanic potentiation refers to the enhancement (potentiation) of muscle contractions or of nerve signals in motor neurons after prolonged, intense stimulation of the related sensory root.

proprioceptive Sensory signals from muscles, tendons and joints.

psychophysics Study of the relationship between stimulus intensity and the intensity of the resultant sensory experience.

roentgenography The use of X-rays to reveal internal structure. The name is derived from Wilhelm Roentgen, the discoverer of X-rays.

sacrum The continuation of the backbone below the lumbar vertebrae, consisting of several vertebrae joined together and making up the central bone of the pelvis. Thus, *sacral*: relating to the sacrum.

soma Greek word for 'body'. Somatic (or 'somatosensory') input refers to sensory signals from all tissues of the body, including skin, viscera, muscles or joints.

somaesthesis Sensory experience derived from the body.

subtemporal decompression See *decompression*.

sudomotor Activity of the sweat glands.

sympathetic nervous system One part of the autonomic nervous system, consisting of a chain of ganglia lying outside and parallel to the spinal cord, and nerve fibres that conduct to viscera, blood vessels and glands.

synapse The relay junction between two neurons. The axon terminals of a neuron release a chemical transmitter that flows across the synapse and influences the dendrites or cell body of an adjacent neuron. The transmitter may excite the cell (or facilitate its excitation by other neurons) or it may inhibit the cell and prevent it from firing (or decrease its firing rate).

thalamus One of the major relay stations of the central nervous system, lying at the top of the brainstem and between the cerebral hemispheres. It relays information projected by the sensory systems to the cortex and by the cortex to motor systems or to other brain areas.

trigeminal nerve The fifth nerve of the head. It carries sensory signals from the skin of the face, parts of the eyes, and a large part of the inner structures and membranes of the mouth and nose.

trophic Relative to nutrition, such as changes in the nutrition of skin tissues after a nerve injury.

vasomotor Activity of the blood vessels.

viscera The specialized internal organs of the abdomen and chest. Singular: *viscus*.

References

ABBOTT, F. V., and MELZACK, R., 'Analgesia produced by stimulation of limbic structures and its relation to epileptiform after-discharges', *Exper. Neurol.*, 62(1978) 720–34.

ABBOTT, F. V., MELZACK, R., and LEBER, B. F., 'Morphine analgesia and tolerance in the tail-flick and formalin tests: dose–response relationships', *Pharmacol. Biochem. Behav.*, 17(1982) 1213–19.

ADAMS, J. E., HOSOBUCHI, Y., and FIELDS, H. L., 'Thalamic syndrome and electrical stimulation of internal capsule', *J. Neurosurg.*, 41(1974) 740–44.

AJEMIAN, I., and MOUNT, B. M. (eds.), *The R.V.H. Manual on Palliative/Hospice Care*, Arno Press, New York, 1980.

ANDERSON, D. G., JAMIESON, J. L., and MAN, S. C., 'Analgesic effects of acupuncture on the pain of ice-water: a double-blind study', *Canad. J. Psychol.*, 28(1974) 239–44.

ANDERSON, T. P., COLE, T. M., GULLICKSON, G., HUDGENS, A., and ROBERTS, A. H., 'Behavior modification of chronic pain: a treatment program by a multi-disciplinary team', *J. clin. Orthop.*, 129(1977) 96–100.

ANGAUT-PETIT, D., 'The dorsal column system. I. Existence of long ascending post-synaptic fibres in the cat's funiculus gracilis', *Exper. Brain Res.*, 22(1975a) 457–70.

ANGAUT-PETIT, D., 'The dorsal column system. II. Functional properties and bulbar relay of the post-synaptic fibres of the cat's fasciculus gracilis', *Exper. Brain Res.*, 22(1975b) 471–93.

BAILEY, A. A., and MOERSCH, F. P., 'Phantom limb', *Canad. Med. Assn J.*, 45(1941) 37–42.

BALAGURA, S., and RALPH, T., 'The analgesic effect of electrical stimulation of the diencephalon and mesencenphalon', *Brain Res.*, 60(1973) 369–81.

BARNETT, H. J. M., HIRSH, J., and MUSTARD, J. F., *Acetylsalicylic Acid: New uses for an old drug*, Raven Press, New York, 1982.

BARR, R. G., 'Pain experience in children: developmental and clinical characteristics'; in P. D. WALL and R. MELZACK (eds.), *Textbook of Pain*, 3rd edn., Churchill Livingston, Edinburgh, 1994, pp. 739–65.

BASBAUM, A. I., 'Conduction of the effects of noxious stimulation by short-fiber multisynaptic systems of the spinal cord in the rat', *Exp. Neurol.*, 40(1973) 699–716.

BASBAUM, A. I., and FIELDS, H. L., 'Endogenous pain control mechanisms: review and hypothesis', *Ann. Neurol.*, 4(1978) 451–62.

BASBAUM, A. I., MARLEY, N. J. E., O'KEEFE, J., and CLANTON, C. H., 'Reversal of morphine and stimulus produced analgesia by subtotal spinal cord lesions', *Pain*, 3(1977) 43–56.

BAXTER, D. W., and OLSZEWSKI, J., 'Congenital insensitivity to pain', *Brain*, 83(1960) 381–93.

BEAVER, D. W., 'Measurement of analgesic efficacy in man'; in J. J. BONICA, U. LINDBLOM and A. IGGO (eds.), *Advances in Pain Research and Therapy*, Vol. 3, Raven Press, New York, 1983, pp. 411–34.

BECKER, D. P., GLUCK, H., NULSEN, F. E., and JANE, J. A., 'An inquiry into the neurophysiological basis for pain', *J. Neurosurg.*, 30(1969) 1–13.

BEECHER, H. K., *Measurement of Subjective Responses*, Oxford University Press, New York, 1959.

BELL, C., SIERRA, G., BUENDIA, N., and SEGUNDO, J. P., 'Sensory properties of neurons in the mesencephalic reticular formation', *J. Neurophysiol.*, 27(1964) 961–87.

BENNETT, G. J., 'Neuropathic pain'; in P. D. WALL and R. MELZACK (eds.), *Textbook of Pain*, 3rd edn., Churchill Livingston, Edinburgh, 1994, pp. 201–24.

BENSON, H., and EPSTEIN, M. D., 'The placebo effect: a neglected asset in the care of patients', *J. Amer. Med. Assn*, 232(1975) 1225–7.

BENSON, H., KOTCH, J. B., CRASSWELLER, K. D., and GREENWOOD, M. M., 'Historical and clinical considerations of the relaxation response', *Amer. Scientist*, 65(1977) 441–5.

BISHOP, G. H., 'Neural mechanisms of cutaneous sense', *Physiol. Rev.* 26(1946) 77–102.

BISHOP, G. H., 'The relation between nerve fiber size and sensory modality: phylogenetic implications of the afferent innervation of the cortex', *J. Nerv. ment. Dis.*, 128(1959) 89–114.

BLENDIS L. M., 'Abdominal pain'; in P. D. WALL and R. MELZACK (eds.), *Textbook of Pain*, 3rd edn., Churchill Livingston, Edinburgh, 1994, pp. 583–95

BLUMBERG, H., and JÄNIG, W., 'Clinical manifestations of reflex sympathetic dystrophy and sympathetically maintained pain'; in P. D. WALL and R. MELZACK (eds.), *Textbook of Pain*, 3rd edn., Churchill Livingston, Edinburgh, 1994, pp. 685–98.

BONICA J. J. (ed.), *The Management of Pain*, 2nd edn., Lea and Febiger, Philadelphia, 1990.

BONICA, J. J., 'Management of myofascial pain syndromes in general practice', *J. Amer. Med. Assn*, 164(1957) 732–8.

BONICA, J. J., 'Organization and function of a pain clinic'; in J. J. BONICA (ed.), *Advances in Neurology*, Vol. 4, Raven Press, New York, 1974a, pp. 433–43.

BONICA, J. J., 'Anesthesiology in the People's Republic of China', *Anesthesiology*, 40(1974b) 175–86.

BONICA, J. J., 'Cancer pain'; in J. J. BONICA (ed.), *Pain*, Raven Press, New York, 1980, pp. 335–62.

BONICA, J. J., 'Current status of postoperative pain therapy'; in T. YOKOTA and R.

DUBNER (eds.), *Current Topics in Pain Research and Therapy*, Excerpta Medica, Amsterdam, 1983, pp. 169–89.

BONICA, J. J. 'Labour pain'; in P. D. WALL and R. MELZACK (eds.), *Textbook of Pain*, 3rd edn., Churchill Livingston, Edinburgh, 1994, pp. 615–41.

BORING, E. G., *Sensation and Perception in the History of Experimental Psychology*, Appleton-Century-Crofts, New York, 1942.

BOTTERELL, E. H., CALLAGHAN, J. C., and JOUSSE, A. T., 'Pain in paraplegia: clinical management and surgical treatment', *Proc. Roy. Soc. Med.*, 47(1954) 281–8.

BOUCKOMS A. J.. 'Limbic surgery for pain'; in P. D. WALL and R. MELZACK (eds.), *Textbook of Pain*, 3rd edn., Churchill Livingston, Edinburgh, 1994, pp. 1171–87.

BOWERS, K. S., 'Pain, anxiety, and perceived control', *J. Consult. Clin. Psychol.*, 32(1968) 596–602.

BOWSHER, D., and ALBE-FESSARD, D., 'The anatomophysiological basis of somatosensory discrimination', *Int. Rev. Neurobiol.*, 8(1965) 35–75.

BREITBART, W., PASSIK, S. D., and ROSENFELD, B., 'Psychiatric and psychosocial aspects of cancer pain'; in P. D. WALL and R. MELZACK (eds.), *Textbook of Pain*, 3rd edn., Churchill Livingston, Edinburgh, 1994, pp. 825–59.

BRENA, S. F., WOLF, S. L., CHAPMAN, S. L., and HAMMONDS, W. D., 'Chronic back pain; electromyographic, motion and behavioural assessments following sympathetic nerve blocks and placebos', *Pain*, 8(1980) 1–10.

BROCKBANK, W., *Ancient Therapeutic Arts*, Heinemann, London, 1954.

BROMAGE, P. R., CAMPORESI, E., and LESLIE, J., 'Epidural narcotics in volunteers: sensitivity to pain and to carbon dioxide', *Pain*, 9(1980) 145–60.

BROMAGE, P. R., and MELZACK, R., 'Phantom limbs and the body schema', *Canad. Anaesth. Soc. J.*, 21(1974) 267–74.

BROWDER, E. J., and GALLAGHER, J. P., 'Dorsal cordotomy for painful phantom limb', *Ann. Surg.*, 128(1948) 456–69.

BROWN, A. G., 'Effects of descending impulses on transmission through the spinocervical tract', *J. Physiol.* (Lond.), 219(1971) 103–25.

BROWN, A. G., ROSE, P. K., and SNOW, P. S., 'Morphology and organization of axon collaterals from afferent fibers of slowing adapting Type I units in cat spinal cord', *J. Physiol.*, 277(1978) 15–27.

BRUCE, M. F. and SINCLAIR, D. C., 'Relationship between tactile thresholds and histology in the human finger', *J. Neurol. Neurosurg. Psychiat.*, 43(1965) 235–42.

BUSHNELL, M. C., DUNCAN, G. H., DUBNER, R.. and HE, L. F., 'Activity of trigeminothalamic neurons in medullary dorsal horn of awake monkeys trained in a thermal discrimination task', *J. Neurophysiol.*, 48(1984) 170–87.

CARLEN, P. L., WALL, P. D., NADVORNA, H., and STEINBACH, T., 'Phantom limbs and related phenomena in recent traumatic amputations', *Neurology*, 28(1978) 211–17.

CASEY, K. L., 'Nociceptive mechanisms in the thalamus of awake squirrel monkey', *J. Neurophysiol.*, 29(1966) 727–50.

CASEY, K. L., 'Somatosensory responses of bulboreticular units in awake cat: relation to escape-producing stimuli', *Science*, 173(1971a) 77–80.

CASEY, K. L., 'Responses of bulboreticular units to somatic stimuli eliciting escape behaviour in the cat', *Int. J. Neurosci.*, 2(1971b) 15–28.

CASEY, K. L., 'Reticular formation and pain: toward a unifying concept'; in J. J. BONICA (ed.), *Pain*, Raven Press, New York, 1980, pp. 93–105.

CASEY, K. L., Personal communication, 1986.

CASEY, K. L., KEENE, J. J., and MORROW, T., 'Bulboreticular and medial thalamic unit activity in relation to aversive behavior and pain'; in J. J. BONICA (ed.), *Pain, Advances in Neurology*, Vol. 4, Raven Press, New York, 1974, pp. 197–205.

CAVANAUGH, J. M., and WEINSTEIN, J. N., 'Low back pain: epidemiology, anatomy and neurophysiology'; in P. D. WALL and R. MELZACK (eds.), *Textbook of Pain*, 3rd edn., Churchill Livingston, Edinburgh, 1994, pp. 441–55.

CERVERO, F., 'Visceral nociception peripheral and central aspects of visceral nociceptive systems'; in A. IGGO, L. L. IVERSEN, and F. CERVERO (eds.), *Nociception and Pain*, The Royal Society, London, 1985, pp. 16–23.

CHAPMAN, C. R., WILSON, M. E., and GEHRIG, J. D., 'Comparative effects of acupuncture and transcutaneous stimulation on the perception of painful dental stimuli', *Pain*, 2(1976) 265–83.

CHAPMAN, S. L., 'A review and clinical perspective on the use of EMG and thermal biofeedback for chronic headaches', *Pain*, 27(1986) 1–43.

CHERNY, N. I., and PORTENOY, R. K., 'Cancer pain: principles of assessment and syndromes'; in P. D. WALL and R. MELZACK (eds.), *Textbook of Pain*, 3rd edn., Churchill Livingston, Edinburgh, 1994a, pp. 787–823.

CHERNY, N. I., and PORTENOY, R. K., 'Practical issues in the management of cancer pain'; in P. D. WALL and R. MELZACK (eds.), *Textbook of Pain*, 3rd edn., Churchill Livingston, Edinburgh, 1994b, pp. 1437–67.

CHERYCROZE, S., and DUCLAUX, R., 'Discrimination of painful stimuli in human beings', *J. Neurophysiol.*, 44(1980) 1–10.

CHOINIÈRE, M., 'Pain of burns'; in P. D. WALL and R. MELZACK (eds.), *Textbook of Pain*, 3rd edn., Churchill Livingston, Edinburgh, 1994, pp. 523–37.

CLARK, W. C., and CLARK, S. B., 'Pain responses in Nepalese porters', *Science*, 209(1980) 410–12.

CO, L. L., SCHMITZ, T. H., HAVDALA, H., REYES, A., and WESTERMAN, M. P., 'Acupuncture: an evaluation in the painful crises of sickle cell anaemia', *Pain*, 7(1979) 181–5.

CODERRE, T. J., KATZ, J., VACCARINO, A. L., and MELZACK, R., 'Contribution of central neuroplasticity to pathological pain: review of clinical and experimental evidence', *Pain*, 52 (1993) 259–85.

CODERRE, T J., ABBOTT, F. V., and MELZACK, R., 'Effects of peripheral antisympathetic treatments in the tail-flick, formalin and autonomy tests', *Pain*, 18(1984) 13–23.

COGHILL, G. E., *Anatomy and the Problem of Behaviour*, Cambridge University Press, Cambridge, 1929.

COHEN, H., 'The mechanism of visceral pain', *Trans. Med. Soc. London*, 64(1944) 65–99.

COHEN, S. R., and MELZACK, R., 'Morphine injected into the habenula and dorsal posteromedial thalamus produces analgesia in the formalin test', *Brain Res.*, 359(1985) 131–9.

COHEN, S. R., and MELZACK, R., 'Habenular stimulation produces analgesia in the formalin test', *Neurosci. Lett.*, 70(1986) 165–9.

COLDING, A., 'The effect of regional sympathetic blocks in the treatment of herpes zoster: a survey of 300 cases', *Acta Anaesth. Scand.*, 13(1969) 133–40.

COLLINS, J. G., and REN, K., 'WDR response profiles of spinal dorsal horn neurons may be unmasked by barbiturate anesthesia', *Pain*, 28(1987) 369–78.

COMINGS, D. E., and AMROMIN, G. D., 'Autosomal dominant insensitivity to pain with hyperplastic myelinopathy and autosomal dominant indifference to pain', *Neurology*, 24(1974) 838–48.

COOK, A. J., WOOLF, C. J., and WALL, P. D., 'Prolonged C-fibre facilitation of the flexion reflex in the rat is not due to changes in afferent terminal or motorneurone excitability', *Neurosci. Lett.*, 70(1986a) 91–6.

COOK, A. J., WOOLF, C. J., WALL, P. D., and MCMAHON, S. B., 'Expansion of cutaneous receptive fields of dorsal horn neurones following C-primary afferent fibre inputs', *Nature*, 325(1986b) 151–3.

CORSSEN, G., HOLCOMB, M. C., MOUSTAPHA, I., LANGFORD, K., VITEK, J. J., and CEBALLOS, R., 'Alcohol-induced adenolysis of the pituitary gland: a new approach to control of intractable cancer pain', *Anesthes, Analges.*, 56(1977) 414–21.

COUSINS, M., 'Acute and postoperative pain'; in P. D. WALL and R. MELZACK (eds.), *Textbook of Pain*, 3rd edn., Churchill Livingston, Edinburgh, 1994, pp. 357–85

COUSINS, M. J., and BRIDENBAUGH, P. O., *Neural Blockade*, Lippincott, Philadelphia, 2nd edn., 1987.

COX, D. J., FREUNDLICH, A., and MEYER, R. C., 'Differential effectiveness of electromyographic feedback, verbal relaxation instructions, and medication placebo with tension headaches', *J. Consult. Clin. Psychol.*, 43(1975) 892–8.

COX, V. C., and VALENSTEIN, E. S., 'Attenuation of aversive properties of peripheral shock by hypothalamic stimulation', *Science*, 149(1965) 323–5.

CRAIG, K. D., 'Emotional aspects of pain'; in P. D. WALL and R. MELZACK (eds.), *Textbook of Pain*, 3rd edn., Churchill Livingston, Edinburgh, 1994, pp. 261–74.

CRONHOLM, B., 'Phantom limbs in amputees', *Acta Psychiat. Neurol. Scand.*, Suppl. 72(1951) 1–310.

DALLENBACH, K. M., 'The temperature spots and end-organs', *Amer. J. Psychol.*, 39(1927) 402–27.

DALLENBACH, K. M., 'Pain: history and present status', *Amer. J. Psychol.*, 52(1939) 331–47.

DAVIS, L., and MARTIN, J., 'Studies upon spinal cord injuries. II. The nature and treatment of pain', *J. Neurosurg.*, 4(1947) 483–91.

DELGADO, J. M. R., 'Cerebral structures involved in transmission and elaboration of noxious stimulation', *J. Neurophysiol.*, 18(1955) 261–75.

DELGADO, J. M. R., ROSVOLD, H. E., and LOONEY, E., 'Evoking conditioned fear by electrical stimulation of subcortical structures in the monkey brain', *J. Comp. Physiol. Psychol.*, 49(1956) 373–80.

DENNIS, S. G., CHOINIÈRE, M., and MELZACK, R., 'Stimulation-produced analgesia in rats: assessment by two pain tests and correlation with self-stimulation', *Exper. Neurol.*, 68(1980a) 295–309.

DENNIS, S. G., and MELZACK, R., 'Pain-signalling systems in the dorsal and ventral spinal cord', *Pain*, 4(1977) 97–132.

DENNIS, S. G., and MELZACK, R., 'Self-mutilation after dorsal rhizotomy in rats: effects of prior pain and pattern of root lesions', *Exper. Neurol.*, 65(1979) 412–21.

DENNIS, S. G., and MELZACK, R., 'Pain modulation by 5-hydroxytryptaminergic agents and morphine as measured by three pain tests', *Exper. Neurol.*, 69(1980) 260–70.

DENNIS, S. G., MELZACK, R., GUTMAN, S., and BOUCHER, F., 'Pain modulation by adrenergic agents and morphine as measured by three pain tests', *Life Sci.*, 26(1980b) 1247–59.

DENNIS, S. G., YEOMANS, J. S., and DEUTSCH, J. A., 'Adaption of aversive brain stimulation. III. Excitability characteristics of behaviorally relevant neural substrates', *Behav. Biol.*, 18(1976) 531–44.

DESCARTES, R., *L'homme* (1664); translated by M. FOSTER, *Lectures on the History of Physiology during the 16th, 17th and 18th Centuries*, Cambridge University Press, Cambridge, 1901.

DEVOR, M., 'The pathophysiology of damaged peripheral nerves'; in P. D. WALL and R. MELZACK (eds.), *Textbook of Pain*, 3rd edn., Churchill Livingston, Edinburgh, 1994, pp. 79–100.

DICK-READ, G., *Childbirth without Fear*, Harper, New York, 1944.

DOSTROVSKY, J. O., MILLAR, J., and WALL, P. D., 'The immediate shift of afferent drive of dorsal column nucleus cells following deafferentation: a comparison of acute and chronic deafferentation in gracile nucleus and spinal cord', *Exper. Neurol.*, 52(1975) 480–95.

DRAKE, C. G., and McKENZIE, K. G., 'Mesencephalic tractotomy for pain', *J. Neurosurg.*, 10(1953) 457–62.

DROSTE, C., GREENLEE, M. W., and ROSKAMM, H., 'A defective angina pectoris pain warning system: experimental findings of ischemic and electrical pain test', *Pain*, 26(1986) 199–209.

DUBNER, R., and BASBAUM, A. I., 'Spinal dorsal horn plasticity following tissue or nerve injury'; in P. D. WALL and R. MELZACK (eds.), *Textbook of Pain*, 3rd edn., Churchill Livingston, Edinburgh, 1994, pp. 225–41.

DUBNER, R., HOFFMAN, D. S., and HAYES, R. L., 'Neuronal activity in medullary dorsal horn of awake monkeys trained in a thermal discrimination task, III. Task-related responses and their functional role', *J. Neurophysiol.*, 46(1981) 444–64.

DUBUISSON, D., *The Descending Control of Substantia Gelatinosa*, University of London (Ph.D. thesis), 1981.

DUBUISSON, D., 'Nerve root damage and arachnoiditis'; in P. D. WALL and R. MELZACK (eds.), *Textbook of Pain*, 3rd edn., Churchill Livingston, Edinburgh, 1994, pp. 711–35.

DUBUISSON, D., and DENNIS, S. G., 'The formalin test: a quantitative study of the analgesic effects of morphine, meperidine, and brain stem stimulation in rats and cats', *Pain*, 4(1977) 161–74.

DUBUISSON, D., and MELZACK, R., 'Classification of clinical pain descriptions by multiple group discriminant analysis', *Exper. Neurol.*, 51(1976) 480–87.

DUGGAN, A. W., HALL, J. G., and HEADLEY, P. M., 'Suppression of transmission of nociceptive impulses by morphine: selective effects of administration in the region of the substantia gelatinosa', *Brit. J. Pharmacol.*, 61(1977) 65–76.

EGBERT, L. D., BATTIT, G. E., WELCH, C. D., and BARTLETT, M. K., 'Reduction of post-operative pain by encouragement and instruction of patients', *New Eng. J. Med.*, 270(1964) 825–7.

ELTON, D., STUART, G. V., and BURROWS, G. D., 'Self-esteem and chronic pain', *J. Psychosom. Res.*, 22(1978) 25–30.

ERIKSSON, M. B. E., SJOLUND, B. H., and NIELZEN, S., 'Long term results of peripheral conditioning stimulation as an analgesic measure in chronic pain', *Pain*, 6(1979) 335–47.

EVANS, F. J., 'Expectancy, therapeutic instructions, and the placebo response'; in L. WHITE, B. TURSKY, and G. E. SCHWARTZ, *Placebo: Theory, Research and Mechanisms*, Guilford Press, New York, 1985, pp. 215–28.

EVERSTINE, D. S., and EVERSTINE, L., *People in Crises: Strategic Therapeutic Interventions*, Brunner/Mazel, New York, 1983.

EWALT, J. R., RANDALL, G. C., and MORRIS, H., 'The phantom limb', *Psychosom. Med.*, 9(1947) 118–23.

FEINMANN, C., 'Pain relief by antidepressants: possible modes of action', *Pain*, 23(1985) 1–8.

FEINSTEIN, B., LUCE, J. C., and LANGTON, J. N. K., 'The influence of phantom limbs'; in P. KLOPSTEG and P. WILSON (eds.), *Human Limbs and Their Substitutes*, McGraw-Hill, New York, 1954, pp. 79–138.

FETZ, E., 'Pyramidal tract effects on the interneurons in the cat lumbar dorsal horn', *J. Neurophysiol.*, 31(1968) 69–80.

FIELDS, H. L., 'Peripheral neuropathic pain; an approach to management'; in P. D. WALL and R. MELZACK (eds.), *Textbook of Pain*, 3rd edn., Churchill Livingston, Edinburgh, 1994, pp. 991–6.

FIELDS, H. L., and BASBAUM, A. I., 'Central nervous system mechanisms of pain modulation'; in P. D. WALL and R. MELZACK (eds.), *Textbook of Pain*, 3rd edn., Churchill Livingston, Edinburgh, 1994, pp. 243–57.

FIELDS. H. L., and HENRICHER, M. H., 'Anatomy and physiology of a nociceptive modulatory system', *Phil. Trans. Roy. Soc.*, B308(1985) 361–74.

FINDLER, G., OLSHWANG, D., and HADANI, M., 'Continuous epidural morphine treatment for intractable pain in terminal cancer patients', *Pain*, 14(1982) 311–15.

FITZGERALD, M., 'Alterations in the inputs of dorsal horn cells produced by capsaicin treatment of one sciatic nerve in the rat', *Brain Res.*, 248(1982) 97–107.

FITZGERALD, M., WALL, P. D., GOEDERT, M., and EMSON, P. C., 'Nerve growth factor counteracts the neurophysiological and neurochemical effects of chronic sciatic nerve injury', *Brain Res.*, 332(1985) 131–41.

FOLTZ, E. L., and WHITE, L. E., 'Pain "relief" by frontal cingulumotomy', *J. Neurosurg.*, 19(1962) 89–100.

FORDYCE, W. E., *Behavioral Methods for Chronic Pain and Illness*, C. V. Mosby, St Louis, Mo., 1976.

FORREST, W. H. BROWN, B. W., BROWN, C. R., DEFALQUE, R., GOLD, M., GORDON, H. E., JAMES, K. E., KATZ, J., MAHLER, D. L., SCHROFF, P., and TEUTSCH, G., 'Dextroamphetamine with morphine for the treatment of postoperative pain', *New Eng. J. Med.*, 296(1977) 712–15.

FOSBURG, M. T., and CRONE, R. K., 'Nitrous oxide analgesia for refractory pain in the terminally ill', *J.A.M.A.*, 250(1983) 511–13.

FOX, E. J., and MELZACK, R., 'Transcutaneous electrical stimulation and acupuncture comparison of treatment for low back pain', *Pain*, 2(1976) 141–8.

FREEMAN, W., and WATTS, J. W., *Psychosurgery in the Treatment of Mental Disorders and Intractable Pain*, C. C. Thomas, Springfield, Ill. 1950.

FREY, M. VON, 'Beitrage zur Sinnesphysiologie der Haut', *Ber. d. kgl. sächs. Ges. d. Wiss., math.-phys. Kl.*, 47(1895) 166–84.

FROMM, G. H., TERRENCE, C. F., and CHATTHA, A. S., 'Baclofen in the treatment of trigeminal neuralgia: double-blind study and long-term follow-up', *Ann. Neurol.*, 15(1984) 240–44.

FROST, F. A., JESSEN, B., and SIGGAARD-ANDERSEN, J., 'A control, double-blind comparison of mepivacaine injection versus saline injection for myofascial pain', *Lancet*, 8 March(1980) 499–501.

GAMSA, A., The role of psychological factors in chronic pain. II. A critical appraisal, *Pain*, 57(1994) 17–29.

GARDNER, W. J., and LICKLIDER, J. C. R., 'Auditory analgesia in dental operations', *J. Amer. Dent. Assn*, 59(1959) 1144–9.

GAW, A. C., CHANG, L. W., and SHAW, L. C., 'Efficacy of acupuncture on osteoarthritic pain', *New Eng. J. Med.*, 293(1975) 375–8.

GHIA, J. N., MAO, W., TOOMEY, T. C., and GREGG, J. M., 'Acupuncture and chronic pain mechanisms', *Pain*. 2(1976) 285–99.

GLOOR, P., 'Inputs and outputs of the amygdala: what the amygdala is trying to tell the rest of the brain'; in K. E. LIVINGSTON and D. HORNYKIEWICZ (eds.), *Limbic Mechanisms*, Plenum Press, New York, 1978, pp. 189–209.

GLYN, J. H., 'Rheumatic pains: some concepts and hypotheses', *Proc. Roy. Soc. Med.*, 64(1971) 354–60.

GOLDSCHEIDER, A., 'Histologische untersuchungen uber die Endigungsweise der Hautsinnesnerven beim Menschen', *Arch. Physiol. Leipzig, Suppl. Bd.*(1886) 191–231.

GOLDSCHEIDER, A., *Uber den Schmerz in Physiologischer und Klinischer Hinsicht*, Hirschwald, Berlin, 1894.

GOMEZ-PEREZ, F. J., RULL, J. A., DIES, H., RODRIGUEZ-RIVERA, J. G., GONZALEZ-BARRANCO, J., and LOZANO-CASTANEDA, O., 'Nortriptyline and fluphenazine in the symptomatic treatment of diabetic neuropathy. A double-blind cross-over study', *Pain*, 23(1985) 395–400.

GOODMAN, L. S., and GILMAN, A., *The Pharmacological Basis of Therapeutics*, Macmillan, New York, 1980.

GOTTLIEB, H., STRITE, L. C., KOLLER, R., MADORSKY, A., HOCKERSMITH, V., KLEEMAN, M., and WAGNER, J., 'Comprehensive rehabilitation of patients having chronic low back pain', *Arch. Phys. Med. Rehabil.*, 58(1977) 101–8.

GRACELY, R. H., 'Psychophysical assessment of human pain'; in J. J. BONICA, J. C. LIEBESKIND, and D. G. ALBE-FESSARD (eds.), *Advances in Brain Research and Therapy*, Vol. 3, Raven Press, New York, 1979, pp. 805–24.

GRACELY, R. H., DUBNER, R., DEETER, W. R., and WOLSKEE, P. J., 'Placebo and naloxone can alter postsurgical pain by separate mechanisms', *Nature*, 306(1983) 264–5.

GRAHAM, C., BOND, S. S., GERKOVICH, M. M., and COOK, M. R., 'Use of the McGill Pain Questionnaire in the assessment of cancer pain: replicability and consistency', *Pain*, 8(1980) 377–87.

GRAHAME, R. (ed.), *Clinics in Rheumatic Diseases, Low Back Pain*, Saunders, Philadelphia, 1980.

GRENNAN, D. M., and JAYSON, M. I. V., 'Rheumatoid arthritis'; in P. D. WALL and R. MELZACK (eds.), *Textbook of Pain*, 3rd edn., Churchill Livingston, Edinburgh, 1994, pp. 397–407.

GRUSHKA, M., and SESSLE, B. J., 'Applicability of the McGill Pain Questionnaire to the differentiation of "toothache" pain', *Pain*, 19(1984) 49–57.

GRUSHKA, M., SESSLE, B. J., and MILLER, R., 'Pain and personality profiles in burning mouth syndrome', *Pain*, 28(1987a) 155–67.

GRUSHKA, M., SESSLE, B. J., and HOWLEY, T. P., 'Psychophysical assessment of tactile, pain and thermal sensory functions in burning mouth syndrome', *Pain*, 28(1987b), 69–184.

GUILBAUD, G., BERNARD, J. F., and BESSON, J. M., 'Brain areas involved in nociception and pain'; in P. D. WALL and R. MELZACK (eds.), *Textbook of Pain*, 3rd edn., Churchill Livingston, Edinburgh, 1994, pp. 113–28.

GUNN, C. C., and MILBRANDT, W. E., 'Early and subtle signs in low back sprain', *Spine*, 3(1978) 267–81.

GYBELS, J. M., and SWEET, W. H., *Neurosurgical Treatment of Persistent Pain*, Karger, Basel, 1989.

HAGBARTH, K. E., and KERR, D. I. B., 'Central influences on spinal afferent conduction', *J. Neurophysiol.*, 17(1954) 295–307.

HALDEMAN, S., 'Manipulation and massage for the relief of back pain'; in P. D. WALL and R. MELZACK (eds.), *Textbook of Pain*, 3rd edn., Churchill Livingston, Edinburgh, 1994, pp. 1251–62.

HALL, K. R. L., and STRIDE, E., 'The varying reponse to pain in psychiatric disorders: a study in abnormal psychology', *Brit. J. Med. Psychol.*, 27(1954) 48–60.

HANNINGTON-KIFF, J. G., 'Sympathetic nerve blocks in painful limb disorders'; in P. D. WALL and R. MELZACK (eds.), *Textbook of Pain*, 3rd edn., Churchill Livingston, Edinburgh, 1994, pp. 1035–52.

HARDY, J. D., WOLFF, H. G., and GOODELL, H., *Pain Sensations and Reactions*, Williams and Wilkins, Baltimore, 1952.

HARTMAN, L. M., and AINSWORTH, K. D., 'Self-regulation of chronic pain', *Canad. J. Psychiat.*, 25(1980) 38–43.

HEAD, H., *Studies in Neurology*, Kegan Paul, London, 1920.

HEBB, D. O., *The Organization of Behavior*, Wiley, New York, 1949.

HEBB, D. O., 'Science and the world of imagination', *Canad, Psychol. Rev.*, 16(1975) 4–11.

HENDERSON, W. R., and SMYTH, G. E., 'Phantom limbs', *J. Neurol. Neurosurg., Psychiat.*, 11(1948) 88–112.

HERZ, A., ALBUS, K., METYS, J., SCHUBERT, P., and TESCHEMACHER, H., 'On the sites for the anti-nociceptive action of morphine and fentanyl', *Neuropharmacol.*, 9(1970) 539–51.

HILGARD, E. R., 'A neodissociation interpretation of pain reduction by hypnosis', *Psychol. Rev.*, 80(1973) 396–411.

HILGARD, E. R., and HILGARD, J., *Hypnosis in the Relief of Pain*, William Kaufmann, Los Altos, Cal., 2nd edn., 1986.

HILL, H. E., KORNETSKY, C. H., FLANARY, H. G., and WIKLER, A., 'Effects of anxiety and morphine on discrimination of intensities of painful stimuli', *J. Clin. Invest.*, 31(1952a) 473–80.

HILL, H. E., KORNETSKY, C. H., FLANARY, H. G., and WIKLER, A., 'Studies of anxiety associated with anticipation of pain. I. Effects of morphine', *Arch. Neurol. Psychiat.*, 67(1952b) 612–19.

HILLMAN, P., and WALL, P. D., 'Inhibitory and excitatory factors influencing the receptive fields of lamina 5 spinal cord cells', *Exper. Brain Res.*, 9(1969) 284–306.

HOKANSON, J. E., DeGOOD, D. E., FORREST, M. S., and BRITTAIN, T. M., 'Availability of avoidance behaviors in modulating vascular-stress responses', *J. Personality Soc. Psychol.*, 19(1971) 60–68.

HORAN, J. J., LAYNG, F. C., and PURSELL, C. H., 'Preliminary study of effects of "in vivo" emotive imagery in dental discomfort', *Percept. Motor Skills*, 42(1976) 105–6.

HOSOBUCHI, Y., ADAMS, J. E., and LINCHITZ, R., 'Pain relief by electrical stimulation of the central gray matter in humans and its reversal by naloxone', *Science*, 177(1977) 183–6.

HOSOBUCHI, Y., ADAMS, J. E., and RUTKIN, B., 'Chronic thalamic stimulation for the control of facial anesthesia dolorosa', *Arch. Neurol.*, 29(1973) 158–61.

HOUCK, C. S., TROSHYNSKI, T., and BERDE, C. B., 'Treatment of pain in children'; in P. D. WALL and R. MELZACK (eds.), *Textbook of Pain*, 3rd edn., Churchill Livingston, Edinburgh, 1994, pp. 1419–34.

HOWE, J. F., LOESER, J. D., and CALVIN, W. H., 'Mechanosensitivity of dorsal root ganglia and chronically injured axons: a physiological basis for the radicular pain of nerve root compression', *Pain*, 3(1977) 25–41.

HUGHES, J., and KOSTERLITZ, H. W., 'Opioid peptides', *Brit. Med. Bull.*, 33(1977) 156–61.

HUTCHINS, H. C., and REYNOLDS, O. E., 'Experimental investigation of the referred pain of aerodontalgia', *J. Dent. Res.*, 26(1947) 3–8.

ISCHIA, S., LUZZANI, A., ISCHIA, A., and PACINI, L., 'Role of unilateral percutaneous cervical cordotomy in the treatment of neoplastic vertebral pain', *Pain*, 19(1984) 123–31.

ISCHIA, S., ISCHIA, A., LUZZANI, A., TOSCANO, D., and STEELE, A., 'Results up to death in the treatment of persistent cervico-thoracic (Pancoast) and thoracic malignant pain by unilateral percutaneous cervical cordotomy', *Pain*, 21(1985) 339–55.

JEANS, M. E., 'Relief of chronic pain by brief, intense transcutaneous electrical stimulation – a double-blind study'; in J. J. BONICA, J. C. LIEBESKIND, and D. G. ALBE-FESSARD (eds.), *Advances in Pain Research and Therapy*, Vol. 3, Raven Press, New York, 1979, pp. 601–6.

JENKINS, W. L., 'Studies in thermal sensitivity: 17. The topographical and functional relations of warmth and cold', *J. Exp. Psychol.*, 29(1941) 511–16.

JENSEN, T. S., KREBS, B., NIELSEN, J., and RASMUSSEN, P., 'Phantom limb, phantom pain and stump pain in amputees during the first six months following limb amputation', *Pain*, 17(1983) 243–56.

JENSEN, T. S., KREBS, B., NIELSON, J., and RASMUSSEN, P., 'Immediate and long-term phantom limb pain in amputees: incidence, clinical characteristics and relationship to pre-amputation limb pain', *Pain*, 21(1985) 267–78.

JENSEN, T. S., and RASMUSSEN, P., 'Phantom pain and other phenomena after amputation'; in P. D. WALL and R. MELZACK (eds.), *Textbook of Pain*, 3rd edn., Churchill Livingston, Edinburgh, 1994, pp. 651–65.

JESSUP, B. A., and GALLEGOS, X., 'Relaxation and biofeedback'; in P. D. WALL and R. MELZACK (eds.), *Textbook of Pain*, 3rd edn., Churchill Livingston, Edinburgh, 1994, pp. 1321–36.

JESSUP, B. A., NEUFIELD, R. W. J., and MERSKEY, H., 'Biofeedback therapy for headache and other pain: an evaluative review', *Pain*, 7(1979) 225–70.

JOHANSSON, R. S., and VALLBO, A. B., 'Tactile sensibility in the human hand: relative and absolute densities of four types of mechanoreceptive units in the glabrous skin area', *J. Physiol.*, 286(1979) 283–300.

JONES, C. M., *Digestive Tract Pain: Diagnosis and Treatment; Experimental Observations*, Macmillan, New York, 1938.

KAO, F. F., *Acupuncture Therapeutics*, Eastern Press, New Haven, Conn., 1973.

KATZ, J., and LEVIN, A. B., 'Treatment of diffuse metastatic cancer pain by instillation of alcohol into the sella turcica', *Anesthesiology*, 46(1977) 115–21.

KATZ, J., and MELZACK, R., 'Pain "memories" in phantom limbs: review and clinical observations', *Pain* 43(1990) 319–36.

KEEFE, F. J., and LEFEBVRE, J. C., 'Behaviour therapy'; in P. D. WALL and R. MELZACK (eds.), *Textbook of Pain*, 3rd edn., Churchill Livingston, Edinburgh, 1994, pp. 1367–80

KEEGAN, J. J., and GARRETT, F. D., 'The segmental distribution of the cutaneous nerves in the limbs of man', *Anat. Rec.*, 102(1948) 409–37.

KEELE, C. A., and ARMSTRONG, D., *Substances Producing Pain and Itch*, Arnold, London, 1964.

KEELE, K. D., *Anatomies of Pain*, Oxford University Press, London, 1957.

KEERI-SZANTO, M., 'Drugs or drums: what relieves post-operative pain?', *Pain*, 6(1979) 217–30.

KENNARD, M. A., and HAUGEN, F. P., 'The relation of subcutaneous focal sensitivity to referred pain of cardiac origin', *Anesthesiology*, 16(1955) 297–311.

312 *References*

KERR, D. I. B., HAUGEN, F. P., and MELZACK, R., 'Responses evoked in the brainstem by tooth stimulation', *Amer. J. Physiol.*, 183(1955) 253–8.

KERR, F. W. L., and LIPPMANN, H. H., 'The primate spinothalamic tract as demonstrated by anterolateral cordotomy and commissural myelotomy'; in J. J. BONICA (ed.), *Pain, Advances in Neurology*, Vol. 4, Raven Press, New York, 1974, pp. 147–56.

KERR, F. W. L., WILSON, P. R., and NIJENSOHN, D. E., 'Acupuncture reduces the trigeminal evoked response in decerebrate cats', *Exper. Neurol.*, 61(1978) 84–95.

KIBLER, R. F., and NATHAN, P. W., 'Relief of pain and paraesthesiae by nerve block distal to a lesion', *J. Neurol. Neurosurg. Psychiat.*, 23(1960) 91–8.

KING, H. E., CLAUSEN, J., and SCARFF, J. E., 'Cutaneous thresholds for pain before and after unilateral prefrontal lobotomy', *J. Nerv. Ment. Dis.*, 112(1950) 93–6.

KOLB, L. C., *The Painful Phantom: Psychology, Physiology and Treatment*, C. C. Thomas, Springfield, Ill., 1954.

KOPELL, H. P., and THOMPSON, W. A. L., *Peripheral Entrapment Neuropathies*, Robert E. Krieger, Huntington, New York, 1976.

KORZENIEWSKA, E., BRINKHUS, H. B., and ZIMMERMANN, M., 'Activities of single neurons in midbrain and thalamus of cats during conditioned nocifensive behavior', *Pain*, 26(1986) 313–29.

KOSAMBI, D. D., 'Living prehistory in India', *Sci. Amer.*, 216(2) (1967) 105–14.

KRAINICK, J. U., THODEN, U., and REICHERT, T., 'Pain reduction in amputees by long term spinal cord stimulation', *J. Neurosurg.*, 52(1980) 346–50.

KRAINICK, J. U., and THODEN, U., 'Spinal cord stimulation'; in P. D. WALL and R. MELZACK (eds.), *Textbook of Pain*, 3rd edn., Churchill Livingston, Edinburgh, 1994, pp. 1219–23.

KRAMES, E. S., WILKIE, D. J., and GERSHOW, J., 'Intrathecal D-Ala²-D-Leu⁵-enkephalin (DADL) restores analgesia in a patient analgetically tolerant to intrathecal morphine sulphate', *Pain*, 24(1986) 205–9.

KREBS, B., JENSEN, T. S., KRONER, K., NIELSEN, J., and JORGENSEN, H. S., 'Phantom limb phenomena in amputees 7 years after limb amputation', *Pain Suppl.*, 2(1984) S85.

KUGELBERG, E., and LINDBLOM, U., 'The mechanism of pain in trigeminal neuralgia', *J. Neurol. Neurosurg. Psychiat.*, 22(1959) 36–43.

LAITINEN, J., 'Acupuncture and transcutaneous electric stimulation in the treatment of chronic sacrolumbalgia and ischialgia', *Amer. J. Chinese Med.*, 4(1976) 169–75.

LAMAZE, F., *Painless Childbirth: Psychoprophylactic Method*, Regnery, Chicago, 1970.

LAMBERT, W. E., LIBMAN, E., and POSER, E. G., 'Effect of increased salience of membership group on pain tolerance', *J. Personality*, 28(1960) 350–57.

LANGER, E., JANIS, I. L., and WOLFER, J. A., 'Reduction of psychological stress in surgical patients', *J. Exper. Soc. Psychol.*, 11(1975) 155–65.

LARBIG, W., *Schmerz: Grundlagen, Forschung; Therapie*, Stuttgart, W. Kohlhammer, 1982.

LARSELL, O., *Anatomy of the Nervous System*, Appleton-Century, New York, 1951.

LASAGNA, L., MOSTELLER, F., VON FELSINGER, J. M., and BEECHER, H. K., 'A study of the placebo response', *Amer. J. Med.*, 16(1954) 770–79.

LEAVITT, F., and GARRON, D. C., 'The detection of psychological disturbance in patients with low back pain', *J. Psychosom. Res.*, 23(1979) 149–54.

LEAVITT, F., and GARRON, D. C., 'Validity of a back-pain classification scale for detecting psychological disturbance as measured by the MMPI', *J. Clin. Psych.*, 36(1980) 186–9.

LE BARS, D., DICKENSON, A. H., and BESSON, J. M., 'Opiate analgesia and descending control systems'; in J. J. BONICA *et al.* (eds.), *Advances in Pain Research and Therapy*, Raven Press, New York, 1983, pp. 341–72.

LEHMANN, J. F., and DE LATEUR, B. J., 'Ultrasound, shortwave, microwave, laser, superficial heat and cold in the treatment of pain'; in P. D. WALL and R. MELZACK (eds.), *Textbook of Pain*, 3rd edn., Churchill Livingston, Edinburgh, 1994, pp. 1237–49.

LERICHE, R., *The Surgery of Pain*, Williams and Wilkins, Baltimore, 1939.

LEVITT, M., and LEVITT, J., 'Sensory hindlimb representation in the SmI cortex of the cat after spinal tractotomies', *Exper. Neurol.*, 22(1968) 276–302.

LEVINE, J. D., GORDON, N. C., SMITH, R., and MCBRYDE, R., 'Desipramine enhances opiate postoperative analgesia', *Pain*, 27(1986) 45–9.

LEVINE, J., and TAIWO, Y., 'Inflammatory pain'; in P. D. WALL and R. MELZACK (eds.), *Textbook of Pain*, 3rd edn., Churchill Livingston, Edinburgh, 1994, pp. 45–56.

LEWIS, T., *Pain*, Macmillan, New York, 1942.

LEWIT, K., 'The needle effect in the relief of myofascial pain', *Pain*, 6(1979) 83–90.

LICHSTEIN, L., and SACKETT, G. P., 'Reactions by differentially raised Rhesus monkeys to noxious stimulation', *Dev. Psychobiol.*, 4(1971) 339–52.

LIEBESKIND, J. C., and PAUL, L. A., 'Psychological and physiological mechanisms of pain', *Ann. Rev. Psychol.*, 28(1977) 41–60.

LINDBLOM, U., and MEYERSON, B. A., 'Influence on touch, vibration and cutaneous pain of dorsal column stimulation in man', *Pain*, 1(1975) 257–70.

LINDBLOM, U., and TEGNER, R., 'Are the endorphins active in clinical pain states? Narcotic antagonism in chronic pain patients', *Pain*, 7(1979) 65–8.

LIPTON, S., MILES, J. B., and WILLIAMS, N. E., 'Pituitary injection of alcohol for inoperable and intractable cancer pain'; in J. J. BONICA, J. C. LIEBESKIND, and D. G. ALBE-FESSARD (eds.), *Advances in Pain Research and Therapy*, Vol. 3, Raven Press, New York, 1979, pp. 905–9.

LIVINGSTON, W. K., *Pain Mechanisms*, Macmillan, New York, 1943.

LIVINGSTON, W. K., 'What is pain?', *Sci. Amer.*, 196(3) (1953) 59–66.

LOBATO, R. D., MADRID, J. L., FATELA, L. V., GOSALO, A., RIVAS, J. J., and SARABIA, R., 'Analgesia elicited by low-dose intraventricular morphine in terminal cancer patient', *Adv. Pain Res. Ther.*, 9(1985) 673–81.

LOESER, J. D., 'Low back pain'; in J. J. BONICA (ed.), *Pain*, Raven Press, New York, 1980, pp. 363–77.

LOESER, J. D., 'Tic douloureux and atypical face pain' in P. D. WALL and R. MELZACK (eds.), *Textbook of Pain*, 3rd edn., Churchill Livingston, Edinburgh, 1994, pp. 699–710.

314   References

LOH, L., NATHAN, P. W., SCHOTT, G. D., and WILSON, P. G., 'Effects of regional guanethidine infusion in certain painful states', *J. Neurol., Neurosurg. Psychiat.*, 43(1980) 446–51.

LOH, L., NATHAN, P. W., and SCHOTT, G. D., 'pain due to lesions of central nervous systems removed by sympathetic block'. *Brit Med. J.*, 282(1981) 1026–8.

LUNDBERG, T., 'Long-term results of vibratory stimulation as a pain relieving measure for chronic pain', *Pain*, 20(1984a) 13–23.

LUNDBERG, T., NORDEMAR, R., and OTTOSON, D., 'Pain alleviation by vibratory stimulation', *Pain*, 20(1984b) 25–44.

LUTHE, W., *Autogenic Therapy*, Vol. 4: *Research and Theory*, Grune and Stratton, New York, 1970.

LYNN, B., 'Cutaneous hyperalgesia', *Brit. Med. Bull.*, 33(1977) 103–8.

MACCARTY, C. S., and DRAKE, R. L., 'Neurosurgical procedures for the control of pain', *Proc. Staff Meetings Mayo Clin.*, 31(1956) 208–14.

MACLEAN, P., 'Psychosomatics', *Hdbk Physiol.*, 3(1958) 1723–44.

MANFREDI, M., BINI, G., CRUCCU, G., ACCORNERO, N., BERARDELLI, A., and MEDOLAGO, L., 'Congenital absence of pain', *Arch. Neurol.*, 38(1981) 507–11.

MANNHEIMER, C., and CARLSSON, C. A., 'The analgesic effect of transcutaneous electrical nerve stimulation (TNS) in patients with rheumatoid arthritis. A comparative study of different pulse patterns', *Pain*, 6(1979) 329–34.

MANNHEIMER, C., CARLSSON, C. A., VEDIN, A., and WILHELMSSON, C., 'Transcutaneous electrical nerve stimulation (TENS) in angina pectoris', *Pain*, 26(1986) 291–300.

MANNHEIMER, C., LUND, S., and CARLSSON, C. A., 'The effect of transcutaneous electrical nerve stimulation (TNS) on joint pain in patients with rheumatoid arthritis', *Scand. J. Rheumatol.*, 7(1978) 13–16.

MARK, V. H., ERVIN, F. R., and YAKOVLEV, P. E., 'Stereotactic thalamotomy', *Arch. Neurol.*, 8(1963) 528–38.

MARSHALL, H. R., *Pain, Pleasure, and Aesthetics*, Macmillan, London, 1894.

MARTIN, P., and MATTHEWS, A. M., 'Tension headaches: a psychophysiological investigation', *J. Psychosom. Res.*, 22(1978) 389–99.

MARTINEZ-URRUTIA, A., 'Anxiety and pain in surgical patients', *J. Consult. Clin. Psychol.*, 43(1975) 437–42.

MARTINS, A. N., RAMIREZ, A., JOHNSTON, J., and SCHWETCHENAU, P. R., 'Double-blind evaluation of chemonucleolysis for herniated lumbar discs; late results', *J. Neurosurg.*, 49(1978) 816–27.

MAYER, D. J., PRICE, D. D., and BECKER, D. P., 'Neurophysiological characterization of the anterolateral spinal cord neurons contributing to pain in man', *Pain*, 1(1975) 51–8.

MAYER, D. J., and WATKINS, L. R., 'The role of endorphins in endogenous pain control systems'; in H. M. EMRICH (ed.), *Modern Problems in Pharmacopsychiatry: The Role of Endorphins in Neuropsychiatry*, S. Karger, Basel, 1981.

MAYER, D. J., WOLFE, T. L., AKIL, H., CARDER, B., and LIEBESKIND, J. C., 'Analgesia from electrical stimulation in the brainstem of the rat', *Science*, 174(1971) 1351–4.

MAZARS, G. J., MERIENNE, J., and CIOLOCA, C., 'Traitement de certain types de douleurs par des stimulations thalamiques implantables', *Neurochimie*, 20(1974) 117–24.

MAZARS, G. L., MERIENNE, L., and CIOLOCA, C., 'Contribution of thalamic stimulation to the pathophysiology of pain'; in J. J. BONICA and D. ALBE-FESSARD (eds.), *Advances in Pain Research and Therapy*, Vol. 1, Raven Press, New York, 1976, pp. 483–5.

MCCAIN, G. A., 'Fibromyalgia and myofascial pain syndromes'; in P. D. WALL and R. MELZACK (eds.), *Textbook of Pain*, 3rd edn., Churchill Livingston, Edinburgh, 1994, pp. 475–93.

MCCARTHY, C., CUSHNAGHAM, J., and DIEPPE, P., 'Osteoarthritis'; in P. D. WALL and R. MELZACK (eds.), *Textbook of Pain*, 3rd edn., Churchill Livingston, Edinburgh, 1994, pp. 387–96.

MCGLASHAN, T. H. EVANS, F. J., and ORNE, M. T., 'The nature of hypnotic analgesia and placebo response to experimental pain', *Psychosom. Med.*, 31(1969) 227–46.

MCGRATH, P. A., 'Alleviating children's pain: a cognitive-behavioural approach'; in P. D. WALL and R. MELZACK (eds.), *Textbook of Pain*, 3rd edn., Churchill Livingston, Edinburgh, 1994, pp. 1403–18.

MCGRATH, P., and UNRUH, A., *Pain in Children and Adolescents*, Elsevier, Amsterdam, 1987.

MCGRATH P. J., and UNRUH, A. M., 'Measurement and assessment of paediatric pain'; in P. D. WALL and R. MELZACK (eds.), *Textbook of Pain*, 3rd edn., Churchill Livingston, Edinburgh, 1994, pp. 303–13.

MCLACHLAN, E. M., and JANIG, W., 'The cell bodies of origin of sympathetic and sensory axons in some skin and muscle nerves of the cat hindlimb', *J. Comp. Neurol.*, 214(1983) 115–30.

MCMAHON, S. B., 'Mechanisms of cutaneous, deep and visceral pain'; in P. D. WALL and R. MELZACK (eds.), *Textbook of Pain*, 3rd edn., Churchill Livingston, Edinburgh, 1994, pp. 129–51.

MCMAHON, S. B., and GIBSON, S., 'Peptide expression is altered when afferent nerves reinnervate in appropriate tissue', *Neurosci. Lett.*, 73(1987) 9–15.

MCMAHON, S. B., and WALL, P. D., 'Plasticity in the nucleus gracilis of the rat', *Exp. Neurol.*, 80(1983) 195–207.

MCMAHON, S. B., and WALL, P. D., 'Receptive fields of rat lamina I projection cells move to incorporate a nearby region of injury', *Pain*, 19(1984) 235–47.

MCMAHON, S. B., and WALL, P. D., 'The distribution and central termination of single cutaneous and muscle unmyelinated fibres in rat spinal cord', *Brain Res.*, 359(1985) 39–48.

MCMURRAY, G. A., 'Experimental study of a case of insensitivity to pain', *Arch. Neurol. Psychiat.*, 64(1950) 650–67.

MEICHENBAUM, D., and TURK, D., 'The cognitive-behavioral management of anxiety, anger, and pain'; in P. O. DAVIDSON (ed.), *The Behavioral Management of Anxiety, Depression, and Pain*, Brunner Mazel, New York, 1976, pp. 1–34.

MELZACK, R., 'Effects of early experience on behavior: experimental and conceptual considerations'; in P. HOCH and J. ZUBIN (eds.), *Psychopathology of Perception*, Grune and Stratton, New York, 1965, pp. 271–99.

MELZACK, R., 'The role of early experience in emotional arousal', *Ann. N. Y. Acad. Sci.*, 159(1969) 721–30.

MELZACK, R., 'Phantom limb pain: implications for treatment of pathological pain', *Anesthesiology*, 35(1971) 409–19.

MELZACK, R., *The Puzzle of Pain*, Basic Books, New York, 1973.

MELZACK, R., 'The McGill Pain Questionnaire: major properties and scoring methods', *Pain*, 1(1975a) 277–99.

MELZACK, R., 'Prolonged relief of pain by brief, intense transcutaneous somatic stimulation', *Pain*, 1(1975b) 357–73.

MELZACK, R. (ed.), *Pain Measurement and Assessment*, Raven Press, New York, 1983.

MELZACK, R., 'The myth of painless childbirth', *Pain*, 19(1984a) 331–7.

MELZACK, R., 'The Short-Form McGill Pain Questionnaire', *Pain*, 30(1987) 191–7

MELZACK, R., 'Labour pain as a model of acute pain'; *Pain*, 53(1993) 117–20.

MELZACK, R., 'Folk Medicine and the sensory modulation of pain'; in P. D. WALL and R. MELZACK (eds.), *Textbook of Pain*, 3rd edn., Churchill Livingston, Edinburgh, 1994, pp. 1209–17.

MELZACK, R., 'Phantom limb pain and the brain'; in B. BROMM and J. E. DESMEADT (eds.), *Pain and the Brain*, Raven Press, New York, 1995, pp. 73–82.

MELZACK, R., ABBOTT, F. V., ZACKON, W., MULDER, D. S., and DAVIS, M. W. L., 'Pain on a surgical ward; a survey of the duration and intensity of pain and the effectiveness of medication', *Pain*, 29(1987) 67–72.

MELZACK, R., BÉLANGER, E., and LACROIX, R., 'Labour pain: effect of maternal position on front and back pain', *J. Pain Sympt. Manag.*, 6(1991) 476–80.

MELZACK, R., and BENTLEY, K. C., 'Relief of dental pain by ice massage of either hand or the contralateral arm', *J. Can. Dent. Assn.*, 106(1983) 257–60.

MELZACK, R., and BROMAGE, P. R., 'Experimental phantom limbs', *Exper. Neurol.*, 39(1973) 261–9.

MELZACK, R., and CASEY, K. L., 'Sensory, motivational, and central control determinants of pain: a new conceptual model'; in D. KENSHALO (ed.), *The Skin Senses*, Thomas, Springfield, Ill., 1968, pp. 423–43.

MELZACK, R., GUITÉ, S., and GONSHOR, A., 'Relief of dental pain by ice massage of the hand', *Canad. Med. Assn J.*, 122(1980a) 189–91.

MELZACK, R., JEANS, M. E., STRATFORD, J. G., and MONKS, R. C., 'Ice massage and transcutaneous electrical stimulation: comparison of treatment for low back pain', *Pain*, 9(1980b) 209–17.

MELZACK, R., and KATZ, J., 'Auriculotherapy fails to relieve chronic pain', *J.A.M.A.*, 251(1984) 1041–3.

MELZACK, R., and KATZ, J., 'Pain measurement in persons in pain'; in P. D. WALL and R. MELZACK (eds.), *Textbook of Pain*, 3rd edn., Churchill Livingston, Edinburgh, 1994, pp. 337–51.

MELZACK, R., KATZ, J., and JEANS, M. E., 'The role of compensation in chronic pain: analysis using a new method of scoring the McGill Pain Questionnaire', *Pain*, 23(1985) 101–12.

MELZACK, R., and LOESER, J. D., 'Phantom body pain in paraplegics: evidence for a central "pattern generating mechanism" for pain', *Pain*, 4(1978) 195–210.

MELZACK, R., and MELINKOFF, D. F., 'Analgesia produced by brain stimulation: evidence of a prolonged onset period', *Exper. Neurol.*, 43(1974) 369–74.

MELZACK, R., MOUNT, B. M., and GORDON, J. M., 'The Brompton Mixture versus morphine solution given orally: effects on pain', *Canad. Med. Assn J.*, 120(1979) 435–8.

MELZACK, R., OFIESH, J. G., and MOUNT, B. M., 'The Brompton Mixture: effects on pain in cancer patients', *Canad. Med. Assn J.*, 115(1976) 125–9.

MELZACK, R., and PERRY, C., 'Self-regulation of pain: the use of alpha-feedback and hypnotic training for the control of chronic pain', *Exper. Neurol.*, 46(1975) 452–69.

MELZACK, R., and PERRY, C., *Psychological Control of Pain*, BMA Audio Cassettes, New York, 1980.

MELZACK, R., ROSE, G., and McGINTY, D., 'Skin sensitivity to thermal stimuli', *Exper. Neurol.*, 6(1962) 300–314.

MELZACK, R., and SCHAFFELBERG, D., 'Low-back pain during labour', *Am. J. Ob. Gyn.*, 156(1987) 901–5.

MELZACK, R., and SCHECTER, B., 'Itch and vibration', *Science*, 147(1965) 1047–8.

MELZACK, R., and SCOTT, T. H., 'The effects of early experience on the response to pain', *J. Comp. Physiol. Psychol.*, 50(1957) 155–61.

MELZACK, R., STILLWELL, D. M., and FOX, E. J., 'Trigger points and acupuncture points for pain: correlations and implications', *Pain*, 3(1977) 3–23.

MELZACK, R., STOTLER, W. A., and LIVINGSTON, W. K., 'Effects of discrete brainstem lesions in cats on perception of noxious stimulation', *J. Neurophysiol.*, 21(1958) 353–67.

MELZACK, R., TAENZER, P., FELDMAN, P., and KINCH, R. A., 'Labour is still painful after prepared childbirth training', *Canad. Med. Assn J.*, 125(1981) 357–63.

MELZACK, R., TERRENCE, C., FROMM, G., and AMSEL, R., 'Trigeminal neuralgia and atypical facial pain: use of the McGill Pain Questionnaire for discrimination and diagnosis', *Pain*, 27(1986) 297–302.

MELZACK, R., and TORGERSON, W. S. 'On the language of pain', *Anesthesiology*, 34(1971) 50–59.

MELZACK, R., and WALL, P. D., 'On the nature of cutaneous sensory mechanisms', *Brain*, 85(1962) 331–56.

MELZACK, R., and WALL, P. D., 'Pain mechanisms: a new theory', *Science*, 150(1965) 971–9.

MELZACK, R., and WALL, P. D., 'Psychophysiology of pain', *Int. Anesthesiol. Clinics*, 8(1970) 3–34.

MELZACK, R., WALL, P. D., and TY, T. C., 'Acute pain in an emergency clinic: latency of onset and descriptor patterns', *Pain*, 14(1982) 33–43.

MELZACK, R., WALL, P. D., and WEISZ, A. Z., 'Masking and metacontrast phenomena in the skin sensory system', *Exper. Neurol.*, 8(1963a) 35–46.

MELZACK, R., WEISZ, A. Z., and SPRAGUE, L. T., 'Stratagems for controlling pain: contributions of auditory stimulation and suggestion', *Exper. Neurol.*, 8(1963b) 239–47.

MENDELL, L. M., 'Physiological properties of unmyelinated fiber projections to the spinal cord', *Exp. Neurol.*, 16(1966) 316–32.

MENDELL, L. M., and WALL, P. D., 'Presynaptic hyperpolarization: a role for fine afferent fibers', *J. Physiol.*, 172(1965) 274–94.

MENDELSON, G., 'Not "cured by a verdict": effect of legal settlement on compensation claimants', *Med. J. Aust.*, 2(1982) 132–4.

MENDELSON, G., 'Compensation pain complaints, and psychological disturbance', *Pain*, 20(1984) 169–77.

MENDELSON, G., 'Chronic pain and compensation: a review', *J. Pain Sympt. Man.*, 1(1986) 135–44.

MENDELSON, G., 'Chronic pain and compensation issues'; in P. D. WALL and R. MELZACK (eds.), *Textbook of Pain*, 3rd edn., Churchill Livingston, Edinburgh, 1994, pp. 1387–1400.

MERSKEY, H., 'The psychological treatment of pain'; in M. SWERDLOW (ed.), *Relief of Intractable Pain*, Elsevier, Amsterdam, 1983, pp. 25–63.

MERSKEY, H. (ed.), 'Classification of chronic pain: descriptions of chronic pain syndromes and definitions of pain terms', *Pain*, Suppl. 3(1986) S1–S225.

MERSKEY, H., 'Pain and psychological medicine'; in P. D. WALL and R. MELZACK (eds.), *Textbook of Pain*, 3rd edn., Churchill Livingston, Edinburgh, 1994, pp. 903–20.

MERSKEY, H., and SPEAR, F. G., *Pain: Psychological and Psychiatric Aspects*, Baillière, Tindall and Cassell, London, 1967.

MEYER, R. A., CAMPBELL, J. N., and RAJA, S. N., 'Peripheral neural mechanisms of nociception'; in P. D. WALL and R. MELZACK (eds.), *Textbook of Pain*, 3rd edn., Churchill Livingston, Edinburgh, 1994, pp. 13–44.

MILLAR, J., and BASBAUM, A. I., 'Topography of the projection of the body surface of the cat to cuneate and gracile nuclei', *Exper. Neurol.*, 49(1975) 281–90.

MILNER, P., *Physiological Psychology*, Holt, Rinehart and Winston, New York, 1970.

MISRA, A. L., PONTANI, R. B., and VADLAMANI, N. L., 'Stereospecific potentiation of opiate analgesia by cocaine: predominant role of noradrenaline', *Pain*, 28(1987) 129–38.

MITCHELL, S. W., *Injuries of Nerves and their Consequences*, Lippincott, Philadelphia, 1872.

MONKS, R., 'Psychotropic drugs'; in P. D. WALL and R. MELZACK (eds.), *Textbook of Pain*, 3rd edn., Churchill Livingston, Edinburgh, 1994, pp. 963–89.

MORICCA, G., 'Chemical Hypophysectomy'; in J. J. BONICA (ed.), *Advances in Neurology*, Vol. 4, Raven Press, New York, 1974, 707–14.

MOULIN, D. E., MAX, M. B., KAIKO, R. F., INTURRISI, C. E., MAGGARD, J., YAKSH, T. L., and FOLEY, K. M., 'The analgesic efficacy of intrathecal D-Ala[2]-D-Leu[5]-Enkephalin in cancer patients with chronic pain', *Pain*, 23(1985) 213–21.

MOULIN, D. E., and COYLE, N., 'Spinal opioid analgesics and local anesthetics in the management of chronic cancer pain', *J. Pain Sympt. Man.*, 1(1986) 79–86.

MOUNT, B. M., 'The problem of caring for the dying in a general hospital: The palliative care unit as a possible solution', *Canad. Med. Assn J.*, 115(1976) 119–21.

MOUNT, B. M., AJEMIAN, I., and SCOTT, J. F., 'Use of the Brompton Mixture in treating the chronic pain of malignant disease', *Canad. Med. Assn J.*, 115(1976) 122–4.

MOUNTCASTLE, V. B., *Medical Physiology*, C. V. Mosby, St Louis, Mo., 1980.

MOUNTCASTLE, V. B., 'The neural mechanisms of cognitive functions can now be studied directly', *Trends Neurosci.*, 9(1986) 505–8.

MOWRER, O. H., and VIEK, P., 'An experimental analogue of fear from a sense of helplessness', *J. Abnorm. Soc. Psychol.*, 43(1948) 193–200.

MULLAN, S., 'Percutaneous cordotomy for pain', *Surg. Clin. N. Amer.*, 46(1966) 3–12.

MÜLLER, J., *Elements of Physiology*, Taylor, London, 1842.

MUSE, M., 'Stress-related, postraumatic chronic pain syndrome: criteria for diagnosis, and preliminary report on prevalence', *Pain*, 23(1985) 295–300.

MUSE, M., 'Stress-related, postraumatic chronic pain syndrome: behavioral treatment approach', *Pain*, 25(1986) 389–94.

NAFE, J. P., 'The pressure, pain and temperature senses'; in C. A. MURCHISON (ed.), *Handbook of General Experimental Psychology*, Clark University Press, Worcester, Mass., 1934.

NASHOLD, B. S., HIGGINS, A. C., and BLUMENKOPF, B., 'Dorsal root entry zone lesions for pain relief'; in R. S. WILKINS and S. S. RENGACHARY (eds.), *Neurosurgery*, Vol. 3, McGraw-Hill, New York, 1985, pp. 2433–7.

NASHOLD, B. S., WILSON, W. P., and SLAUGHTER, D. G., 'Sensations evoked by stimulation in the midbrain of man', *J. Neurosurg.*, 30(1969) 14–24.

NATHAN, P. W., 'Reference of sensation at the spinal level', *J. Neurol. Neurosurg. Psychiat.*, 19(1956) 88–100.

NATHAN, P. W., 'Pain traces left in the central nervous system'; in C. A. KEELE and R. SMITH (eds.), *The Assessment of Pain in Man and Animals*, Livingstone, London, 1962, 129–34.

NATHAN, P. W., 'Results of antero-lateral cordotomy for pain in cancer', *J. Neurol. Neurosurg. Psychiat.*, 26(1963) 353–62.

NATHAN, P. W., 'Painful legs and moving toes: evidence on the site of the lesion', *J. Neurol. Neurosurg. Psychiat.*, 41(1978) 934–9.

NATHAN, P. W., and WALL, P. D., 'Treatment of post-herpetic neuralgia by prolonged electrical stimulation', *Brit. Med. J.*, 3(1974) 645–7.

NAUNYN, B., 'Uber die Auslosung von Schmerzemfindung durch summation sich zeitlich folgender sensibelen Erregungen', *Arch. Exper. Pathol. Pharmakol.*, 25(1889) 272–305.

NAUTA, W. J. H., 'Hippocampal projections and related neural pathways to the midbrain in the cat', *Brain*, 81(1958) 319–40.

NEWHAM, D. J., EDWARDS, R. H. T., and MILLS, K. R., 'Skeletal muscle pain'; in P. D. WALL and R. MELZACK (eds.), *Textbook of Pain*, 3rd edn., Churchill Livingston, Edinburgh, 1994, pp. 423–40.

NOBACK, C. R., and SCHRIVER, J. E., 'Encephalization and the lemniscal systems during phylogeny', *Ann. N.Y. Acad. Med.*, 167(1969) 118–28.

NOORDENBOS, W., *Pain*, Elsevier Press, Amsterdam, 1959.

NOORDENBOS, W., and WALL, P. D., 'The failure of nerve grafts to relieve pain following nerve injury', *J. Neurol. Neurosurg. Psychiat.*, 44(1981) 1008–73.

NUSSBAUMER, J. C., and WALL, P. D., 'Expansion of receptive fields in the mouse cortical barrelfield after administration of capsaicin to neonates or local application on the infraorbital nerve in adults', *Brain Res.*, 360(1985) 1–9.

O'KEEFE, J., and NADEL, L., *The Hippocampus as a Cognitive Map*, Oxford University Press, New York, 1978.

OLDS, M. E., and OLDS, J., 'Approach-escape interactions in the rat brain', *Amer. J. Physiol.*, 203(1962) 803–10.

OLDS, M. E., and OLDS, J., 'Approach-avoidance analysis of rat diencephalon', *J. Comp. Neurol.*, 120(1963) 259–95.

OLESEN, J., 'The pathophysiology of migraine'; in F. C. ROSE (ed.), *Handbook of Clinical Neurology*, Vol. 48, revised series, Elsevier, Amsterdam, 1986, pp. 59–83.

OLSHWANG, D., SHAPIRO, A., PERLBERG, S., and MAGORA, F., 'The effect of epidural morphine on ureteral colic and spasm of the bladder', *Pain*, 18(1984) 97–101.

ONG, B., SINGER, G., and WALLACE, M., 'Pain sensations produced by algogens in humans'; in C. PECK, and M. WALLACE, (eds.) *Problems in Pain*, Pergamon, Oxford, 1980, pp. 98–110.

PAVLOV, I. P., *Conditioned Reflexes*, Humphrey Milford, Oxford, 1927.

PAVLOV, I. P., *Lectures on Conditioned Reflexes*, International Publishers, New York, 1928.

PERL, E. R., 'Afferent basis of nociception and pain: evidence from the characteristics of sensory receptors and their projections to the spinal dorsal horn'; in J. J. BONICA (ed.), *Pain*, Raven Press, New York, 1980, pp. 19–45.

PERL, E. R., 'Pain and nociception'; in *Handbook of Physiology, sect. 1, vol. 3*, Am. Physiol. Soc., Bethesda, 1984, pp. 915–75.

PERL, E. R., 'Unraveling the story of pain'; in H. L. FIELDS, R. DUBNER and F. CERVERO (eds.), *Advances in Pain Research and Therapy*, Raven Press, New York, 1985, pp. 1–29.

PERRY, C., 'Cognitive patterns in hypnosis', Paper presented at the 88th Ann. Conf. Amer. Psychol. Assoc., Montreal, 1980.

PERRY, S. W., CELLA, D. F., FALKENBERG, J., HEIDRICH, G., and GOODWIN, C., 'Pain perception in burn patients with stress disorders', *J. Pain Sympt. Man.*, 2(1987) 29–32.

PESCHANSKI, M., and BESSON, J.-M., 'A spino-tectal pathway', *Neuroscience*, 12(1984) 165–78.

PHILIPS, H. C., 'Changing chronic pain experience', *Pain*, 32(1988) 165–72.

PIKOFF, H., 'Is the muscular model of headache still viable? A review of conflicting data', *Headache*, 24(1984) 186–98.

PILOWSKY, I., 'Pain and illness behaviour: assessment and management'; in P. D. WALL and R. MELZACK (eds.), *Textbook of Pain*, 3rd edn., Churchill Livingston, Edinburgh, 1994, pp. 1309–19.

POMERANZ, B., CHENG, R., and LAW, P., 'Acupuncture reduces electrophysiological and behavioral responses to noxious stimuli: pituitary is implicated', *Exper. Neurol.*, 54(1977) 172–8.

POMERANZ, B., WALL, P. D., and WEBER, W. V., 'Cord cells responding to fine myelinated afferents from viscera, muscle and skin', *J. Physiol.*, 199(1968) 511–32.

PORTENOY, R. K., and FOLEY, K. M., 'Chronic use of opioid analgesics in non-malignant pain: report of 38 cases', *Pain*, 25(1986) 171—86.

PRICE, D. D., and MAYER, D. J., 'Physiological laminar organization of the dorsal horn of *M. mulatta*', *Brain Res.*, 79(1974) 321–5.

PRIETO, E. J., HOPSON, L., BRADLEY, L. A., BYRNE, M., GEISINGER, K. F., MIDAX, D., and MARCHISELLO, P. J., 'The language of low back pain: factor structure of the McGill Pain Questionnaire', *Pain*, 8(1980) 11–19.

PROCACCI, P., ZOPPI, M., PADELETTI, L., and MARESCA, M., 'Myocardial infarction without pain: a study of sensory function of the upper limbs', *Pain*, 2(1976) 309–13.

PROCACCI, P., ZOPPI, M., and MARESCA, M., 'Heart and vascular pain'; in P. D. WALL and R. MELZACK (eds.), *Textbook of Pain*, 3rd edn., Churchill Livingston, Edinburgh, 1994, pp. 541–54.

REXED, B., 'The cytoarchitectonic organization of the spinal cord in the cat', *J. Comp. Neurol.*, 96(1952) 415–95.

REYNOLDS, D. V., 'Surgery in the rat during electrical analgesia induced by focal brain stimulation', *Science*, 164(1969) 444–5.

REYNOLDS, D. V., 'Reduced response to aversive stimuli during focal brain stimulation: electrical analgesia and electrical anaesthesia'; in D. V. REYNOLDS and A. E. SJOBERG (eds.), *Neuroelectric Research*, Thomas, Springfield, Ill. 1970, 151–67.

REYNOLDS, O. E., and HUTCHINS, H. C., 'Reduction of central hyperirritability following block anesthesia of peripheral nerve', *Amer. J. Physiol.*, 152(1948) 658–62.

RICHLIN, D. M., JAMRON, L. M., and NOVICK, N. L., 'Cancer pain control with a combination of methadone, amitriptyline, and non-narcotic analgesic therapy: a case series analysis', *J. Pain Sympt. Man.*, 2(1987) 89–94.

ROBERTS, A. H., and REINHARDT, L., 'The behavioral management of chronic pain: long-term follow-up with comparison groups', *Pain*, 8(1980) 151–62.

ROCHE, P. A., GIJSBERS, K., BELCH, J. J. F., and FORBES, C. D., 'Modification of haemophiliac haemorrhage pain by transcutaneous electrical nerve stimulation', *Pain*, 21(1985) 43–8.

ROSE, J. E., and MOUNTCASTLE, V. B., 'Touch and Kinesthesis', *Hdbk Physiol.*, 1(1959) 387–429.

RUBINS, J. L., and FRIEDMAN, E. D., 'Asymbolia for pain', *Arch. Neurol. Psychiat.*, 60(1948) 554–73.

RUFFINI, A., 'Les dispositifs anatomiques de la sensibilité cutanée sur les expansions nerveuses de la peau chez l'homme et quelques autres mammifères', *Rev. Gen. Histol.*, 1(1905) 421–510.

RUSSELL, W. R., and SPALDING, J. M. K., 'Treatment of painful amputation stumps', *Brit. Med. J.*, 2(1950) 68–73.

RYBSTEIN-BLINCHIK, E., 'Effects of different cognitive strategies on chronic pain experience', *J. Behav. Med.*, 2(1979) 93–101.

SAUNDERS, C., 'Care of the dying', *Nursing Times*, 72(1976) 3–24.

SAUNDERS, C. (ed.), *The Management of Terminal Disease*, Edward Arnold, London, 1978.

SAUNDERS, C., 'Pain and impending death'; in P. D. WALL and R. MELZACK (eds.), *Textbook of Pain*, 3rd edn., Churchill Livingston, Edinburgh, 1994, pp. 861–68.

SCADDING, J. W., 'Peripheral neuropathies'; in P. D. WALL and R. MELZACK (eds.), *Textbook of Pain*, 3rd edn., Churchill Livingston, Edinburgh, 1994, pp. 667–83.

SCHOENEN, J., 'Organisation Neuronale de la Moelle Epinière de l'Homme', thesis, Faculty of Medicine, Université de Liège, 1980.

SCHOENEN, J., and MAERTENS DE NOORDHOUT, A., 'Headache' in P. D. WALL and R. MELZACK (eds.), *Textbook of Pain*, 3rd edn., Churchill Livingston, Edinburgh, 1994, pp. 495–521.

SCHOTT, G. D., 'Mechanisms of causalgia and related clinical conditions', *Brain*, 109(1986) 717–38.

SCHREINER, L., and KLING, A., 'Behavioral changes following rhinencephalic injury in cat', *J. Neurophysiol.*, 15(1953) 643–59.

SCHWEITZER, A., *On the Edge of the Primeval Forest*, Adam and Charles Black, London, 1953.

SCHWETSCHENAU, P. R., RAMIREZ, A., JOHNSTON, J., BARNES, E., WIGGS, C., and MARTINS, A. N., 'Double-blind evaluation of intradiscal chymopapain for herniated lumbar discs', *J. Neurosurg.*, 45(1976) 622–7.

SEMMES, J., and MISHKIN, M., 'Somatosensory loss in monkeys after ipsilateral cortical ablation', *J. Neurophysiol.*, 28(1965) 473–86.

SHEALY, C. N., MORTIMER, J. T., and RESWICK, J. B., 'Electrical inhibition of pain by stimulation of the dorsal columns', *Anesth. Analg.*, 46(1967) 489 91.

SHEEHAN, P. W., and PERRY, C. W., *Methodologies of Hypnosis: A Critical Appraisal of Contemporary Paradigms of Hypnosis*, Lawrence Erlbaum Associates, Hillsdale, N.J., 1976.

SHERER, C. L., CLELLAND, J. A., O'SULLIVAN, P., DOLAYS, P. M., and CANAN, B., 'The effect of two sites of high frequency vibration on cutaneous pain threshold', *Pain*, 25(1986) 133–8.

SHERMAN, R. A., SHERMAN, C. J., and GALL, N. G., 'A survey of current phantom limb pain treatment in the United States', *Pain*, 8(1980) 85–99.

SHERMAN, R. A., SHERMAN, C. J., and PARKER, L., 'Chronic phantom and stump pain among American veterans: results of a survey', *Pain*, 18(1984) 83–95.

SHERRINGTON, C. S., 'Cutaneous sensations'; in E. A. SCHÄFER (ed.), *Textbook of Physiology*, Pentland, London, 1900, pp. 920–1001.

SHERRINGTON, C. S., *Integrative Action of the Nervous System*, Scribner, New York, 1906.

SILVER, B. V., and BLANCHARD, E. G., 'Biofeedback and relaxation training in the treatment of psychophysiological disorders: Or, are the machines really necessary?', *J. Behav. Med.*, 1(1978) 217–39.

SIMMEL, M. L., 'On phantom limbs', *Arch. Neurol. Psychiat.*, 75(1956) 637–47.

SIMMEL, M. L., 'The reality of phantom sensations', *Soc. Res.*, 29(1962) 337–56.

SIMONS, D. G., 'Muscle pain syndromes, Part I', *Amer. J. Phys. Med.*, 54(1975) 289–311.

SIMONS, D. G., 'Muscle pain syndromes. Part II', *Amer. J. Phys. Med.*, 55(1976) 15–42.

SINCLAIR, D. C., 'Cutaneous sensation and the doctrine of specific nerve energies', *Brain*, 78(1955) 584–614.

SINCLAIR, D. C., *Mechanisms of Cutaneous Sensation*, Oxford University Press, London, 1982.

SJOLUND, B. H., and ERIKSSON, M. B. E., 'Endorphins and analgesia produced by peripheral conditioning stimulation'; in J. J. BONICA, D. ALBE-FESSARD and J. C. LIEBESKIND (eds.), *Advances in Pain Research and Therapy*, Vol. 3, Raven Press, New York, 1979, pp. 587–99.

SLOAN, P. A., 'Nitrous oxide/oxygen analgesia in palliative care', *J. Palliative Care*, 2(1986) 43–8.

SMYTHE, H. A., 'Nonarticular rheumatism and psychogenic musculoskeletal syndromes'; in D. J. MCCARTY (ed.), *Arthritis and Allied Conditions*, Lea and Febiger, Philadelphia, 1979, pp. 881–91.

SNYDER, S., 'Brain peptides as neurotransmitters', *Science*, 209(1980) 976–83.

SOLA, A. E., 'Upper extremity pain'; in P. D. WALL and R. MELZACK (eds.), *Textbook of Pain*, 3rd edn., Churchill Livingston, Edinburgh, 1994, pp. 457–74.

SOLA, A. E., and WILLIAMS, R. L., 'Myofascial pain syndromes', *Neurology*, 6(1956) 91–5.

SOPER, W. Y., 'Analgesia induced by brain stimulation: interaction of site and parameters of stimulation on the distribution of analgesic fields', McGill University (Ph.D. thesis), Montreal, 1979.

SOPER, W. Y., and MELZACK, R., 'Stimulation-produced analgesia: evidence for somatotopic organization in the midbrain', *Brain Res.*, 51(1982) 307–11.

SOUREK, K., 'Commissural myelotomy', *J. Neurosurg.*, 31(1969) 524–7.

SPANOS, N. P., CARMANICO, S. J., and ELLIS, J. A., 'Hypnotic analgesia'; in P. D. WALL and R. MELZACK (eds.), *Textbook of Pain*, 3rd edn., Churchill Livingston, Edinburgh, 1994, pp. 1349–66.

SPIEGEL, E. A., KLETZKIN, M., and SZEKELEY, E. G., 'Pain reactions upon stimulation of the tectum mesencephali', *J. Neuropath, Exper. Neurol.* 13(1954) 212–20.

SPIEGEL, E. A., and WYCIS, H. T., 'Present status of stereoencephalotomies for pain relief', *Confinia Neurologica*, 27(1966) 7–17.

SPILLANE, J. D., NATHAN, P. W., KELLY, R. E., and MARSDEN, C. D., 'Painful legs and moving toes', *Brain*, 94(1971) 541–56.

STEINMAN, J. L., KOMISARUK, B. R., YAKSH, T. L., and TYEE, G. M., 'Spinal cord monoamines modulate the antinociceptive effects of vaginal stimulation in rats', *Pain*, 16(1983) 155–66.

STERLING, P., 'Referred cutaneous sensation', *Exper. Neurol.*, 41(1973) 451–6.

STERNBACH, R. A., 'Congenital insensitivity to pain: a critique', *Psychol. Bull.*, 60(1963) 252–64.

STERNBACH, R. A., *Pain: A Psychophysiological Analysis*, Academic Press, New York, 1968.

STERNBACH, R., A., *Pain Patients: Traits and Treatment*, Academic Press, New York, 1974.

STERNBACH, R. A., and TIMMERMANS, G., 'Personality changes associated with reduction of pain', *Pain*, 1(1975) 177–81.

STERNBACH, R. A., and TURSKY, B., 'On the psychophysical power function in electric shock', *Psychosom. Sci.*, 1(1964) 217–18.

STERNBACH, R. A., and TURSKY, B., 'Ethnic differences among housewives in psychophysical and skin potential responses to electric shock', *Psychophysiology*, 1(1965) 241–6.

STEVENS, S. S., CARTON, A. S., and SHICKMAN, G. M., 'A scale of apparent intensity of electric shock', *J. Exper. Psychol.*, 56(1958) 328–34.

STEWART, D., THOMSON, J., and OSWALD, D., 'Acupuncture analgesia: an experimental investigation', *Brit. Med. J.*, 1(1977) 67–70.

SUNDERLAND, S., *Nerves and Nerve Injuries*, E. and S. Livingstone, Edinburgh, 1978.

SUNSHINE, A., and OLSON, N. Z., 'Nonnarcotic analgesics'; in P. D. WALL and R. MELZACK (eds.), *Textbook of Pain*, 3rd edn., Churchill Livingston, Edinburgh, 1994, pp. 923–42.

SWANSON, D. W., MARUTA, T., and SWENSON, W. M., 'Results of behavior modification in the treatment of chronic pain', *Psychosom. Med.*, 41(1979) 55–61.

SWANSON, D. W., SWENSON, W. M., MARUTA, T., and MCPHEE, M. C., 'Program for managing chronic pain', *Proc. Staff Meetings Mayo Clinic*, 51(1976) 401–8.

SWEET, W. H., 'Pain', *Hdbk Physiol.*, 1(1959) 459–506.

SWEET, W. H., General discussion; in J. J. BONICA (ed.), *Pain*, Raven Press, New York, 1980, 379–80.

TAENZER, P. A., *Self-control of Postoperative Pain: Effects of Hypnosis and Waking Suggestion*, unpublished doctoral dissertation, McGill University, Montreal, 1983.

TAENZER, P. A., MELZACK, R., and JEANS, M. E., 'Influence of psychological factors on postoperative pain, mood and analgesic requirements', *Pain*, 24(1986) 331–42.

TAMSEN, A., HARTVIG, P., FAGERLUND, C., and DAHLSTROM, B., 'Patient-controlled analgesic therapy. II. Individual analgesic demand and analgesic concentrations of pethidine in postoperative pain', *Clin. Pharmacokinet.*, 7(1982) 164–75.

TAN, S.-Y., 'Cognitive and cognitive-behavioural methods for pain control: a selective review', *Pain* 12(1982) 201–28.

TAUB, A., 'Local, segmental and supraspinal interaction with a dorsolateral spinal cutaneous afferent system', *Exper. Neurol.*, 10(1964) 357–74.

TAUB, H. A., BEARD, M. C., EISENBERG, L., and MCCORMACK, R. K., 'Studies of acupuncture for operative dentistry', *J. Amer. Dent. Assn*, 95(1977) 555–61.

TAYLOR, C. B., ZLUTNICK, S. I., CORLEY, M. J., and FLORA, J., 'The effects of detoxification, relaxation, and brief supportive therapy on chronic pain', *Pain*, 8(1980) 319–29.

TERENIUS, L., 'Endogenous peptides and analgesia', *Ann. Rev. Pharmacol.*, 18(1978) 189–205.

TERENIUS, L., 'Endorphins in chronic pain'; in J. J. BONICA, J. C. LIEBESKIND and D. G. ALBE-FESSARD (eds.), *Advances in Pain Research and Therapy*, Vol. 3, Raven Press, New York, 1979, pp. 459–71.

THORSTEINSSON, G., STONNINGTON, H. H., STILLWELL, G. K., and ELVEBACK, L. R., 'Transcutaneous electrical stimulation: a double-blind trial of its efficacy for pain', *Arch. Phys. Med. Rehabil.*, 58(1977) 8–13.

TRAVELL, J. G., and RINZLER, S. H., 'Relief of cardiac pain by local block of somatic trigger areas', *Proc. Soc. Exper. Biol. Med.*, 63(1946) 480–82.

TRAVELL, J. G., and RINZLER, S. H., 'The myofascial genesis of pain', *Postgrad. Med.*, 11(1952) 425–34.

TRAVELL, J. G., and SIMONS, D. G., *Myofacial Pain and Dysfunction: the Trigger Point Manual*, Williams and Wilkins, Baltimore, 1983.

TSUBOKAWA, T., YAMAMOTO, T., KATAYAMA, Y., HIRAYAMA, T., and SIBUYA, H., 'Thalamic relay nucleus stimulation for relief of intractable pain. Clinical results and beta-endorphin immunoreactivity in the cerebrospinal fluid', *Pain*, 18(1984) 115–26.

TURK, D. C., and GENEST, M., 'Regulation of pain: the application of cognitive and behavioral techniques for prevention and remediation'; in P. C. KENDALL and S. D. HOLLON (eds.), *Cognitive-Behavioral Interventions: Theory, Research, and Procedures*, Academic Press, New York, 1979, pp. 287–318.

TURK, D. C., and MEICHENBAUM, D., 'A cognitive-behavioural approach to pain management'; in P. D. WALL and R. MELZACK (eds.), *Textbook of Pain*, 3rd edn., Churchill Livingston, Edinburgh, 1994, pp. 1337–48.

TURK, D. C., MEICHENBAUM, D. H., and BERMAN, W. H., 'Application of biofeedback for the regulation of pain: a critical review', *Psychol. Bull.*, 86(1979) 1322–38.

TURK, D. C., and MELZACK, R., (eds.), *Handbook of Pain Assessment*, Guilford Press, New York, 1992.

TURNBULL, I. M., 'Brain stimulation': in P. D. WALL and R. MELZACK (eds.), *Textbook of Pain*, 2nd edn., Churchill Livingstone, Edinburgh, 1984, pp. 706–14.

TURNBULL, I. M., SHULMAN, R., and WOODHURST, W. B., 'Thalamic stimulation for neuropathic pain', *J. Neurosurg.*, 52(1980) 486–93.

TURNER, J. A., and CHAPMAN, C. R., 'Psychological interventions for chronic pain: a critical review. I. Relaxation training and biofeedback', *Pain*, 12(1982) 1–21.

TWYCROSS, R., 'Clinical experience with diamorphine in advanced malignant disease', *Int. J. Clin. Pharmacol. Therap. Toxicol.*, 9(1974) 184–98.

TWYCROSS, R. G., 'Relief of pain'; in C. M. SAUNDERS (ed.), *The Management of Terminal Disease*, Edward Arnold, London, 1978, pp. 65–92.

TWYCROSS, R. G., 'Opioids'; in P. D. WALL and R. MELZACK (eds.), *Textbook of Pain*, 3rd edn., Churchill Livingston, Edinburgh, 1994, pp. 943–62.

UDDENBERG, N., 'Functional organization of long, second-order afferents in the dorsal funiculus', *Exper. Brain Res.*, 4(1968) 377–82.

URBAN, B. J., and NASHOLD, B. S., 'Percutaneous epidural stimulation of the spinal cord for relief of pain', *J. Neurosurg.*, 48(1978) 323–8.

VALLBO, A. B., and HAGBARTH, K. E., 'Activity from skin mechanoreceptors recorded percutaneously in awake human subjects', *Exper. Neurol.*, 21(1968) 270–89.

VAN BUREN, J., and KLEINKNECHT, R. A., 'An evaluation of the McGill Pain Questionnaire for use in dental pain assessment', *Pain*, 6(1979) 23–33.

VAN HEES, J., and GYBELS, J., 'C nociceptor activity in human nerve during painful and non-painful skin stimulation', *J. Neurol. Neurosurg. Psychiat.*, 44(1981) 600–607.

VANE, J. R., 'Inhibition of prostaglandin synthesis as a mechanism of action for aspirin-like drugs', *Nature New Biol.*, 231(1971) 232–5.

VEILLEUX, S., and MELZACK, R., 'Pain in psychotic patients', *Exp. Neurol.*, 52(1976) 535–43.

VERHAGEN, W. I. M., HORSTINK, M. W. I. M., and NOTERMANS, S. L. H., 'Painful arm and moving fingers', *J. Neurol. Neurosurg. Psychiat.*, 48(1985) 384–9.

VIERCK, C. J., HAMILTON, D. M., and THORNBY, J. I., 'Pain reactivity of monkeys after lesions to the dorsal and lateral columns of the spinal cord', *Exper. Brain Res.*, 13(1971) 140–58.

VIERCK, C. J., LINEBERRY, C. G., LEE, P. K., and CALDERWOOD, H. W., 'Prolonged hypalgesia following "acupuncture" in monkeys', *Life Sci.*, 15(1974) 1277–89.

WALL, P. D., 'Cord cells responding to touch, damage and temperature of skin', *J. Neurophysiol.*, 23(1960) 197–210.

WALL, P. D., 'Presynaptic control of impulses at the first central synapse in the cutaneous pathway', *Progr. Brain Res.*, 12(1964) 92–118.

WALL, P. D., 'The laminar organization of dorsal horn and effects of descending impulses', *J. Physiol.*, 188(1967) 403–23.

WALL, P. D., 'The sensory and motor role of impulses travelling in the dorsal columns towards cerebral cortex', *Brain*, 93(1970) 505–24.

WALL, P. D., 'The placebo and the placebo response'; in P. D. WALL and R. MELZACK (eds.), *Textbook of Pain*, 3rd edn., Churchill Livingston, Edinburgh, 1994, pp. 1297–1308.

WALL, P. D., and EGGER, M. D., 'Formation of new connections in adult rat brains after partial deafferentation', *Nature*, 232(1971) 542–5.

WALL, P. D., FITZGERALD, M., and WOOLF, C. J., 'Effects of capsaicin on receptive fields and on inhibitions in rat spinal cord', *Exp. Neurol.*, 78(1982) 425–36.

WALL, P. D., FREEMAN, J., and MAJOR, D., 'Dorsal horn cells in spinal and in freely moving rats', *Exp. Neurol.*, 19(1967) 519–29.

WALL, P. D., and GUTNICK, M., 'Ongoing activity in peripheral nerves. II. The physiology and pharmacology of impulses originating in a neuroma', *Exper. Neurol.*, 43(1974) 580–93.

WALL, P. D., and MCMAHON, S. B., 'Microneuronography and its relation to perceived sensation', *Pain*, 21(1985) 209–29.

WALL, P. D., NATHAN, P. W., and NOORDENBOS, W., 'Ongoing activity in peripheral nerve. I. Interactions between electrical stimulation and ongoing activity', *Exper. Neurol.*, 38(1973) 90–98.

WALL, P. D., and SWEET, W. H., 'Temporary abolition of pain', *Science*, 155(1967) 108–9.

WALL, P. D., WAXMAN, S., and BASBAUM, A. I., 'Ongoing activity in peripheral nerve. III. Injury discharge', *Exper. Neurol.*, 45(1974) 576–89.

WALL, P. D., and WOOLF, C. J., 'What we don't know about pain', *Nature*, 287(1980) 185–6.

WALL, P. D., and WOOLF, C. J., 'Muscle but not cutaneous C-afferent input produces prolonged increases in the excitability of the flexion reflex in the rat', *J. Physiol.*, 356(1984) 443–58.

WALL, P. D., and WOOLF, C. J., 'The brief and the prolonged facilitatory effects of unmyelinated afferent input on the rat spinal cord are independently influenced by peripheral nerve injury', *Neuroscience*, 17(1986) 1199–206.

WAND-TETLEY, J. I., 'Historical methods of counter-irritation', *Ann. Phys. Med.*, 3(1956) 90–98.

WATERSTON, D., 'Observations on sensation: the sensory functions of the skin for touch and pain', *J. Physiol. London*, 77(1933) 251–7.

WATTS, C., 'Chemonucleolysis'; in R. H. WILKINS and S. S. RENGACHARY (eds.), *Neurosurgery*, Vol. 3, McGraw-Hill, New York, 1985, pp. 2260–64.

WEDDELL, G., 'Somesthesis and the chemical senses', *Ann. Rev. Psychol.*, 6(1955) 119–36.

WEISENBERG, M., 'Cognitive aspects of pain'; in P. D. WALL and R. MELZACK (eds.), *Textbook of Pain*, 3rd edn., Churchill Livingston, Edinburgh, 1994, pp. 275–89.

WEISENBERG, M., WOLF, Y., MITTWOCH, T., MIKULINCER, M., and AVIRAM, O., 'Subject versus experimenter control in the reaction to pain', *Pain*, 23(1985) 187–200.

WHIPPLE, B., and KOMISARUK, B. R., 'Elevation of pain threshold by vaginal stimulation in women', *Pain*, 21(1985) 357–67.

WHITE, J. C., and SWEET, W. H., *Pain and the Neurosurgeon*, C. C. Thomas, Springfield, Illinois, 1969.

WOLF, S., and WOLFF, H. G., 'Pain arising from the stomach and mechanisms underlying gastric symptoms', *Assn Res. Nerv. Ment. Dis.*, 23(1943) 289–301.

WOOLF, C. J., 'Evidence for a central component of post-injury hypersensitivity', *Nature*, 306(1983) 686–8.

WOOLF, C. J., 'The dorsal horn; state-dependent sensory processing and the generation of pain'; in P. D. WALL and R. MELZACK (eds.), *Textbook of Pain*, 3rd edn., Churchill Livingston, Edinburgh, 1994, pp. 101–12.

WOOLF, C. J., and THOMPSON J. W., 'Stimulation fibre-induced analgesia: transcutaneous electrical nerve stimulation (TENS) and vibration'; in P. D. WALL and R. MELZACK (eds.), *Textbook of Pain*, 3rd edn., Churchill Livingston, Edinburgh, 1994, pp. 1191–208.

WOOLF, C. J., and WALL, P. D., 'Chronic peripheral nerve section diminishes the primary afferent A-fibre mediated inhibition of rat dorsal horn neurones', *Brain Res.*, 242(1982) 77–85.

WOOLF, C. J., and WALL, P. D., 'A dissociation between the analgesic and antinociceptive effects of morphine', *Neurosci. Lett.*, 64(1986) 238.

WYNN PARRY, C. B., 'Pain in avulsion lesions of the brachial plexus', *Pain*, 9(1980) 41–53.

YAKSH, T. L., (ed.), *Spinal Afferent Processing*, Plenum, New York, 1986.

YAKSH, T. L., and MALMBERG, A. B., 'Central pharmacology of nociceptive transmission'; in P. D. WALL and R. MELZACK (eds.), *Textbook of Pain*, 3rd edn., Churchill Livingston, Edinburgh, 1994, pp. 165–200.

YOUNG, R. F., and RINALDI, P. C., 'Brain stimulation for relief of chronic pain'; in P. D. WALL and R. MELZACK (eds.), *Textbook of Pain*, 3rd edn., Churchill Livingston, Edinburgh, 1994, pp. 1225–33.

ZBOROWSKI, M., 'Cultural components in responses to pain', *J. Soc. Issues*, 8(1952) 16–30.

ZIMMERMANN, M., 'Ethical guidelines for investigations of experimental pain in conscious animals': in P. D. WALL and R. MELZACK (eds.), *Textbook of Pain*, 2nd edn., Churchill Livingstone, Edinburgh, 1984, pp. 205–6.

ZOHN, D. A., and MENNELL, J. M., *Musculoskeletal Pain: Diagnosis and Physical Treatment*, Little, Brown, Boston, 1976.

Index